Carroll & Brown

my
pregnancy
& baby

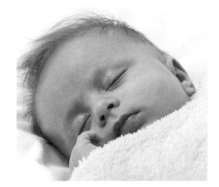

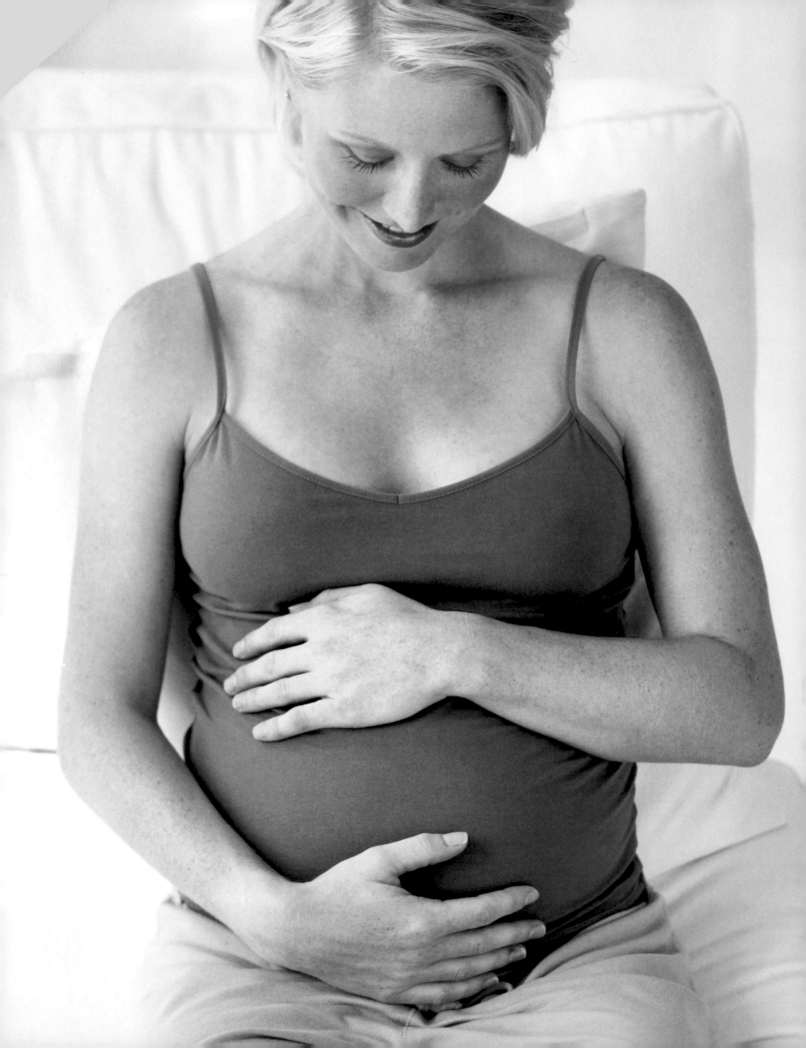

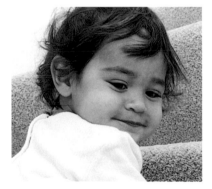 Carroll & Brown

my pregnancy & baby

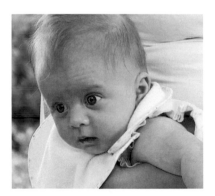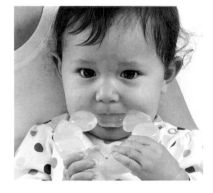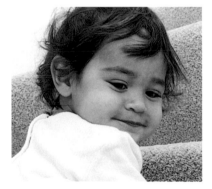

your guide to a **happy** and **healthy pregnancy** and the **care** of a **baby** up to **three** years of age

CARROLL & BROWN PUBLISHERS LIMITED

First published in 2011 in the United Kingdom by

Carroll & Brown Publishers Limited
20 Lonsdale Road
London NW6 6RD

Editor Amy Carroll
Managing Art Editor Emily Cook
Photographer Jules Selmes

Copyright © Carroll & Brown Limited 2011

A CIP catalogue record for this book is available
from the British Library.

ISBN 978 1 904 760 810 1

10987654321

Reproduced by RALI, Spain
Printed and bound in China

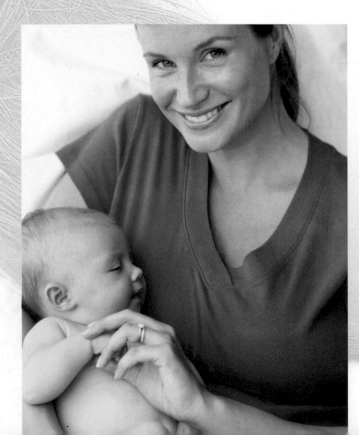

Contents

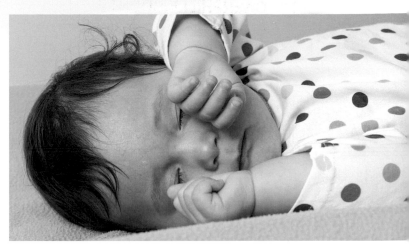

Foreword

Women are made to have babies. If you are one who has undertook to do so, you are about to embark on the most transformative experience of your life. In choosing this book to be your pregnancy and baby care companion, you have placed yourself in safe hands. In it you will find all the guidance you need so that your instincts and desires to do the best for yor baby (or babies) can prevail. You already know much of what you should be doing to safeguard your baby and yourself – but what you may not, you will undoubtedly find within.

You will always be your baby's greatest protector, and this starts even before you fall pregnant, with your care to follow a healthy diet and fitness programme and your avoidance of

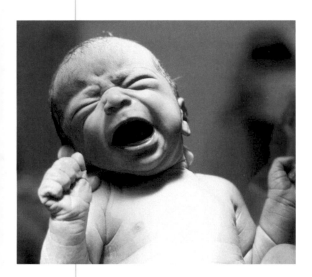

potential hazards. Once your baby is here, you'll know her better than any one, and will be the first to understand her needs and respond to them. It is with the desire of supporting and strengthening you in seeking to do the best you can for your baby that this book has been written. Rather than imparting information from 'on high', it seeks to work in partnership with your ideas and thoughts about having, and caring for, your baby. It will provide you with the all the information you need to make informed decisions thus encouraging you to do the right thing. The *If nothing else I will...* features, the checklists and *Off the menu* and *Experts advise* boxes will make it easy for you to follow best practice. The special 'lift up and look' pregnancy calendar will provide surprising glimpses of your baby's development in utero. The extensive pages on safety, first aid and health issues will ensure that you can prevent accidents or conditions worsening and act quickly and correctly if something untoward happens or your child becomes ill.

The knowledge of many pregnancy experts has been distilled in the creation of this book though the 'voice' that speaks is, in effect, that of an average woman. Her baby is a girl. As all fetuses begin as female (until male hormones fashion a boy) and we are thought to have a common ancestor, known as Eve, this seems appropriate. However, mums expecting boys can rest assured that unless indicated otherwise, all the information pertains to them as well.

No two pregnancies are the same – even if experienced by the same mother – so don't be afraid of using the book to record your own unique experiences and reactions. After all, it's your pregnancy and baby!

The Editors

PART I My pregnancy

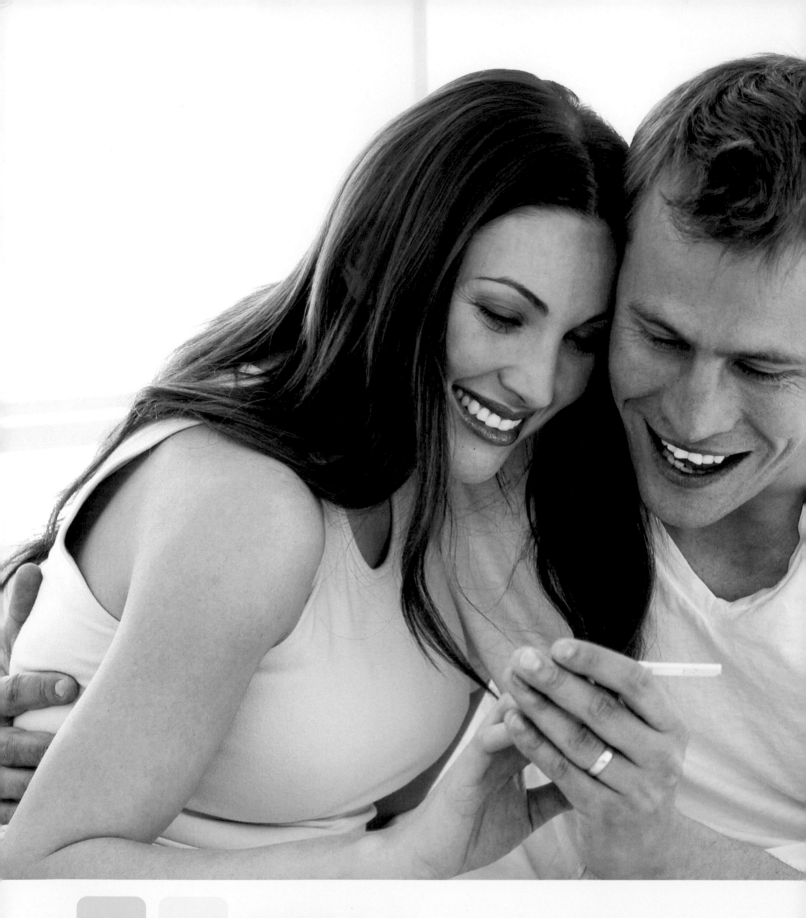

PART I My pregnancy

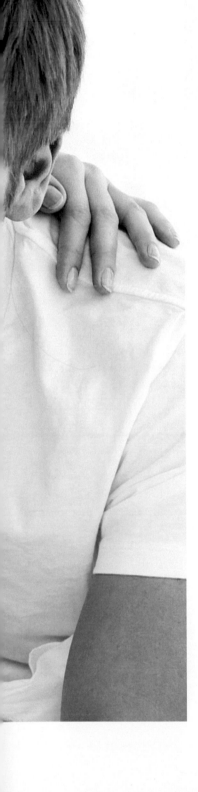

I'm pregnant!

Finding out I was pregnant was definitely one of the most excitng moments I ever experienced. The immediate thrill, however, was almost instantly tempered by anxieties about my preparedness and suitability to be a parent. Luckily, these negative thoughts quickly dissipated as I thought about the miraculous things that had already taken place without my being aware of them – one of my eggs had been fertilised and a new life had begun – and of the many months to come with their manifold new developments for me and my baby.

Early days

I've been trying for a baby and think I've succeeded at last in falling pregnant. My body feels different from usual but I've not experienced all the tell-tale signs. A home pregnancy test should let me know definitively, but if I have irregular periods or my pregnancy is too early to detect, the test may turn out negative. If I still feel that I may be pregnant, I can repeat the test in 5–7 days. I also can ask my doctor to perform a blood test or examine me internally.

PREGNANCY TESTING KITS

Several kinds of tests are available but they all check the presence of hCG (human chorionic gonadotropin), which is a hormone excreted by the developing placenta. I've chosen a test that can be used from the first day of a missed period. The test is most accurate with the first urine I pass in the morning, as this is the most concentrated, so even tiny amounts of hCG can be picked up. This test requires that I first pass the urine into a clean container and then squeeze a few drops from the dropper provided onto a window on an oblong stick; another type depends on my holding a stick in my urine flow. The result should appear within minutes and I can read it by looking for a coloured line in a window on the stick. Often there is also a line indicating that the test has been carried out correctly.

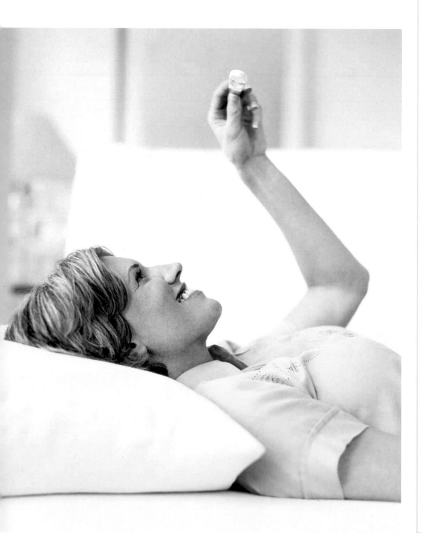

AM I PREGNANT?

The following are the classical signs and symptoms of pregnancy though they may appear at different times.

☐ I missed my period this month.

☐ My breasts feel tender and they've increased in size.

☐ I've been feeling sick in the morning and sometimes at night as well. I've vomited a couple of times.

☐ I'm feeling really tired and find it hard getting out of bed in the morning and am ready to get back in just after I get back in the evening.

☐ I'm having to urinate more frequently than usual.

☐ At the same time, I find that I'm constipated.

☐ Particular smells and tastes have become off putting. In fact, there's a strange metallic taste in my mouth and my coffee tastes odd.

☐ My moods are fluctuating a lot; sometimes I feel really weepy and overly emotional.

	1	2	3	4	5	6	7	8	9	10	11	12	13	14	15	16	17	18	19	20	21	22	23	24	25	26	27	28	29	30	31
January	1	2	3	4	5	6	7	8	9	10	11	12	13	14	15	16	17	18	19	20	21	22	23	24	25	26	27	28	29	30	31
Oct/Nov	8	9	10	11	12	13	14	15	16	17	18	19	20	21	22	23	24	25	26	27	28	29	30	31	1	2	3	4	5	6	7
February	1	2	3	4	5	6	7	8	9	10	11	12	13	14	15	16	17	18	19	20	21	22	23	24	25	26	27	28			
Nov/Dec	8	9	10	11	12	13	14	15	16	17	18	19	20	21	22	23	24	25	26	27	28	29	30	1	2	3	4	5			
March	1	2	3	4	5	6	7	8	9	10	11	12	13	14	15	16	17	18	19	20	21	22	23	24	25	26	27	28	29	30	31
Dec/Jan	6	7	8	9	10	11	12	13	14	15	16	17	18	19	20	21	22	23	24	25	26	27	28	29	30	31	1	2	3	4	5
April	1	2	3	4	5	6	7	8	9	10	11	12	13	14	15	16	17	18	19	20	21	22	23	24	25	26	27	28	29	30	
Jan/Feb	6	7	8	9	10	11	12	13	14	15	16	17	18	19	20	21	22	23	24	25	26	27	28	29	30	31	1	2	3	4	
May	1	2	3	4	5	6	7	8	9	10	11	12	13	14	15	16	17	18	19	20	21	22	23	24	25	26	27	28	29	30	31
Feb/Mar	5	6	7	8	9	10	11	12	13	14	15	16	17	18	19	20	21	22	23	24	25	26	27	28	1	2	3	4	5	6	7
June	1	2	3	4	5	6	7	8	9	10	11	12	13	14	15	16	17	18	19	20	21	22	23	24	25	26	27	28	29	30	
Mar/Apr	8	9	10	11	12	13	14	15	16	17	18	19	20	21	22	23	24	25	26	27	28	29	30	31	1	2	3	4	5	6	
July	1	2	3	4	5	6	7	8	9	10	11	12	13	14	15	16	17	18	19	20	21	22	23	24	25	26	27	28	29	30	31
Apr/May	7	8	9	10	11	12	13	14	15	16	17	18	19	20	21	22	23	24	25	26	27	28	29	30	1	2	3	4	5	6	7
August	1	2	3	4	5	6	7	8	9	10	11	12	13	14	15	16	17	18	19	20	21	22	23	24	25	26	27	28	29	30	31
May/Jun	8	9	10	11	12	13	14	15	16	17	18	19	20	21	22	23	24	25	26	27	28	29	30	31	1	2	3	4	5	6	7
September	1	2	3	4	5	6	7	8	9	10	11	12	13	14	15	16	17	18	19	20	21	22	23	24	25	26	27	28	29	30	
Jun/Jul	8	9	10	11	12	13	14	15	16	17	18	19	20	21	22	23	24	25	26	27	28	29	30	1	2	3	4	5	6	7	
October	1	2	3	4	5	6	7	8	9	10	11	12	13	14	15	16	17	18	19	20	21	22	23	24	25	26	27	28	29	30	31
Jul/Aug	8	9	10	11	12	13	14	15	16	17	18	19	20	21	22	23	24	25	26	27	28	29	30	31	1	2	3	4	5	6	7
November	1	2	3	4	5	6	7	8	9	10	11	12	13	14	15	16	17	18	19	20	21	22	23	24	25	26	27	28	29	30	
Aug/Sept	8	9	10	11	12	13	14	15	16	17	18	19	20	21	22	23	24	25	26	27	28	29	30	31	1	2	3	4	5	6	
December	1	2	3	4	5	6	7	8	9	10	11	12	13	14	15	16	17	18	19	20	21	22	23	24	25	26	27	28	29	30	31
Sept/Oct	7	8	9	10	11	12	13	14	15	16	17	18	19	20	21	22	23	24	25	26	27	28	29	30	1	2	3	4	5	6	7

CALCULATING MY DELIVERY DATE

Pregnancy is dated from the first day of my last menstrual period (LMP) and averages out at 280 days. The chart above will show the estimated date of delivery (EDD). To use it, I first have to look at the numbers in bold to find the date of the start of my last menstrual period. Then I look at the number in the line directly below it, which represents my EDD. As the date of my LMP was on 1 November, my baby will be due on 8 August the following year. This is just a general guide, however, as the chart is designed for women who have regular 28-day menstrual cycles and the date will need adjusting according to the length of a woman's cycle. If you have a 26-day cycle, for example, count on 9 months plus 5 days from your LMP – or 278 days. If you have a 32-day cycle, count on 9 months plus 11 days from your LMP – or 284 days – and so on.

EXPECTING TWINS (OR MORE)

In the UK, there are over 12,000 multiple births a year, and one in every 34 babies is a twin. Twins and other multiple births are increasing due to fertility treatment. As part of the process, drugs are routinely used to stimulate the release of more than one egg. About a third of twins are identical – technically monozygotic – and two-thirds are nonidentical – technically dizygotic – twins. Identical twins develop when, as in a normal conception, an egg is fertilised by a single sperm. The fertilised egg then splits in two, causing two separate embryos to develop – if it splits into three, triplets result, and so on. Identical twins may or may not share a placenta and amniotic sac, but each twin has his or her own umbilical cord. These babies will have an identical genetic make-up and will be the same sex. They will also have the same hair and eye colour, and be of the same blood type.

Nonidentical twins – also called fraternal twins – are produced when more than one egg is released at ovulation. This could be two eggs from one ovary, or one egg from each ovary. Each egg is fertilised by a different sperm and two genetically different babies are conceived. They can be the same sex or boy and girl, and will look as much alike or different as any other two siblings.

In the case of triplets, quads and more, there can be any combination of identical and nonidentical children (see also page 17).

Antenatal care

HEALTHCARE PROVIDERS

Antenatal care is offered by most general practitioners (GPs) – shared with the local hospital for a hospital birth, or by a community midwife. Generally, I will see my GP and community midwife for the majority of my checks-ups and will usually only attend hospital for one or two and my scans. In some areas of the United Kingdom, if my pregnancy is likely to be straightforward, I'd be looked after entirely by midwives. They would undertake all my antenatal care and my delivery – either in hospital or at home – as well as providing postnatal care. Or, I may choose to go privately and be seen by an obstetrician – a doctor who specialises in pregnancy, labour and birth. In this case, I would be seen by a consultant obstetrician at a private hospital for all my antenatal care, delivery and postnatal care. Private midwifery teams are also available to undertake all my care. With the latter, I would usually deliver my baby at home.

If I had a pre-existing medical condition, a previous complicated pregnancy or delivery, or if there are factors that could make my pregnancy 'high-risk', my antenatal care will be under a consultant obstetrician at the hospital.

VISITS AND APPOINTMENTS

Throughout my pregnancy, I will be seen on a regular basis and various tests and examinations (see pages 26–29) will be done to check that my health and that of my baby is as expected. After my booking visit, I will have shorter visits, about once a month, until 28 weeks of prenancy when the visits will increase to every two weeks until 36 weeks, when they'll occur weekly.

Booking appointment

At this long visit, from 8–12 weeks after my LMP, I will have a number of tests, answer a lot of questions and be told my EDD.

My doctor or midwife will want to know about my past medical history (and my partner's), family background and lifestyle in order to assess any potential health risks to my baby. If there is a history of genetic disease in the family, I will have to undergo additional blood tests. My weight and height may be

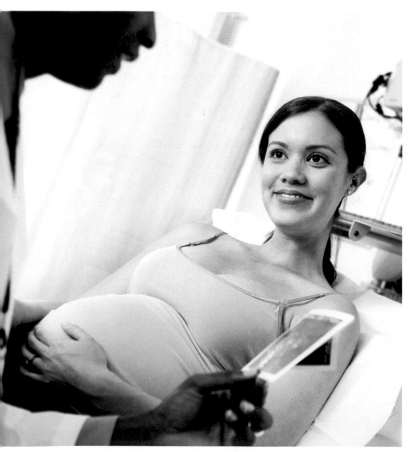

measured; the latter being a rough guide to the size of my pelvis. My heart and lungs will be examined. Not normally a part of a booking appointment, I might have to be examined internally if my doctor is concerned about something.

I will have a urine test to check for sugar or protein in the urine – signs that diabetes or an infection may be present. My blood pressure will be measured and some blood taken to assess my blood group and Rhesus status as well as determine whether I am anaemic, have hepatitis B or syphilis and whether I am immune to rubella. I will be asked whether I want an HIV test.

If I haven't had a cervical smear within three years, I'll be offered one.

Subsequent visits

Different screening tests, including both the early/dating and anomaly scans may be scheduled at or between visits, but at each visit, my blood pressure will be checked and urine tested for protein (for an early diagnosis of pre eclampsia). My caregiver will listen for my baby's heartbeat and he or she will palpate my abdomen in order to assess her growth.

CHECKS ON MY BABY

To follow the growth of my baby, my caregiver will palpate my abdomen at each visit and will measure the fundal height – the distance from the top of my uterus to my pelvic bone. The distance lengthens (stretching to the sternum) as my baby grows and so gives an estimate of her size for her age. It should be roughly equal to the number of weeks of my pregnancy, though sometimes the measurement is given in centimetres if assessed with a tape measure. If my baby is thought to be either too big or too small for my dates, an ultrasound scan will be done for a more accurate measurement.

From 16 weeks, my caregiver will listen to my baby's heartbeat at every visit.

After 35 weeks, my abdomen may be checked at each visit to ascertain my baby's position for birth (see page 91).

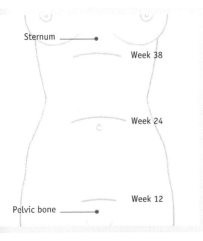

Sternum

Week 38

Week 24

Week 12

Pelvic bone

Fundal height

If I do nothing else I will ...

ATTEND ALL ANTENATAL VISITS
Good antenatal care can ensure a healthy pregnancy and baby. The tests, examinations and team will:

✔ **Assess my general health.** Any existing medical problems, such as high blood pressure will be uncovered and, if present, will be monitored at subsequent visits and I'll be advised on how the condition may change as a result of my pregnancy and how it may affect my baby.

✔ **Check on my wellbeing.** My antenatal team can monitor my physical condition and emotional and mental outlook.

✔ **Check on my baby's wellbeing.** The various tests will monitor her normal development and growth. If anything unusual is found, I'll be offered other tests to confirm the problem and determine the cause. I will then have the options explained and be helped to take whatever steps are necessary to safeguard my baby's health.

✔ **Detect complications.** Blood and urine tests can uncover 'hidden' problems such as Rhesus incompatibility or diabetes so that these can be treated successfully. I should also be offered help in coping with less serious but common pregnancy complaints such as nausea and swollen feet.

✔ **Prepare me for the birth.** My team will not only help my partner and me make informed choices about our choice of birth experience, but should support us both throughout labour and delivery.

✔ **Educate and prepare me for parenthood.** My caregiver should be able to advise me on parenting classes to attend.

Dates for my diary

Visits to a caregiver and the timing of antenatal tests can vary, depending on the GP or hospital and personal circumstances. The chart sets out the range of suitable dates and indicates possible procedures.

APPOINTMENTS

Place: Date/Time:
_____   _____
_____   _____

Place: Date/Time:
_____   _____
_____   _____

Place: Date/Time:
_____   _____
_____   _____

Place: Date/Time:
_____   _____
_____   _____

Place: Date/Time:
_____   _____
_____   _____

Place: Date/Time:
_____   _____
_____   _____

Place: Date/Time:
_____   _____
_____   _____

Place: Date/Time:
_____   _____
_____   _____

Place: Date/Time:
_____   _____
_____   _____

Place: Date/Time:
_____   _____
_____   _____

Place: Date/Time:
_____   _____
_____   _____

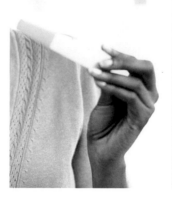

WEEKS 8–12

Booking appointment scheduled • A physical examination, blood pressure check and routine blood and urine tests will be carried out • Blood testing for genetic conditions may be performed • Due date established

WEEK 16

Antenatal appointment to discuss booking test results • Blood pressure check and blood test for Down's syndrome may be offered • Baby's heartbeat will be listened for • Anomaly scan may be performed • Amniocentesis can be performed • Serum screening including alpha-fetoprotein (AFP) test can be performed

WEEK 18

Serum screening including alpha-fetoprotein (AFP) test can be performed • Anomaly scan may be performed • Amniocentesis can be performed

WEEK 26 & 27*

Glucose tolerance test may be performed • Fetal blood sampling can be performed

* End of second trimester

WEEK 36

Antenatal appointment • Blood pressure and signs of pre-eclampsia check • Urine test • Baby's heartbeat will be listened for • Test for Group B Strep may be offered • Fetal blood sampling can be performed

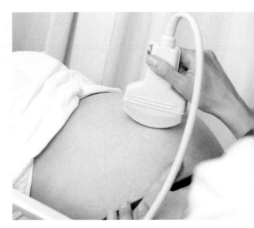
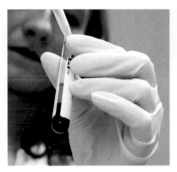
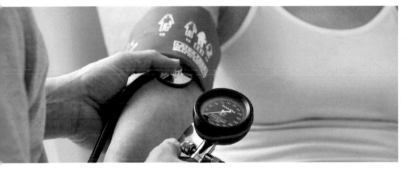
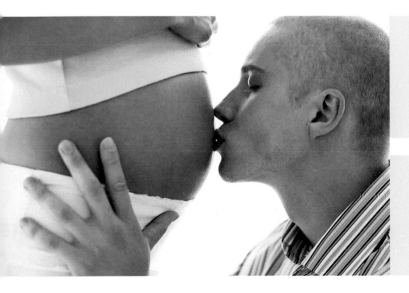
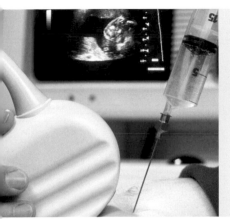

🔴 1ST TRIMESTER   ⚪ 2ND TRIMESTER   ⚪ 3RD TRIMESTER

WEEKS 11 & 12*

Early/dating scan and nuchal translucency test may be performed • Chorionic villus sampling can be performed • Serum screening can be performed

* End of first trimester

WEEK 13–15

Early/dating scan and nuchal translucency test may be performed • Chorionic villus sampling can be performed • Serum screening can be performed

WEEK 17

Serum screening including alpha-fetoprotein (AFP) test can be performed • Amniocentesis can be performed

WEEKS 20–23

Antenatal appointment • Blood pressure and signs of pre-eclampsia check • Baby's heartbeat will be listened for • Serum screening including alpha-fetoprotein (AFP) test can be performed • Anomaly scan may be performed • Fetal blood sampling can be performed

WEEK 24

Antenatal appointment • Blood pressure and signs of pre-eclampsia check • Baby's heartbeat will be listened for • Fetal blood sampling can be performed

WEEKS 28, 30, 32 & 34

Antenatal appointment • Blood pressure and signs of pre-eclampsia check • Baby's heartbeat will be listened for • Blood test for anaemia and/or glucose screen may be offered • Fetal blood sampling can be performed

WEEKS 37–40

Antenatal appointment • Blood pressure and signs of pre-eclampsia check • Urine test • Baby's heartbeat will be listened for • Baby's size and position assessed • Fetal blood sampling can be performed

The first few weeks

During the first four weeks of pregnancy, only the last two are concerned with a baby's gestation. Convention means that pregnancy is dated from the start date of the last menstrual period (LMP), although the majority of women ovulate around two weeks after this. For this reason, there is normally a 2-week gap when comparing pregnancy dates with that of the baby's gestation.

WEEK 3

Conception occurs when one of the millions of sperm released in a man's ejaculation travels through the vagina, up the cervix and uterus and towards the fallopian tube to meet a waiting egg. The sperm is nourished by chemicals released at the time of ejaculation as well as from the vagina. When the 'lucky' sperm penetrates the egg, it burrows through the outer layer (corona radiata) and into the zona pellucida to connect to the nucleus, forming a new cell. The new cell will contain 46 chromosomes – 23 from each parent – enough genetic information for a new life.

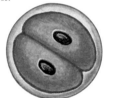

GENDER

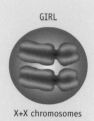

GIRL

X+X chromosomes

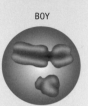

BOY

X+Y chromosomes

Whether a baby is a boy or girl is determined during conception. Sperm can contain a single X (girl) or Y (boy) chromosome, while eggs only contain a single X chromosome. When a sperm with an X chromosome fertilises an egg, the baby will be a girl. When a sperm with a Y chromosome fertilises an egg, the baby will be a boy.

Zygote

The egg, once fertilised, is called a zygote. Between 12–20 hours after fertilisation, the zygote begins to divide in two, replicating its DNA. As the zygote divides, it travels along the fallopian tube towards the uterus, pushed along by feelers in the tube.

CONCEPTION

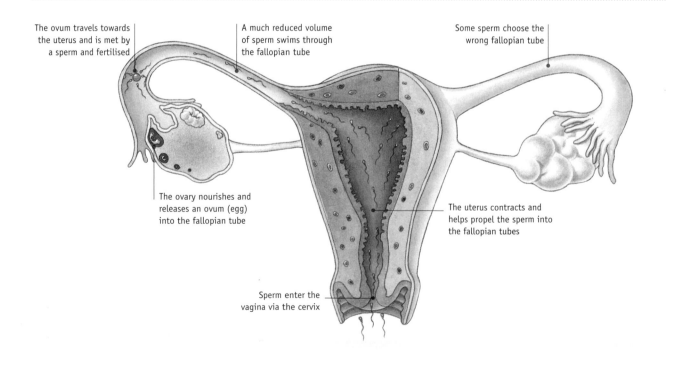

The ovum travels towards the uterus and is met by a sperm and fertilised

A much reduced volume of sperm swims through the fallopian tube

Some sperm choose the wrong fallopian tube

The ovary nourishes and releases an ovum (egg) into the fallopian tube

The uterus contracts and helps propel the sperm into the fallopian tubes

Sperm enter the vagina via the cervix

Morula

The zygote continues to divide and subdivide until it becomes a tiny, solid ball the size of a pinhead consisting of 16–32 cells, and is known as a morula. The morula continues to travel towards the uterus, dividing in 15-hour intervals. Once it reaches the uterus (in about 90 hours), it will have 64 cells. A few of these cells will become the embryo; the other cells will become the placenta and membranes of the uterus.

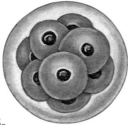

Blastocyst

The morula slowly transforms from a solid into a fluid-filled ball of cells. In this stage it is called a blastocyst. The surface of the blastocyst is made of a single layer of large, flat cells called trophoblast cells. These cells will later become the placenta. The inner cluster of cells contained in the blastocyst will develop into the embryo.

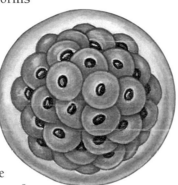

WEEK 4
Implantation

When the blastocyst arrives in the uterus, it is composed of hundreds of cells. It begins to attach itself to the uterine wall by using projections of trophoblast cells, which burrow into the endometrium. The cells grow into the chorionic villi, which will later develop into the placenta. Enzymes are then released which pierce the lining of the uterus and cause tissue to break down, providing nourishing blood cells on which the chorionic villi feed. It takes 13 days for the blastocyst to firmly implant itself.

Once the blastocyst implants, its cells begin to separate into layers. The top layer becomes the embryo and amniotic cavity and the lower layer becomes the yolk sac. Then the embryo forms into three layers: the inner (yellow) layer quickly develops into the lungs, liver, digestive system and pancreas; the middle (pink) layer starts to form the skeleton, muscles, kidneys, blood vessels and heart; and the outer (blue) layer houses the nervous system, teeth and skin.

TWINS

If two eggs are released and fertilised by two different sperm simultaneously, two babies – non-identical or fraternal twins – will be conceived. These babies can be of different sexes and each baby has his or her own placenta. Such twins are only as similar as any two siblings.

If, however, a sperm fertilises a single egg and that egg then splits in two, two identical embryos will be formed. Since they originate from the same egg, identical twins share all chromosomes, are always the same sex and look alike. They may also share a placenta and amniotic sac, although they will have individual umbilical cords.

With triplets and quadruplets, there is a range of possibilities. The siblings may be identical or non-identical, or any combination of identical and non-identical babies.

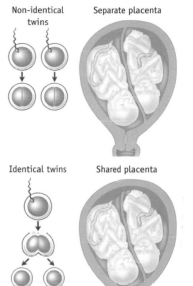

Non-identical twins | Separate placenta

Identical twins | Shared placenta

DEVELOPMENT OF THE EMBRYO

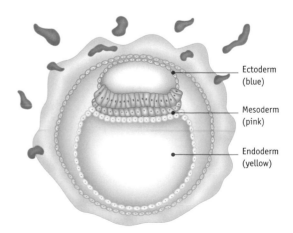

Ectoderm (blue)

Mesoderm (pink)

Endoderm (yellow)

PREGNANCY CALENDAR

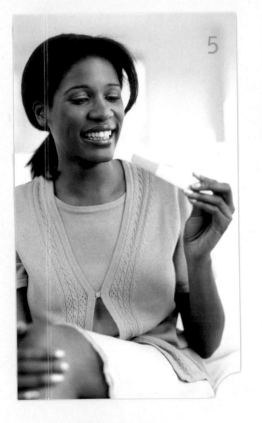

5

MOTHER-TO-BE WEEK 6

After missing my period last week, an over-the-counter pregnancy test confirmed that I'm pregnant – not surprising as my breasts have become tender and full and I feel very tired. In the last few days, I've felt nauseous – particularly in the morning – so I'm now eating small meals and mild-tasting foods to try to settle my stomach. I scheduled an appointment with my doctor.

MOTHER-TO-BE WEEK 7

I'm aware of some internal changes – my heart seems to be beating faster and my senses of smell and taste appear more acute. The walls of my uterus and cervix have softened to allow for implantation and my cervical mucus has thickened to form a plug in my cervical canal, sealing off my uterus until I go into labour.

MOTHER-TO-BE WEEK 11

I've gained around 1 kg, but it is common to lose weight in early pregnancy – particularly if morning sickness is severe. Fatigue is still a problem, yet I find it diffcult to sleep. I'm also feeling warmer than usual and am thirstier – a result of the increased amount of blood being pumped around my body. Small bumps, called Montgomery's tubercles, have appeared on my nipples.

MOTHER-TO-BE WEEK 12

I saw baby on ultrasound – it was fantastic! I also had a nuchal fold translucency test to check for Down's. My morning sickness has stopped and while my skin feels softer due to increased hormone levels, I still break out. I also need to urinate more frequently – I guess my growing uterus is pressing on my bladder.

MOTHER-TO-BE WEEK 13

This is the first week of my second trimester; I'm feeling good and the risk 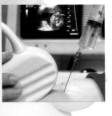 of miscarriage has been reduced. My mood swings have lessened. I had a Chorionic Villus Sampling test to diagnose any possible chromosomal problems or genetic diseases in baby.

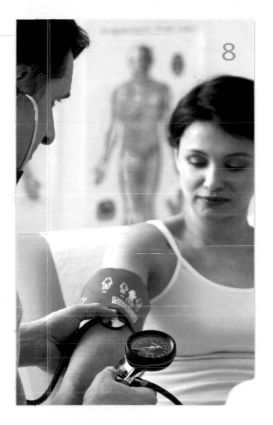

8

MOTHER-TO-BE WEEK 9

At my first antenatal visit, I had a physical examination, blood pressure check and routine blood and urine tests. My uterus has doubled in size and although I don't show yet, my clothes feel a little snug around my waist. My hair is becoming thicker and needs more frequent washing, while my face looks smoother and plumper, and I do get the occasional spot.

MOTHER-TO-BE WEEK 10

My mood swings have increased and I am easily irritated due to hormonal changes and anxiety. Changes in blood pressure have also made me feel faint and dizzy occasionally, especially when I move suddenly. I eat plenty of protein and healthy snacks to get an energy boost.

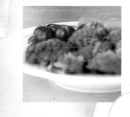

MOTHER-TO-BE WEEK 14

I'm finally showing a bump so have started thinking about maternity clothes. Sometimes I become constipated, which is due to my higher levels of progesterone and the growing uterus putting pressure on my bowels. I've started drinking more water and eating more fibre-rich vegetables and fruit. My placenta is fully formed and producing the necessary hormones. I feel more energetic recently.

MOTHER-TO-BE WEEK 15

The hormones that support pregnancy also cause changes in my skin, hair and gums so I moisturise more regularly and massage my gums to improve blood circulation. I've also noticed changes in skin pigmentation. I have another check-up next week and I will get my earlier blood test results and may be able to hear my baby's heartbeat using an ultrasound monitor.

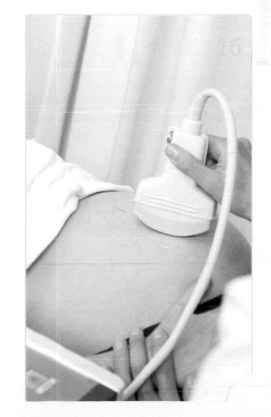

16

PREGNANCY CALENDAR

MOTHER-TO-BE WEEK 17

My breasts are sensitive and I've been fitted for a larger bra. My uterus has moved higher and no longer presses on my bladder so I've stopped urinating so often. The greater volume of circulating blood puts pressure on small blood vessels, resulting in the occasional nosebleed. Also, my hands and feet swell sometimes due to water retention.

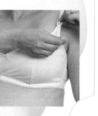

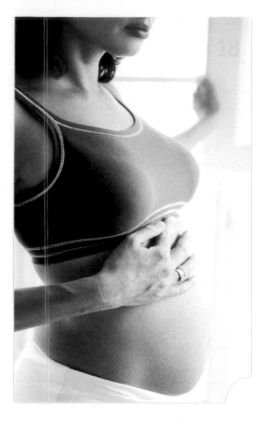

MOTHER-TO-BE WEEK 19

I felt baby move for the first time – really exciting! My energy levels are back to normal and my libido has increased (extra oestrogen heightens blood flow to my pelvis). Everyone says I'm positively blooming – I hope they don't mean this because my hips and buttocks have gotten larger! I have been doing gentle exercises to help me cope with the pregnancy and prepare for labour.

MOTHER-TO-BE WEEK 23

I have been getting bouts of heartburn and indigestion due to my enlarging abdomen so tend to eat several small snacks throughout the day and walk after meals to aid digestion. My hair has become thicker since the shedding cycle has stopped and occasionally my breasts leak a small amount of colostrum.

MOTHER-TO-BE WEEK 24

I've been getting irregular, painless Braxton-Hicks contractions, which help my body prepare for labour. To strengthen my pelvic floor muscles, I have started to Kegel exercises. It's becoming more difficult to go about my normal tasks, as certain movements become more awkward and the pressure on my stomach has led to heartburn after heavy meals. I need to get plenty of rest.

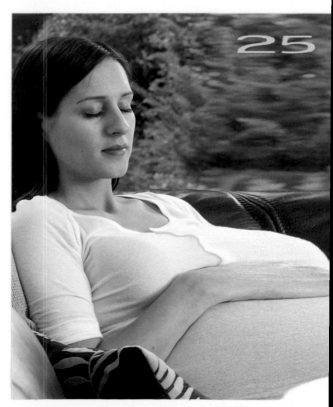

MOTHER-TO-BE WEEK 20

I had a scan during a check-up for the doctor to see baby and check on her development. My bump is more noticeable and gaining weight has changed my posture and gravity. Some back pain has developed since I tend to lean backwards and lying in bed has become uncomfortable. Putting pillows between my knees and under my bump is more comfortable.

MOTHER-TO-BE WEEK 21

My weight gain is causing me to perspire more often and I often feel tummy pain as the ligaments around my uterus stretch. A brownish line has appeared running down my abdomen. I can now feel the top of my uterus in my abdomen, right below my navel (which is sticking out). My expanding uterus puts pressure on my lungs and sometimes I feel breathless.

MOTHER-TO-BE WEEK 22

I have leg cramps often, which are especially bad at night. I have been walking in bare feet and stretching and extending my legs and feet to ease the cramps. Whenever I can, I keep them raised. My appetite has increased, but I try to avoid unhealthy foods and snacks though have the occasional craving for something 'sinful'.

MOTHER-TO-BE WEEK 26

I'm getting stretch marks around my tummy and breasts as my abdomen expands and have started feeling postural pains in my back, along with pains under my ribs. I'm experimenting with pelvic tilts, massage and side lying to see what can help. I have started looking for childbirth classes in my area.

MOTHER-TO-BE WEEK 27

I have occasional episodes of stress incontinence, where I urinate when laughing or sneezing, so I wear panty-liners and continue to work on my pelvic floor exercises. I'm becoming more forgetful, so I carry around a small notebook filled with reminders and leave myself lots of notes around the house.

MOTHER-TO-BE WEEK 28

From this week I will have ante natal checks every two weeks until 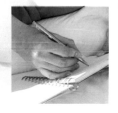 week 36. During my check-ups I will have my iron and glucose levels tested. Due to my increasing size, I have been experiencing some more discomfort – constipation, cramp, breathlessness and backache. On the plus side, I'm more aware of baby's movements and sleep patterns.

PREGNANCY CALENDAR

MOTHER-TO-BE WEEK 29

More colostrum (my baby's first food) is leaking from my breasts. I just put some pads in my bras. I've been eating healthy snacks to increase my calorie intake by 250–300 calories a day and started writing my birth plan to ensure I get the birth I want.

MOTHER-TO-BE WEEK 30

My uterus is once again pressing against my bladder, which means I have started urinating more often so it's hard to get a good night's sleep. This, coupled with increasing back pain, fatigue, breathlessness, swelling and constipation, have left me exhausted. I drink warm milk at night to help me sleep and try to get rest during the day.

MOTHER-TO-BE WEEK 31

I am slower and clumsier recently, in fact, I've become completely uncoordinated. My weight has affected my balance and my joints are loosened due to pregnancy hormones, so I have to be careful on stairs or in the rain and while getting out of bed. I have to remember to roll on to my side before getting up.

MOTHER-TO-BE WEEK 35

The amount of blood in my body increased in my first two trimesters, but now my blood volume will remain the same until I give birth. My Braxton Hicks contractions are occurring more frequently, but this isn't the onset of true labour. I feel very cramped and heavy and try not to stand too long.

MOTHER-TO-BE WEEK 36

I now need checks weekly until the birth. My pelvic area and legs are painful due to my expanding pelvic joints and baby's weight. I've been resting and I make sure to change position often. My breasts have become larger and heavier and the Braxton Hicks contractions continue. By next week my hospital bag will be packed.

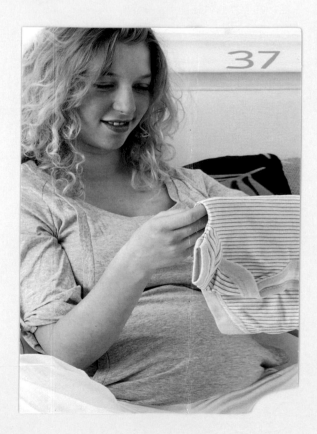

37

MOTHER-TO-BE WEEK 32

My uterus is approaching its highest position. The top sits about 12 cm 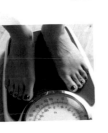 from my belly button. I have gained 8.6 kg – not just from the baby, but also from the placenta, amniotic fluid, increased blood volume, enlarged breasts and uterus. My internal organs have become displaced, but this is normal.

MOTHER-TO-BE WEEK 33

It suddenly became easier to breathe because baby has permanently turned head down. While this also eases my indigestion, it feels painful when she kicks upwards. Fluid retention is making my fingers and ankles swell. I have stopped doing unnecessary work but am buying baby clothes and equipment.

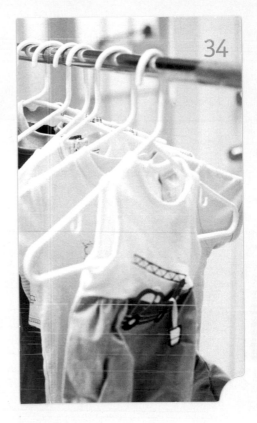
34

MOTHER-TO-BE WEEK 38

I have been feeling tired and anxious about the birth, which has made me irritable, so I'm taking time to calm myself by practising some meditation. I look a little flushed, too, since my circulation is working extra hard. Baby is far down in my pelvis, so walking is uncomfortable, and I have to make frequent trips to urinate.

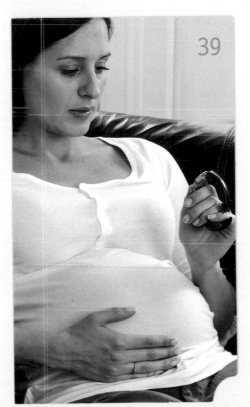
39

MOTHER-TO-BE WEEK 40

I am due to give birth this week, but although I started experiencing false labour contractions (stronger than Braxton Hicks contractions), these are irregular and stop once I move around. It is likely that I will give birth at a later date. I've actually stopped gaining weight, but all the pressure on my pelvis and abdomen is making me very uncomfortable.

The birth

Although the birth canal is only some 23 cm long, it will take many hours for it to be formed and for my baby to negotiate it. Initially sealed by the cervix, the uterus must open out into the vagina to create the birth canal, which needs to stretch to accommodate my baby.

At the same time, my baby's head will be moulded to enable her to safely make her way through. Nobody knows what triggers the birth process, but when I feel cramp-like sensations arising in my uterus, I will know labour has started.

THE BIRTH CANAL STARTS TO BE FORMED

Contractions occur when the uterine muscles tighten and shorten. Cramp-like sensations come in waves: they begin, build in intensity, peak and then ease off. Their purpose is to push baby's head against my cervix so that this thick, sealed exit gradually thins (effaces) and opens up (dilates).

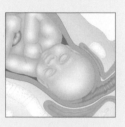

Baby starts out with her head facing up on or near my cervix. As labour progresses, she turns to the side, with the widest part of her head in the widest part of my pelvis.

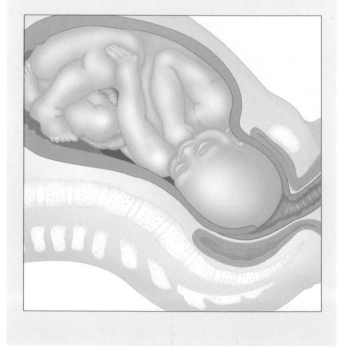

THE FIRST STAGE OF LABOUR ENDS

When my baby's head has acted sufficiently on the cervix so it is transformed into a soft, thin opening – at 10 cm it is fully dilated – and cups my baby's head like the rim of a teacup with her head filling the centre (known as properly engaged), the first stage of labour is finished. Now, my uterus, cervix and vagina seamlessly form the birth canal.

Baby now has her chin on her chest and her head and upper body begin to twist further to face my back.

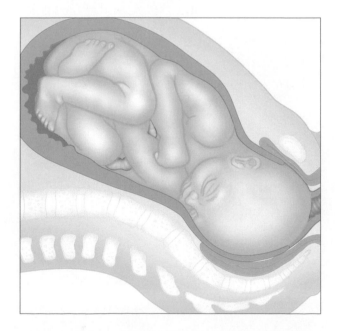

THE 'PUSHING' STAGE BEGINS

An intense urge to push replaces the wave-like sensations of contractions, and to aid her expulsion, my baby joins in the birth process. She uses her feet to push herself away from the wall of my uterus and wriggles her head through my cervix into my vagina. As she goes under my pubic bone and through the opening in the pelvic floor muscles, her skull bones overlap, easing her passage. She also turns her chin down so her head is at its narrowest when passing through the pelvis. She has 'crowned' when her head can be seen at the opening to my vagina.

THE HEAD AND BODY ARE DELIVERED

Once the top of her head has appeared at the vaginal opening, it takes only a few more contractions for me to push baby's head out of my body. With the next contraction her shoulders are born – one before the other – while she keeps her arms held close to her body. Once her shoulders are through, the rest of her body slips out quickly.

Once her head has emerged, baby turns to straighten her neck, so she's facing my side again.

Baby has completed a 90° rotation and is now facing my back.

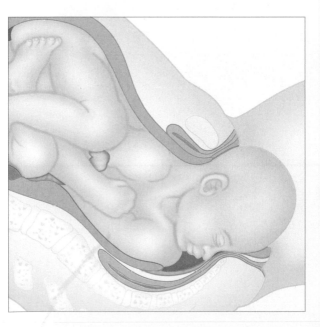

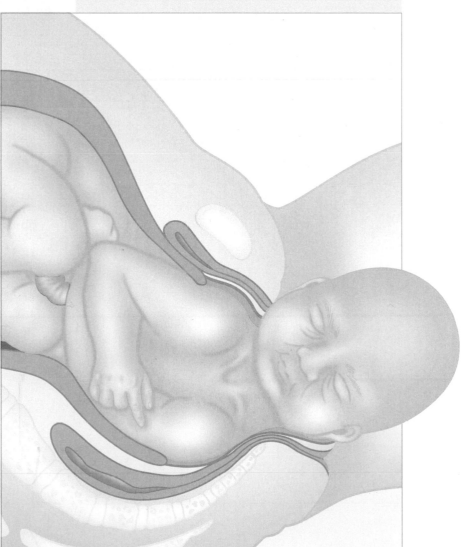

Tests and procedures

ULTRASOUND SCANS

Pain-free and harmless, this technology uses sound waves and their echoes to create a picture of the uterus and developing baby. Before 8–10 weeks of pregnancy, scans can be performed using a probe that is inserted into the vagina; later on, a transducer is moved across the abdomen. 3D versions are possible, which produce a life-like picture of baby and 4D scans show movement. Doppler scans trace the blood flow between the placenta and baby through the umbilical cord and may be done during the anomaly scan (see page 27) to check on any placental problems.

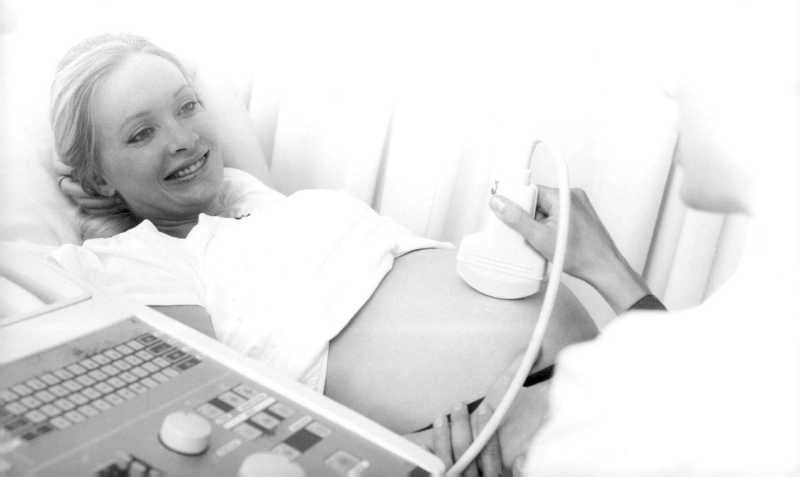

NHS patients are routinely offered at least two scans during pregancy. More scans and/or other tests may be recommended if a problem is found. Gel is spread over the abdominal skin and the transducer is moved on the gel. The sound waves travel through liquid such as the amniotic fluid, but are reflected (bounced back) by more solid structures such as the heart, brain and uterine wall. The quality is variable.

Early/dating scan

Usually carried out between 11–14 weeks, the scan helps:

- Locate the pregnancy.
- Establish an accurate due date. (Scans done after 20 weeks are less reliable.)
- Check the number of babies. If twins or more are present, it can show whether the babies share a placenta or not.
- Check the health of the uterus and ovaries.
- Assess the risk of Down's syndrome. A special fluid-filled area behind a baby's neck – the nuchal translucency – can be measured. If this is thicker than average, the risk of Down's syndrome is increased.

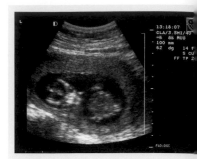

2D ultrasound

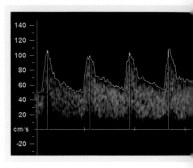

Doppler ultrasound

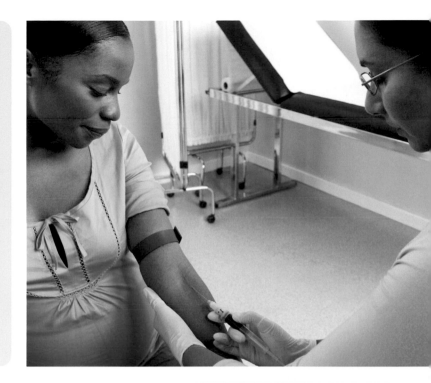

Anomaly scan

This more detailed scan is performed at around 16–22 weeks to check the following:

- Fetal anatomy.
- Gestational age.
- Growth rate.
- Amount of amniotic fluid.
- Location of the placenta.
- The baby's gender.

MATERNAL BLOOD TESTS

Early in pregnancy my blood will be tested to screen for anaemia, to check my blood group and Rhesus factor status, and to assess my immunity or previous exposure to infections including rubella, Hepatitis B, syphilis and HIV. Later in pregnancy I may have blood testing to assess my baby's risk of Down's syndrome.

If my partner or I have a family history of an inherited disease such as Tay-Sachs, sickle cell disease, cystic fibrosis or thalassaemia, I may be offered a blood test to help assess whether my baby is at risk.

DOWN'S SYNDROME SCREENING

The risk of a baby having Down's syndrome – a chromosomal abnormality which is associated with severe learning difficulties – can be estimated by a combination of ultrasound examination (nuchal transparency screening) and serum testing. The latter looks at specific substances in the maternal blood (alpha-fetoprotein (AFP), human chorionic gonadotropin (hCG), Papp-A and inhibin A), which have come from the baby and the placenta and that are raised with Down's syndrome and with some neural tube defects. These tests will pick up more than 75 per cent of women whose babies are at risk. An actual diagnosis can be achieved only by looking at the baby's chromosomes through amniocentesis or chorionic villus sampling.

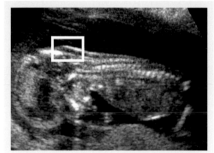

In nuchal transparency screening, a fluid-filled space in the fetal neck is measured.

In the United Kingdom, women who are aged 35 or older – or who will be at their due date – are offered the chance to undergo one of these invasive antenatal tests to check for abnormalities. A woman's risk of having a baby with a chromosomal abnormality increases significantly after she reaches 35 and the risk of miscarriage from the procedure itself is roughly equal to the chance that her baby has a chromosomal abnormality. Most babies with Down's syndrome, however, are born to women under 35, because women aged under 35 have the most babies.

Any woman under 35 who wants to have her baby tested for chromosomal abnormalities should be able to do so, as long as the risks and benefits of the testing are thoroughly understood.

Chorionic villus sampling (CVS)

Typically done between 10–13 weeks, tiny, finger-like pieces of tissue known as chorionic villi, which make up the placenta are removed in one of two ways: by withdrawing placental tissue containing chorionic villi using a flexible catheter inserted through the cervix (transcervical CVS) or using a hollow needle inserted through the abdomen (transabdominal CVS). Ultrasound is used to guide the doctor to the right

location and to avoid causing injury to the baby as the procedure is performed. The tissue, which develops from cells arising out of the fertilised egg and has the same chromosomes and genetic make-up as the developing baby, is then processed in a laboratory and a karyotype (a picture of the chromosomes) is prepared. This is checked to see whether the chromosomes are normal in number and structure. The results may be available in a week, although it can take 2–3 weeks for a full report to be issued.

Amniocentesis

Usually done at 15–20 weeks, a thin needle is inserted through the abdomen and the uterine wall into the amniotic sac to withdraw 15–20 cc (1–2 tbsp) of amniotic fluid from the uterus, which contains chromosomal cells from the baby. An ultrasound scan is used to identify a 'pocket' of amniotic fluid away from the baby. The amniotic fluid cells taken are then incubated and cultured and results are usually available in 1–2 weeks. The test will show whether the 23 chromosome pairs are present and that their structures are normal. A preliminary, more rapid test called a fluorescent in situ hybridisation (FISH) takes 24–48 hours for a result, and may be used if there is a high suspicion of a chromosomal abnormality like Down's syndrome or trisomy 13 (Patau syndrome) or 18 (Edward's syndrome).

Amniocentesis later in pregnancy tests for:
• Infections.
• Rh sensitisation.
• Abnormalities.
• Premature labour.
• The maturity of the fetal lungs.

FETAL BLOOD SAMPLING

Usually performed after week 18 of pregnancy, fetal blood is withdrawn from the umbilical cord for rapid chromosomal diagnosis when a fast result is critical. Also known as percutaneous umbilical blood sampling (PUBS) or cordocentesis, the test is performed under ultrasound guidance and is similar to an amniocentesis, except that the needle is directed into the umbilical cord instead of into the amniotic fluid. It usually takes 3 days for the results to come through. It is sometimes carried out in order to diagnose:
• Some fetal infections.
• Fetal anaemia.
• Hydrops, in which fluid accumulates abnormally in the baby.

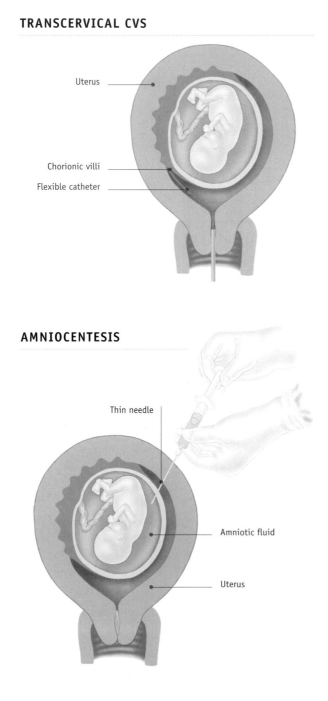

TRANSCERVICAL CVS

Uterus

Chorionic villi

Flexible catheter

AMNIOCENTESIS

Thin needle

Amniotic fluid

Uterus

Monitoring my baby

Although I could see my baby bobbing up and down on the ultrasound, I didn't actually feel her moving until I was just about 20 weeks pregnant. I wasn't certain even then that the flutterings I was feeling were really her moving around.

Once she gets bigger, I will be able to feel her movements more distinctly, although they will happen less frequently. Obviously by then she will have less room in my uterus to move around. In late pregnancy, I should feel quite strong kicks to my ribs and bladder and I will sometimes see as well as feel her moving around; she will push against the skin on my abdomen.

Once I get used to her movements, I should notice that my baby may become more active in response to certain foods I eat – sweets and other sugary food will obviously give her some energy, so there may sometimes be a burst of movement after eating – and also in response to my emotions. She may jump around during a film that enthralls me or become active during a classical concert – particularly if cymbals clash. I should feel her move most at night and when I'm resting during the day, probably because I'll be lying down, relaxed and quiet, and free from distractions.

PATTERNS OF ACTIVITY

Just like a newborn, my unborn baby will have regular sleeping and waking periods. For about 80 per cent of the time she will sleep, but this can be divided into active and inactive sleep. In active sleep, she may dream as she moves her limbs about. During about 12 per cent of the time she'll be awake, but only for part of this time will she be active. The rest of the time, she'll change from being asleep to being awake.

From week 28 onwards, I will be asked to record my baby's movements on a kick chart in order to check on her wellbeing. My caregiver has said I should be able to count at least 10 movements in a 12-hour period and I should immediately report any significant decrease in my baby's movements.

SAMPLE KICK-COUNT SHEET														
TIME	WEEK 39							WEEK 40						
	M	T	W	T	F	S	S	M	T	W	T	F	S	S
9 am														
9.30 am														
10 am														
10.30 am														
11 am														
11.30 am														
12 pm														
12.30 pm														
1 pm														
1.30 pm			▓											
2 pm														
2.30 pm	▓													
3 pm										▓				
3.30 pm				▓										
4 pm									▓					
4.30 pm														
5 pm							▓							
5.30 pm														
6 pm														
6.30 pm														
7 pm														
7.30 pm														
8 pm														
8.30 pm														
9 pm														
If fewer than ten movements by 9 pm, record total number here														
9														
8														
7								▓						
6														
5														
4														
3														
2														
1														

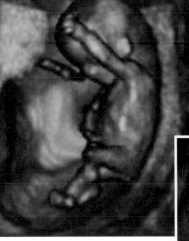

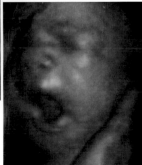

Many different types of movements have been identified in the early part of pregnancy. As well as whole body and limb movements such as rolling over, kicking and 'walking', a fetus also holds on to the umbilical cord, sucks, yawns and hiccups.

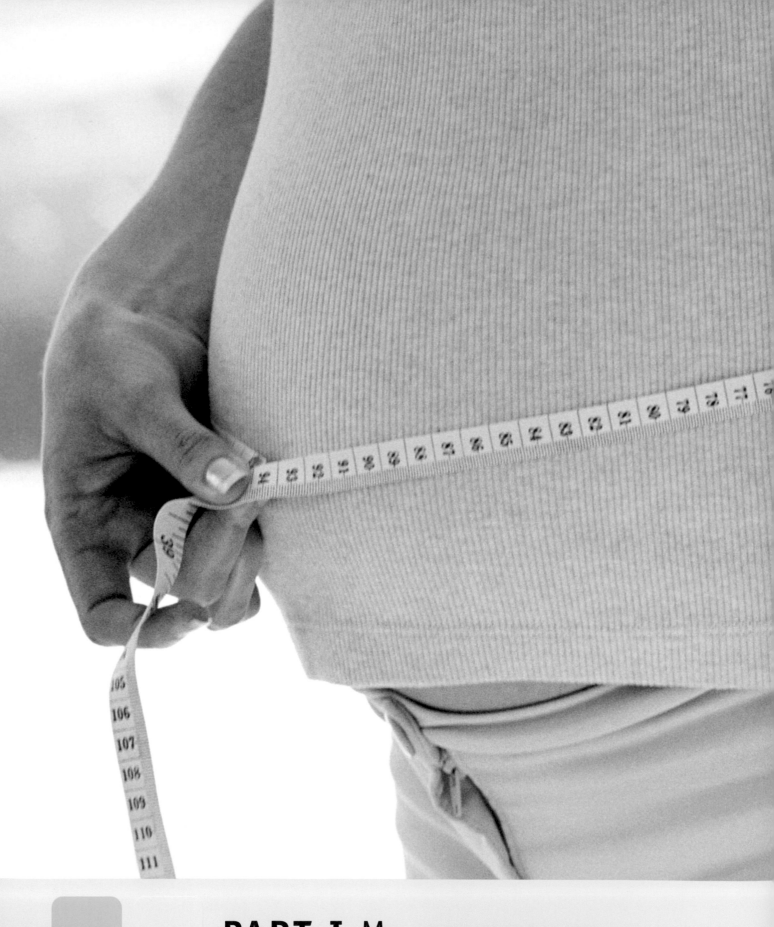

PART I My pregnancy

My pregnant body

There are lots of internal adjustments going on as my body starts to nourish and protect my growing baby, but I'm mainly aware of them by my growing fatigue and changing moods. What I'm most aware of and excited about, however, is my enlarging abdomen. Now everyone can see that I'm expecting a baby and others can share in my joy and anticipation. I will have to make adjustments to my daily care routines and my partner will have to adjust to my changing silhouette.

Pregnancy-related changes

Right from the start I feel different being pregnant, but a lot of the expected changes will only manifest later on and some I'm aware of because of their effects. For example, I am often hungry late at night and this is because my baby is being constantly supplied with nutrients while I eat just my three regular meals. If I eat more frequent smaller meals and snacks, this may help.

LARGER BREASTS

One of the first changes I noticed was the appearance of and sensations in my breasts. Almost immediately, they became fuller and more tender. Now that I'm in the second trimester, my nipples look more prominent and they, and the immediate area around them (areole), have become noticeably darker with more prominent glands. These changes are a result of the pregnancy hormones enlarging the milk ducts that will be used when breastfeeding. In time, further changes will occur.

My breasts will develop more prominent veins as their blood supply increases, and near term, they may secrete colostrum, which is a clear or golden-coloured liquid that will be baby's first milk.

EXPANDING BELLY

In order to accommodate my growing baby and her support system, my belly gradually enlarges. Baby is responsible for about 39 per cent of my weight gain with the placenta, amniotic fluid and enlarging uterus making up 31 per cent. The rest is made up of additional blood and breast tissue.

The placenta nourishes my baby, supplying her with oxygen and removing waste products, and it generates vital pregnancy hormones. My baby is connected to the placenta via the umbilical cord, which is made up of a vein and two arteries. Although my blood and my baby's never actually mixes, my baby is totally

MILK PRODUCTION

Alveoli are clusters of cells in the lobules that produce and store milk. Milk travels from the alveoli through ducts to sinuses, which release milk through openings in the nipple. Sucking sends signals to the brain telling it to release oxytocin, which triggers milk to flow (the let-down reflex). Colostrum, the first fluid, contains a larger amount of protein than mature breast milk and all the minerals, fats and vitamins a baby needs in the first few days. It is also rich in antibodies to protect a baby from infections and clears out the meconium (the first dark green stools) from a baby's bowels. It is followed by transitional milk – a mixture of colostrum and mature milk – and then mature milk, which is both thirst-quenching and highly nutritious.

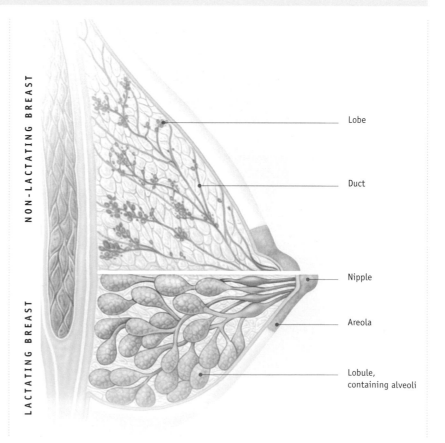

NON-LACTATING BREAST

LACTATING BREAST

Lobe

Duct

Nipple

Areola

Lobule, containing alveoli

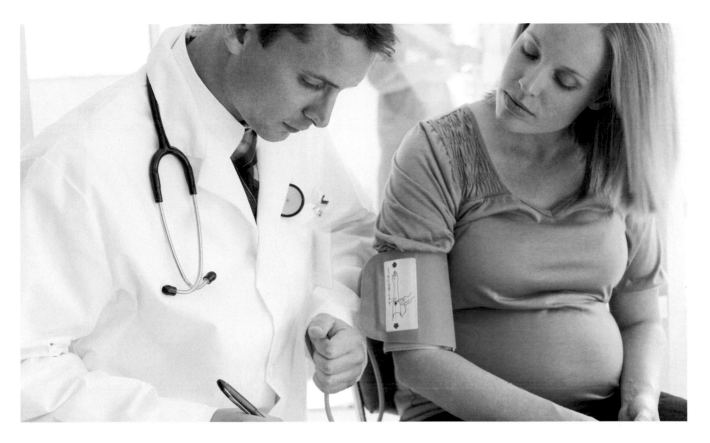

dependent on me for her vital nutrients, antibodies and oxygen and to have her waste products removed. Everything I take in, my baby takes in as well, which is why I must eat a healthy, balanced diet and avoid any substances that could harm her (see page 60).

SKIN PIGMENTATION

Pigmentation changes are common in pregnancy. Existing moles, blemishes and freckles frequently darken, and a dark line can appear running from the pubic bone up to the navel (linea nigra). A mask-like area on the face can appear dark in fair-skinned women and light in dark-skinned women (chloasma), and this becomes worse on exposure to the sun. High levels of oestrogen can cause concentrations of blood vessels to appear as tiny red spots (spider angiomas) anywhere on the body. Pregnancy also has a variable effect on acne; if present, it may

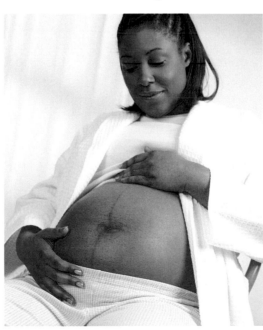

cause it to improve or worsen, and where it is not, it can cause it to arise! Dark pink or red streaks, known as stretch marks, may appear where the skin enlarges.

HORMONAL EFFECTS

Released by the developing placenta as it begins to implant within the uterus, human chorionic gonadrotropin (hCG) triggers the other hormonal activity needed to maintain pregnancy and prevents menstruation. It is thought to be partly responsible for the nausea and vomiting that occur in the first trimester.

Progesterone maintains the functions of the placenta, strengthens the pelvic walls in preparation for labour and relaxes certain ligaments and muscles. This relaxant effect can cause some unwelcome side effects, however; when bowel muscles become sluggish, constipation as well as an uncomfortable feeling of 'fullness' after eating can occur.

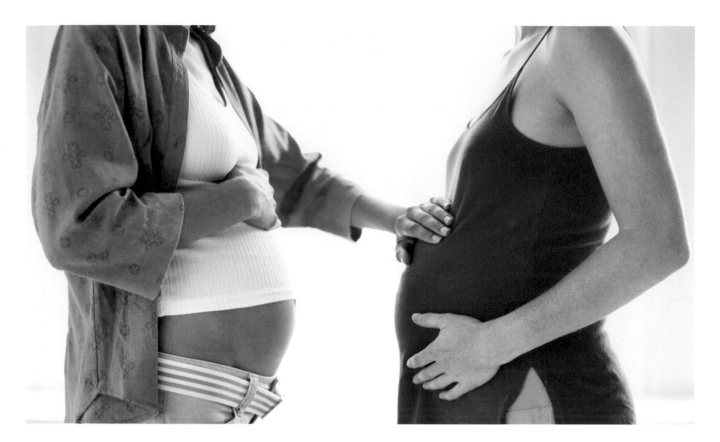

Progesterone also relaxes the sphincter (ring of muscle) between the oesophagus and the stomach; this can, at times, result in heartburn. It also causes veins to dilate, which can lead to varicose veins. Progesterone also helps to stimulate and develop the duct system in my breasts, which is why they feel tender.

Oestrogen helps to prepare the lining of the uterus for pregnancy, increasing the number of blood vessels and glands present within the uterus. It is responsible for some increase in blood volume, which can lead occasionally to bleeding gums or nosebleeds. Its most noticeable effect is an increased flushing, or redness of the skin. Both oestrogen and progesterone have a profound effect on emotions (see page 35).

There are a number of other hormones whose actions are not readily apparent and two that are: relaxin encourages my cervix, pelvic muscles and ligaments and joints to relax in preparation for birth, which is why I need to take care when exercising, and oxytocin, which will cause my milk to flow when breastfeeding.

CIRCULATION CHANGES

Starting from the beginning of pregnancy, blood volume increases to provide an adequate blood supply to my developing baby, enlarging uterus and growing placenta, so much so that by week 30, I'll have 50 per cent more blood circulating within my bloodstream. However, some women's blood counts decrease during pregnancy because their blood cells don't increase in proportion to plasma, and they suffer what is called 'dilutional anaemia'.

I've been told that my heartbeat may become a little faster as it adapts to pregnancy. No one knows for certain why the heart rate increases now; one theory is that it's nature's way of making sure that the extra blood volume gets circulated throughout the body.

Some pregnant women also suffer from low blood pressure, so when they stand up quickly, they may feel dizzy or faint. Others may find their blood pressure increases. This is usually picked up at a routine check and will need to be monitored closely as it is one of the signs of pre-eclampsia, a dangerous condition.

RESPIRATORY CHANGES

Towards the end of pregnancy, breathlessness is likely because my growing baby will prevent my lungs from fully expanding. If I get short of breath, I will need to sit down and breathe steadily, consciously pushing my lungs up and down. If, however, I suddenly develop severe shortness of breath or get a sudden chest pain, I'll seek medical attention at once.

EMOTIONAL CHANGES

Pregnancy hormones can result in a newfound serenity, whereby one's focus turns inwards to form a protective cocoon around baby, or they can produce a roller coaster of emotions: sadness turning into floods of tears; a new sensitivity to the sufferings of others and joy so intense that it, too, spills over into tears.

Even though I was desperate to have a baby, once the pregnancy was confirmed, some doubts and worries began to arise – like wondering how my body would cope with pregnancy and childbirth, whether I might miscarry and if I was really capable of taking care of another human being. After the first rush of emotions, things have settled down and I am more relaxed and trusting of my body. Seeing my tiny but complete baby moving around or sucking her thumb during an ultrasound scan makes me feel reassured, and like others, my antenatal testing (see pages 26–29) does worry me a bit, even though it's designed to provide reassuring information. I try to bear in mind that testing can detect problems early so that my baby has the best chance of being born healthy.

When you first discover that you're pregnant, you may feel delighted that you're having a longed-for baby, triumphant that you're fertile or tender and close to your partner, since it was your physical union that created your baby. However, because of your circumstances, you may see pregnancy as an enormous problem. If you don't feel ready for a baby, your natural response may be anxiety or even panic. Hopefully, this book will help to reassure you and make you feel more comfortable and prepared.

Changing appearance

Emotional reactions to pregnancy are highly individual and unpredictable, but it's almost impossible not to have a strong reaction to one's changing body. Some women who are conscious of their figures feel disturbed by their increasing size during pregnancy. I don't know why they feel embarrassed about their bumps; they aren't getting fat, they're growing a baby!

When I first fell pregnant, I was frustrated that there was nothing to see. Only in my third month did my clothes begin to feel tight and when my tummy did protrude, about the fourth month, I was excited that my pregnancy was clearly visible. Some people even asked to touch my bump. I didn't mind, though I know some women think touching would be invading their space. In these last months, I can hardly believe that my body can go on growing and my bump is so firm.

If I do nothing else I will ...

TRY TO QUELL MY FEARS

Being positive is good for my baby and me. To make sure I don't worry unnecessarily, I will take the following steps:

✓ **Discuss with my caregiver** anything that causes me concern – such as whether any of the antenatal testing I am advised to undergo is harmful to my baby.

✓ **Talk to my mum** and other close relatives or friends about their pregnancy and childbirth experiences.

✓ **Sign up for antenatal classes,** so I can meet other pregnant women and find out what they think about things and what they are experiencing.

✓ **Use positive thinking** whenever problems arise.

✓ **Give up any bad habits** (drinking, smoking, etc.) that could have an impact on my developing baby.

✓ **Try meditation** to relax my mind and body; in times of stress, anxiety, pain or discomfort, simply taking 3 deep breaths and saying "relax" on each long, slow out-breath should bring instant comfort.

Managing common complaints

The 'side effects' of pregnancy are many but generally not serious. However, if my recommended preventative strategies don't work sufficiently and something becomes a real problem, consult your caregiver. He or she may prescribe medication for the problem.

MORNING SICKNESS

Like 80 per cent of women, I suffered from nausea early on and the nausea and vomiting was not limited to mornings. I was lucky that my morning sickness went away by the end of my first trimester. Other women find it continues but becomes much less severe once the first 3 months have passed. Sometimes I felt like vomiting or found the nausea extremely unpleasant and at times debilitating. I was fortunate that the queasiness didn't usually get out of control and I knew it was harmless to me and my baby. Though I'd lost some weight early on, it really wasn't a problem.

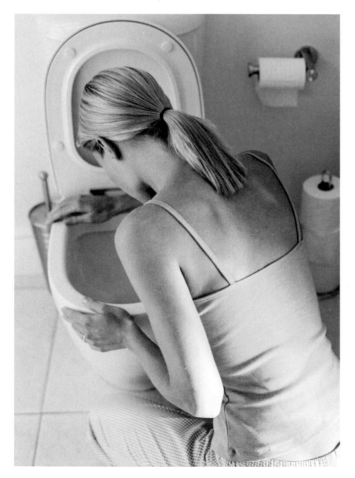

My solutions for combatting nausea include:

✓ Eating small, frequent meals so that you never have an empty stomach. You don't need to worry overly much about eating a balanced diet, but just snack frequently on dry, carbohydrate-rich nibbles throughout the day.

✓ Keeping well hydrated with water or juices; cut down on caffeinated drinks (see also page 50).

✓ Learning accupressure points that can relieve nausea.

✓ Taking ginger in the form of tea, tablets and biscuits.

✓ Switching toothpaste brands when nausea gets worse when tooth brushing.

FATIGUE

I can't believe how exhausted I felt when first pregnant, but this was probably due to all the changes taking place, including the dramatic rise in my hormone levels. Now, as I enter my second trimester, the tiredness is slowly easing but it will return in late pregnancy. This is only to be expected as I will then be carrying around a lot of extra weight.

EXPERTS ADVISE

Excessive vomiting

If you lose a fair amount of weight, can't keep down food or liquids or feel dizzy or faint, tell your caregiver right away. He or she will want to rule out hyperemesis gravidarum – a serious condition involving excessive vomiting leading to a need for rehydration by intravenous drip (see page 66).

I find that fatigue is helped by:

✓ Getting as much rest as possible. I sit with my feet up whenever I can and go to bed early.

✓ Being realistic about what I can do. I expect my partner and others to help with household chores, run errands and do the shopping.

✓ Eating a healthy pregnancy diet (see page 48) and avoiding caffeine and sweets. Sweets provide a quick energy lift but leave me feeling more fatigued as my blood sugar level drops.

✓ Exercising gently every day.

CONSTIPATION

About half of pregnant women suffer from hard and difficult-to-pass stools as a result of pregnancy hormones making waste matter pass more sluggishly through the intestines and bowel, complicated by the expanding uterus squashing the intestines. Taking iron supplements can make the problem worse.

In order to prevent constipation, I:

✓ Eat plenty of high-fibre foods such as bran cereals, fruit and vegetables.

✓ Drink plenty of fluids such as watered-down fruit juice, milk and water.

✓ Put prunes on the menu. I eat a few or drink a glass of prune juice every day.

✓ Exercise regularly. Exercise encourages the bowels to become more active and promotes daily bowel movements.

VARICOSE VEINS AND HAEMORRHOIDS (PILES)

The expanding uterus puts pressure on major blood vessels, producing swollen and enlarged veins in the leg and around the anus (haemorrhoids). A woman is more likely to get varicose veins if they run in her family. The swollen veins are usually painless, but occasionally may ache and haemorrhoids may bleed. Varicose veins usually regress after delivery, but sometimes not completely, and haemorrhoids may appear only as a result of delivery.

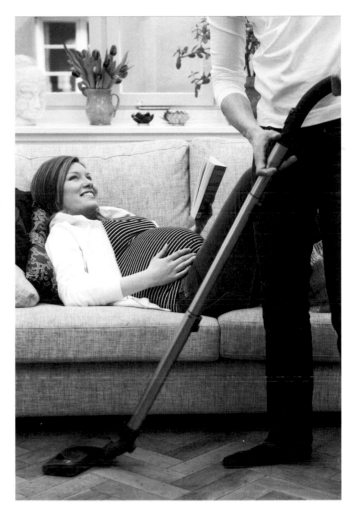

To ensure that I avoid swollen veins, I:

✓ Try to take several rest periods throughout the day and elevate my legs whenever possible.

✓ Wear support stockings. Ask your caregiver about special prescription elastic stockings.

✓ Take measures against constipation (see opposite) and do not strain during bowel movements.

✓ Exercise every day. I also exercise my pelvic floor muscles (see Kegel exercises, page 56) regularly, to improve circulation to that area.

✓ Sit in a warm bath 2–3 times a day if I get muscle spasms.

✓ Soothe the perineal area with witch hazel or special pads.

✗ Don't stand still or sit for long periods of time. If I have to sit, I move my legs around from time to time to stimulate circulation and flex my feet to keep the blood from pooling.

✗ Avoid tights or socks with tight elastic tops that grip around one part of my leg.

HEARTBURN

This burning sensation in the upper part of the abdomen, near the breastbone, is the result of stomach acids being pushed up into the lower oesophagus (the tube connecting the mouth to your stomach). Heartburn is common during pregnancy because pregnancy hormones slow digestion and relax the sphincter muscle between the oesophagus and the stomach, which normally prevents the upward movement of stomach acids.

To combat the effects of heartburn, I try:

✓ Eating small, frequent meals.

✓ Taking a safe-for-pregnancy antacid after meals and at bedtime.

✓ Munching on dry cream crackers when I feel heartburn to neutralise the wind.

✓ Sleeping with my head elevated on several pillows.

✗ Not eating spicy, fatty or greasy foods or eating anything just before bedtime (heartburn occurs most readily when lying down).

FLUID RETENTION (OEDEMA) AND SWELLING

During pregnancy, body fluids increase and tissues swell so that three out of four pregnant women will develop oedema at some point. Usually the swelling appears in feet and ankles, hands and fingers. It's most noticeable at the end of the day or after prolonged standing or sitting and in warm weather. Swelling could be a sign of pre-eclampsia, so I will mention it at my check-ups.

To alleviate any swelling, I will:

✓ Take regular breaks from standing and sit with my legs elevated.

✓ Keep swollen hands elevated above my heart rather than held down by my sides.

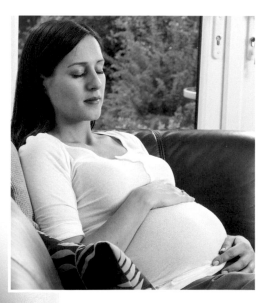

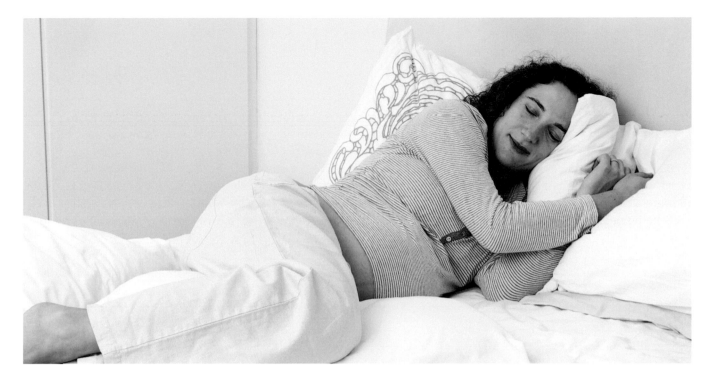

✓ Wear support stockings or ask about special prescription elastic stockings.

✓ Drink plenty of fluids to help to expel excess fluid.

✗ Not stand for long periods.

✗ Not wear tight clothing or shoes.

✗ Not restrict my salt intake unless my blood pressure is high.

STRESS INCONTINENCE

During the last months of pregnancy, I may begin to leak a little urine when I cough, sneeze, laugh or move around. Known as stress incontinence, this is perfectly normal and is caused by the growing uterus putting pressure on my bladder. However, as urine loss can be a sign of a urinary tract infection or a continuous fluid loss be a sign of ruptured membranes (see page 96), I will notify my caregiver if I continue to lose large or frequent amounts of fluid.

I can help prevent stress incontinence by:

✓ Practising pelvic floor exercises (see Kegel exercises page 56) regularly to help to strengthen my muscles and support the urinary sphincter.

DIFFICULTY SLEEPING

During the last few months of pregnancy, insomnia can occur due to an inability to find a comfortable sleeping position as well as to normal anxiety about having a baby.

In order to help ensure a good night's sleep, I will:

✓ Invest in a number of pillows to tuck under my bump, and under and between my legs, making it easier to find a comfortable position.

✓ Take a warm, relaxing bath before going to bed.

✓ Drink warm milk. Warming the milk releases tryptophan, a naturally occurring amino acid that makes one feel sleepy.

✓ Get plenty of fresh air. I will make sure there's a window open so that I am not sleeping in a stuffy environment.

✓ Try to exercise on a regular basis.

✗ Not eat a heavy meal before bedtime. I will eat earlier in the evening and then have a light snack before bed, if I get peckish.

In the bedroom

In some ways, since I became pregnant, my partner and I have grown closer – sharing experiences with and expectations about our baby. However, the hormonal changes going on in my body with all their accompanying side effects – low energy levels, morning sickness, backache, change in sex drive and sore breasts to name but a few – do seem to get on top of me sometimes and it's hard not to feel irritable and annoyed when my partner expects me to act as I did before I was pregnant – especially in the bedroom – instead of appreciating that pregnancy can put you off preparing meals and having sex!

I also worry about how our life together will change once our little one is here although we've already discussed the financial implications and how we're going to manage, at least for a while, on just one salary.

If I do nothing else I will ... ✓

WORK ON MY RELATIONSHIP
In order to make sure we remain a happy couple, I will:

✓ **Talk with my partner** about anything that may be worrying him as well as me. It's important that we can provide each other with mutual support.

✓ **Continue to spend time together.** Whether we're out and about doing things we both enjoy or simply relaxing together, this will be the last months on our own as a couple and we should make the most of it!

✓ **Make sure he shares in the pregnancy.** Having my partner come to some of my antenatal procedures and childbirth preparation classes, reading books together and discussing issues like baby's name makes him feel part of the pregnancy and me as if I'm not doing everything alone.

✓ **Go to bed early.** While having an early night won't guarantee I'll feel like sex, it's more likely I'll be more in the mood for intimacy if I'm not completely exhausted before retiring.

✓ **Encourage my partner** when he shares my work load. If I praise him for taking over some chores, he'll more readily do so when the baby is here.

✓ **Not go to bed angry.** If I have problems with my partner, I'll make sure to resolve them before we go to sleep.

SHOWING AFFECTION
Like most other things, pregnant women have different reactions to sexual intercourse. Emotional closeness can lead to particularly tender, loving sex, which is intensified by physical changes (see opposite page) but in the early weeks, if they experience nausea and extreme tiredness, many women won't feel in the mood.

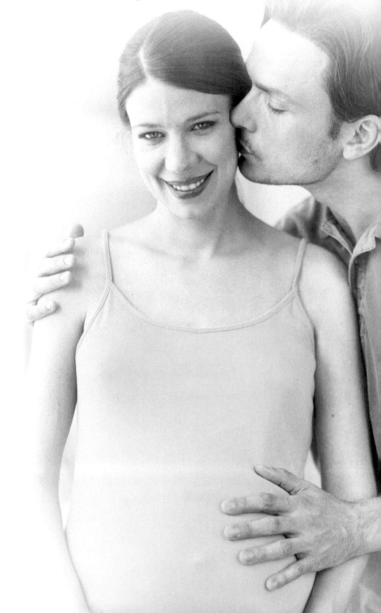

No sex, please...

Generally, there is no risk to your unborn baby when you make love. If you have a history of miscarriages, however, you may want to avoid penetrative sex until you are beyond the first 12 weeks. Likewise, if you've previously had a premature delivery or are experiencing signs of early labour, it may be best to avoid sex in the last trimester, as it could trigger the onset of labour. You should also avoid sex in late pregnancy if your membranes have broken or if you have any bleeding.

CHANGES IN SEXUAL RESPONSE

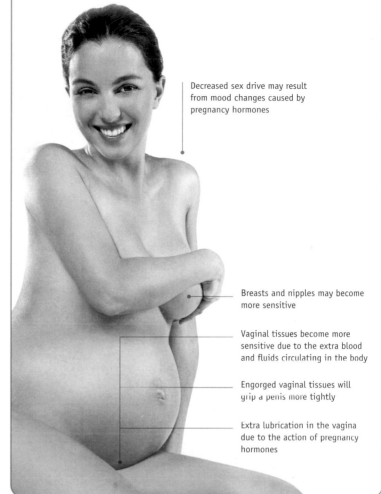

Decreased sex drive may result from mood changes caused by pregnancy hormones

Breasts and nipples may become more sensitive

Vaginal tissues become more sensitive due to the extra blood and fluids circulating in the body

Engorged vaginal tissues will grip a penis more tightly

Extra lubrication in the vagina due to the action of pregnancy hormones

However, once this stage passes, most feel liberated in their lovemaking, as there's no longer pressure to become pregnant or any need for birth control. Some pregnant women describe being in an almost constant state of arousal, particularly in the second trimester, and many women experience more intense orgasms than before they became pregnant, with the vaginal tissues remaining swollen long after orgasm. This may mean, however, that they can feel somewhat unsatisfied after sex – a sensation that can be eased with masturbation.

After the fourth month of pregnancy it's not a good idea to spend too much time lying on one's back, so the missionary position is out and women-on-top and side-by-side positions will be more comfortable. A lubricant may be necessary to avoid the possibility of abrasions and soreness, as the vagina is extra sensitive.

In any event, sex doesn't have to mean full intercourse. If you prefer or need to avoid penetrative sex, extended foreplay can be tried though if your partner is masturbating you, he should use a lubricant – saliva, if nothing else – to avoid causing abrasions. Vaginal secretions may taste stronger during oral sex, which can come as a surprise to some partners.

Of course, there are other ways of enjoying intimacy – simple kisses, cuddles and stroking or sharing a bath together. Massage is a welcome luxury during pregnancy, especially if you're feeling uncomfortable and finding it difficult to relax (see page 94).

SEXUAL PROBLEMS

Pregnancy doesn't always mean satisfying and carefree sex. Some women feel uncomfortable, tired or dislike their new shape, and don't feel at all sexy. Tender breasts, particularly in early and late pregnancy, may be too sore to be caressed by a partner and in late pregnancy may leak colostrum, which a woman or her partner might find off-putting.

Some men feel daunted by their partner's changing body or anxious about hurting her or their baby. A partner might start to see you more as a mother figure than a lover, and this could disturb his usual response. Some men are put off sex by the very proximity of their babies, who seem to be 'witnessing' the whole performance (though this is not, in fact, the case).

It's all too possible in pregnancy for one partner to feel rejected by the other – not because there's less love between you, but because the usual patterns of expressing it are disturbed. If I feel turned off sex for any reason, I know it's important to talk about it, to be specific about what has changed for me, but also to express all the positive feelings that remain unchanged.

9 months of looking good

TAKING CARE OF MY SKIN

Due to the greater volume of blood circulating in my body, combined with the slight rise in body temperature, my skin has the characteristic pregnancy 'glow' and its texture has become softer and more velvety as it plumps out and retains more moisture. However, it also has become a bit unpredictable; it feels unusually greasy, though some of my pregnant friends find their skins are drier than normal, and spots or acne are not uncommon. My daily skincare routine – cleansing with a suitable non-soap product, a mild astringent followed by a moisturiser – may need to be adjusted to accommodate these changes and I may have to keep making minor adjustments as my pregnancy progresses. I may have to start using a cleanser for oilier skin, for example. I find facials a great way to relax and they won't worsen any pregnancy-related skin changes, but as my skin is more sensitive than usual, I'll have to check with the therapist that her products are suitable to use in pregnancy.

If I develop spider angiomas (tiny broken blood vessels) on my cheeks or chloasma (see Skin pigmentation page 33), I'll use a good quality concealer to even out my skin colour; most of these marks will fade after delivery.

My lips, however, are drier than usual, so I use a moisturising lip balm regularly – on its own or under lipstick – to stop them from cracking.

My increased blood flow makes me feel warmer than I'm used to and, as a result, I'm sweating more easily. However, when I take my daily bath or shower, I need to use warm water rather than hot, as hot water opens my pores and makes me even more likely to sweat. When my skin feels dry, instead of soap, I use a light aqueous cream. Clothes made of natural fibres help me to stay cooler than those of synthetic fibres. I also wear cotton underwear and tights with cotton-lined gussets.

The skin on my abdomen and breasts is being stretched considerably and it feels dry and itchy. Massaging my tummy with a moisturising cream or oil may help to ward off stretch marks and is a great way to communicate with my baby. I also rub some on my breasts as well but not so much that they become soft and damp as this can make them feel sore. Sometimes, when I'm home alone, I expose them to the air. I also have an occasional body massage but I see someone

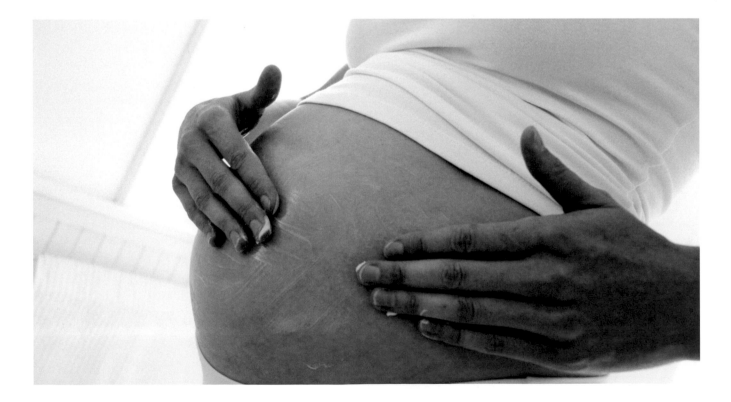

who specialises in pregnancy massage and uses appropriate oils.

Stretch marks

My thighs, stomach and breasts are the most likely places to develop stretch marks. There's no certain way of preventing them, nor any miracle cure for them once they have arrived, but doing the following can help:

- Not gaining too much weight. Too much rapid weight gain won't give my skin a chance to adapt, so it will stretch to accommodate my new shape.
- Wearing a well-fitting bra that supports my breasts throughout my pregnancy. If my breasts become very large, wearing the bra while sleeping can also help.
- Massaging my skin morning and night with cocoa butter or almond oil extract to keep it supple and itch-free.

Sun protection

Hormones will make my skin more susceptible to the effects of the sun, so that it may burn much more quickly than before. I need to use a foundation or moisturising cream containing sunscreen daily, and cover all my exposed skin with sun cream with a sun protection factor (SPF) of at least 15 before I leave the house. Wearing a hat in strong sunshine is also important.

LOOKING AFTER MY HAIR

The same factors that improve my complexion may affect my hair – it can grow faster and hair loss lessens so that my hair looks thicker and more lustrous than usual. Some pregnant women, however, are less lucky and find that their hair becomes greasy or unusually dry or lifeless. No matter whether my hair improves or worsens, the situation is only temporary; any extra hair will disappear within six months of baby's birth and its condition will revert to what it was before.

- If it becomes greasy, I'll need to wash it frequently with a specially formulated shampoo and not brush it too vigorously, as this will encourage the sebaceous glands in the scalp to produce even more oil.
- If, on the other hand, my hair becomes dry and flyaway, I'll use a hot-oil treatment or deep conditioner once a week. Mousse can add volume, improve 'bad-hair days' and keep my style in place. Again, I won't brush my hair too much as this will encourage split ends.
- I'll also find an easily manageable hair style because as my pregnancy progresses, and certainly once my

baby is born, I won't want to cope with anything complicated.
- If I have any treatments – colouring or perming – I need to be aware that hormones may make my hair react differently now. I could end up with a colour I wasn't expecting or with frizzy rather than wavy hair.

CARING FOR MY TEETH AND GUMS

Good dental hygiene is very important throughout pregnancy. My circulating pregnancy hormones will probably cause my gums to swell slightly, making them more susceptible to bleeding during brushing and flossing, and to plaque and bacteria. I need to brush my teeth and floss at least twice a day, ideally after meals, and to massage my gums gently with my fingertips after brushing to encourage blood circulation. A soft-bristled brush is less likely to cause my gums to bleed.

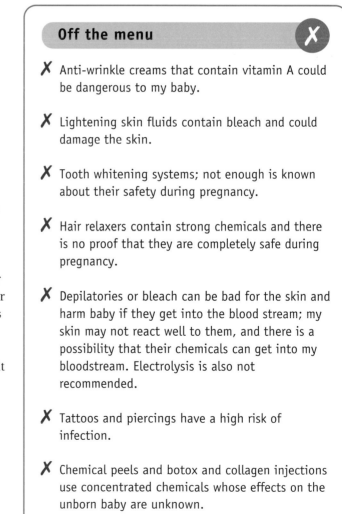

Off the menu ✗

✗ Anti-wrinkle creams that contain vitamin A could be dangerous to my baby.

✗ Lightening skin fluids contain bleach and could damage the skin.

✗ Tooth whitening systems; not enough is known about their safety during pregnancy.

✗ Hair relaxers contain strong chemicals and there is no proof that they are completely safe during pregnancy.

✗ Depilatories or bleach can be bad for the skin and harm baby if they get into the blood stream; my skin may not react well to them, and there is a possibility that their chemicals can get into my bloodstream. Electrolysis is also not recommended.

✗ Tattoos and piercings have a high risk of infection.

✗ Chemical peels and botox and collagen injections use concentrated chemicals whose effects on the unborn baby are unknown.

- When I can't brush after eating, a stick of sugar-free chewing gum will help to prevent plaque build-up.
- I'll need to see my dentist once every 6 months and to be sure to tell him or her I'm pregnant. X-rays and extensive treatment should be avoided at this time.

TAKING CARE OF MY BACK

As my pregnancy progresses, my centre of gravity shifts forward, which can result in bad posture, upper back and shoulder pain and lower back discomfort. To prevent the stresses and strains that can cause

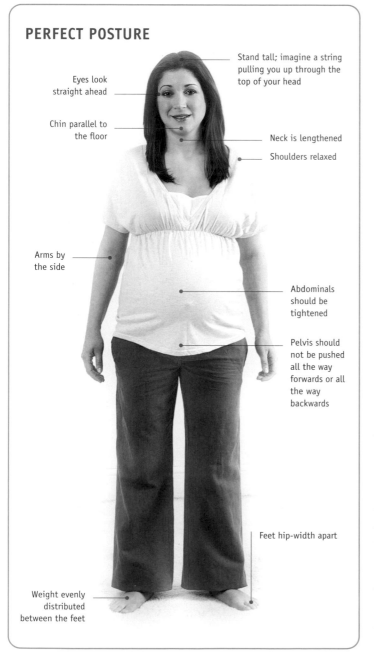

PERFECT POSTURE

Stand tall; imagine a string pulling you up through the top of your head

Eyes look straight ahead

Chin parallel to the floor

Neck is lengthened

Shoulders relaxed

Arms by the side

Abdominals should be tightened

Pelvis should not be pushed all the way forwards or all the way backwards

Feet hip-width apart

Weight evenly distributed between the feet

problems, I'll need to maintain good posture while performing my everyday activities. Pilates and other core stability exercises can help greatly with posture.

- To prevent any back pain, I always sit on chairs with good back support and, when possible, keep my knees elevated above my hips. I also sleep on my side on a firm mattress. I find keeping a pillow between my legs and under my bump supports my back.
- When lifting, I try not to strain my back. I keep my feet shoulder-width apart and bend at the knees. As I lift, I push up with my thighs keeping my back straight. When carrying bags, I keep the weight evenly distributed – either dividing the load into two bags and carrying one in each hand or using a small backpack carried on both shoulders.
- I wear low-heeled shoes.

MY PREGNANCY WARDROBE

It probably won't become overly obvious until about week 20 (week 14 in subsequent or multiple pregnancies) that I'm pregnant, but as my bump grows my clothes will start to feel uncomfortable when my tummy is squeezed or my breasts enlarge. I can still wear many of my existing clothes – opening the zips on some trousers – and I've borrowed some of my partner's larger shirts. However, maternity clothes are specially designed to flatter pregnant women. Skirts and dresses are usually longer at the front than the back so that the growing bump does not cause a wavy hemline. Tucks and darts are positioned to ensure that clothes continue to hang well as my bump enlarges. Ribbed panels and special stretch material can accommodate the expanding bump without distorting more fitted styles. Fastenings are usually adjustable, often with several holes and buttons sewn on with elastic thread. As a result, a small selection of such clothes will grow with me and continue to look good until the end of pregnancy and even through the first few weeks, or even months, after the birth, if necessary, while my figure gradually reverts to its pre-pregnancy state.

As I'm planning to breastfeed, I need to choose tops, dresses and nightdresses that give easy and discreet access to my breasts – those with ample material or ties or buttons down the front are ideal.

Maternity bras

Unsupported or badly supported breasts are more likely to develop stretch marks or to sag because they contain no muscles and are supported solely by the muscles on the chest wall. By the end of 9 months, my breasts may be up to two cup sizes larger than before, and the measurement around my chest, below my breasts, will probably increase as my ribs expand to accommodate my growing baby.

After the birth – and once I've have stopped breastfeeding – my breasts will reduce in size, but probably won't be the same size and shape as they were before pregnancy. It's vital that I look after them well.

MY TO DO LIST

Buying the following special maternity items can help make me look and feel better during pregnancy and the first weeks following birth.

☐ **Tights:** Maternity tights have extra material in front to accommodate my bump and the waistband sits high enough to keep my tights up. Maternity support tights – available in light, medium or firm – can be helpful If Imy feet ache feet or I have varicose veins (see page 37). It's advisable to slip them on before geting out of bed in the morning.

☐ **Knickers:** Mini maternity briefs fit snugly under my bump, while full maternity briefs have ample material to fit over it. Maternity support knickers, which incorporate a semi-rigid back panel, can help relieve backache.

☐ **Swimsuit:** A maternity one will 'grow' along with me and my baby.

☐ **Bras:** I need to buy a new maternity bra each time my breast size increases or when I feel uncomfortable and cramped inside my existing one. As I'm planning to breastfeed, from around 36 weeks, I should invest in a nursing bra that allows me to expose one breast at a time to feed my baby. Drop-cup, where each cup unhooks from the shoulder strap; zip-cup, where the cups unzip under the breast and front opening, where each cup is attached to the centre of the bra by a hook-and-eye fastening are all available. Bra tops are also available with maternity features.

I need to replace any existing bras that don't offer good support or squeeze my breasts in any way or make me feel uncomfortable and cramped. If my breasts become particularly large and heavy, a sleep bra (a lightweight maternity bra worn through the night) will help to make me feel more comfortable and I'll have to buy a nursing bra since I'll be breastfeeding – one that I can open and close easily with one hand – the other will be occupied holding my baby. I need to choose bras that have:

• Wide, adjustable shoulder straps. These distribute the weight more evenly.
• A high proportion of cotton. Natural fibres allow my skin to breathe.
• A broad band of elastic under the cups. This will support my breasts as they become heavier.
• An adjustable back. The ideal is to have 4 hook-and-eye fastenings, so that I can loosen my bra as my ribcage expands.
• No underwiring. The stiff wire can pinch and damage my breast tissues.

Footwear

It's not unusual for feet to swell, so I may need shoes in a larger size than usual. Like many pregnant women, I find that trainers are the most comfortable form of footwear, particularly those with good foot and ankle support. As a rule, I shouldn't wear the same pair of shoes two days in a row, but to swap between at least two pairs to allow each pair time to breathe and dry out.

• Ideally, I should go barefoot in the house as much as I can, to exercise the muscles in my feet and improve my circulation.
• In addition to maternity tights, I will choose cotton or cotton-rich socks, which allow my skin to breathe. They musn't be they too tight for my feet or legs. Shorter socks, such as ankle socks, will ensure that the veins in my legs aren't compressed.

In choosing suitable shoes I need to seek out:

• Comfortable, low-heeled shoes. High heels will throw my posture out, making me thrust my bump forwards and possibly leading to backache. Completely flat styles won't help my balance either.
• Breatheable materials. Leather and canvas are more suitable than patent leather, nylon, rubber or PVC.
• Loafers, slip-ons or pumps. Lace-up or buckle styles will be hard to put on in the later stages of pregnancy, when I won't be able to bend easily to do them up.

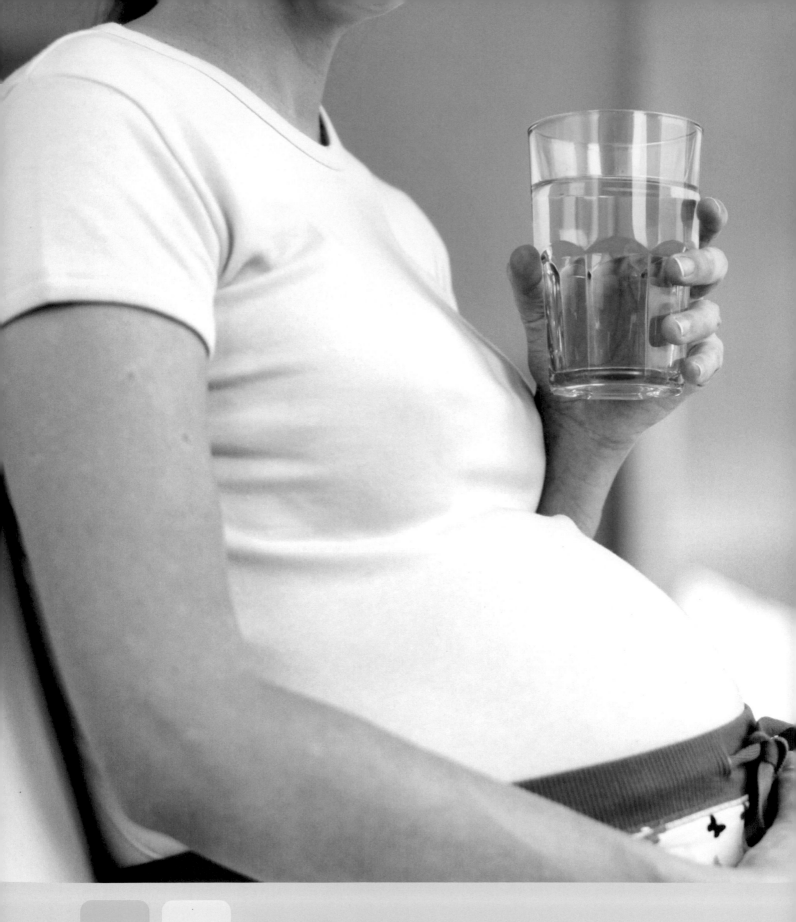

PART I My pregnancy

Making my body a safe haven

To ensure that my baby is able to grow and develop in supportive surroundings, it's important that I take care with what I eat and drink and how I keep it in shape. There are also substances and activities I should avoid – both at home and in other environments – as well as being aware of conditions and situations that could prove hazardous to my baby or me.

My pregnancy diet

My daily diet differs little from that which I used to eat for all-round health. It basically consists of the five major food groups eaten in different proportions. However, there are certain foods that I should avoid to protect myself and my baby.

VEGETABLES AND FRUIT

A third of my diet should be comprised of vegetables and fruit – of as many different types as possible.They will provide me with vital vitamins (A, B and C) as well as iron and fibre. The vitamins and iron will help my baby's body to develop properly in the womb, while fibre (see opposite page) will aid my digestion and prevent constipation.

I should eat at least five portions a day, which could be fresh, dried, frozen or tinned – and more vegetables than fruit. A portion can be 3 tbsp cut-up or cooked vegetables, 4 tbsp fresh greens, a medium pear or two small satsumas; two tinned pear or peach halves; 30 g dried apricots; 150-ml glass of pure vegetable or fruit juice (one per day). In order to preserve the nutrients in vegetables, I must lightly steam them or eat them raw but well washed.

BREAD, RICE, POTATOES, PASTA AND CEREALS

Another third of my diet should be composed of starchy foods, which, in addition to the above, include noodles, maize, millet, oats, sweet potatoes, yams and cornmeal. Also known as complex carbohydrates, these foods are important sources of vitamins B and E, folic acid, minerals and fibre. Starchy foods are needed to maintain my blood sugar levels and help me feel energised for long periods of time.

A portion of starchy food can be two slices of wholemeal bread, 4 tbsp cooked rice or 6 tbsp cooked pasta. Wholemeal instead of processed (white) varieties are best because they are more nutritious and contain the most fibre.

I must try to avoid unhealthy toppings, fillings and sauces, as they contain high levels of fat and calories and don't contribute any essential nutrients.

MEAT, POULTRY, FISH, EGGS AND LENTILS

Protein foods are essential for my baby and me since they contain essential vitamins and minerals, such as iron and zinc, which help my baby's cells, tissues and

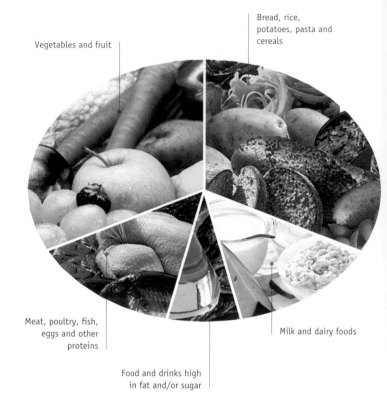

Vegetables and fruit

Bread, rice, potatoes, pasta and cereals

Meat, poultry, fish, eggs and other proteins

Milk and dairy foods

Food and drinks high in fat and/or sugar

organs develop. It is important that I eat 2–3 portions a day. Because my body cannot make some of the amino acids that build protein, I need to eat foods that contain the amounts needed. As well as in meat, poultry, fish and eggs, proteins are also found in pulses, nuts and cheese, which is important if I want to rely on meatless meals some of the time (see also Vegetarian or Vegan Mum, page 52). A portion of protein can be 115 g fish, 85 g meat or 140 g cooked lentils.

The best choices are lean meats and skinless poultry (the fat and skin are high in unhealthy saturated fat), as well as oily fish. All contain calcium and omega-3 fatty acids that help in the development of my baby's eyes and brain. However, I need to limit oily fish including tuna to two portions a week (though I can eat up to 4 170-g portions of tinned tuna) because they can contain chemicals that could hurt my baby (see Off the menu, page 50). I also try to eat cooked shellfish and white fish twice a week.

Nuts, pulses and beans contain iron, potassium and zinc, but have fewer essential amino acids, so I need to eat a variety of these along with cereals and legumes to get the appropriate amount.

MILK AND DAIRY FOODS

Milk, cheese and yogurt contain protein, vitamins A and B and calcium, which are necessary to ensure that my baby develops healthy teeth and bones and my own stay protected. Soya-based versions are available for vegans and those who are lactose intolerant. I try to eat three portions of low-fat versions in order to receive the necessary nutrients and calcium whilst avoiding saturated fat and extra calories. Portions consist of ½ pint milk, 140 g of yogurt or 40 g of cheese.

Calcium requires vitamin D in order to be absorbed properly, so I also eat eggs or canned oily fish in addition to my prescribed supplement.

SUGAR, FATS, SALT AND OILS

Dressings and spreads, creams, chocolate, crisps, chips, pastries, ice cream and carbonated drinks should make up less than 30 per cent of my daily calories. I try to limit these treats to rare occasions, as they contain few nutrients and excessive amounts of sugar and fat, all of which can be detrimental to my baby's health as well as my own. Processed foods are also high in sugars and fats, which can lead to tooth decay, excess weight gain and obesity. Fat and salt can lead to health problems such as obesity, clogged arteries, high blood pressure and heart disease. Therefore, I avoid chips, meats with large amounts of fat and other fried or fatty foods.

However, there are healthy sources for the small amounts of sugar and fat – which are necessary to maintain energy, healthy skin and hair – and essential fatty acids. The sugar found naturally in fruit and milk is acceptable because these foods also provide needed nutrients and vitamins. Olive or rapeseed oil contains beneficial monounsaturated fatty acids; sunflower, sesame and corn oils provide the polyunsaturated fatty acid omega-6.

FIBRE

This is necessary to sustain a healthy digestive system, keep my blood sugar levels constant and prevent constipation. There are two types of fibre – soluble and insoluble – both of which I need in my diet. Soluble fibre helps me feel full for longer and to allow for sugars to be steadily released into the bloodstream. Fibre can be found in apples, pears, rye bread, oats and legumes. Insoluble fibre acts as a preventative for constipation by allowing foods to travel through my body faster and then removing waste products in stools. It is found in beans, wholegrain cereals, lentils, leafy green vegetables and fruit.

If I do nothing else I will ...

EAT TO ENSURE MY BABY'S HEALTH

A few changes to my ordinary diet are all that's needed. I must try to:

✓ **Eat 5 portions** of vegetables and fruit a day.

✓ **Make starchy carbohydrates the largest part of my meals.** Bread, cereal, pasta, grains and rice will provide me with lots of needed energy.

✓ **Stay aware of the amount of alcohol** that I drink – having no more than 2 small drinks a week – and not getting drunk.

✓ **Limit or avoid caffeine.**

✗ **Not add any extra salt** to my meals; a diet high in salt (greater than 6 g) can lead to increased blood pressure – a risk factor for pre-eclampsia.

✗ **Not miss any meals** as my baby needs a constant supply of nutrients.

WATER AND OTHER LIQUIDS

Water is essential for numerous processes. My baby requires water in order to receive nutrients from my blood and the additional blood that I make requires sufficient levels of fluid. Fluids also can prevent constipation (see page 37).

I try to drink 2 litres, or 6–7 glasses daily. I can drink a range of liquids, such as water, fruit or vegetable juices or reduced fat milk or commercially sold herbal teas, but it is best that I drink mostly water.

Alcohol

I need to limit my alcohol intake to a glass or two of wine a week – or none at all – and to drink only when eating food. Many health professionals state that not drinking at all would be safest, but there are no known health problems caused by having fewer than 2 units a week. Drinking more than 2 alcohol units a day or binge drinking can have serious consequences for my baby; she will not get the nutrients she needs because my appetite will be suppressed and this will affect placental function resulting in a low birth weight,

Certain foods and food preparation techniques (see page 53) may contain or spread organisms harmful to my baby and me. Potential illnesses include salmonellosis, listeriosis and toxoplasmosis (see page 60), food and mercury poisoning and worms.

✗ Liver and liver-based products. These contain high levels of vitamin A (retinol) that can cause malformations in my baby.

✗ Raw fish (sushi). Supermarket versions that are pasteurised are safe to eat, but worms are often found in restaurant dishes or those prepared at market stalls or at home.

✗ Large fish like king mackerel, tilefish, swordfish, shark and marlin. These very often contain mercury or dangerous bacteria.

✗ Oily fish including mackerel, salmon, herring, sardines, pilchards, fresh tuna and trout, if eaten more than 2 times a week. Oily fish store dangerous chemicals, including mercury.

✗ Shellfish that is raw or undercooked; it can cause food poisoning.

✗ Meat (tartare dishes) and eggs that are undercooked. Raw or undercooked meat and poultry can result in toxoplasmosis. Mayonnaise, mousses and ice creams may result in salmonella.

✗ Milk that is unpasteurised including sheep or goat's milk; there is a risk of salmonella.

✗ Cheese made from unpasteurised milk including goat's and sheep's and feta and blue-veined or mould rinds. These can cause listeriosis, which can lead to miscarriage or stillbirth unless they are cooked at high temperatures.

✗ Peanuts. New reasearch into the rise of peanut allergy in children suggests that all pregnant women should avoid them; previous advice was to do so only if the father or I have a nut allergy.

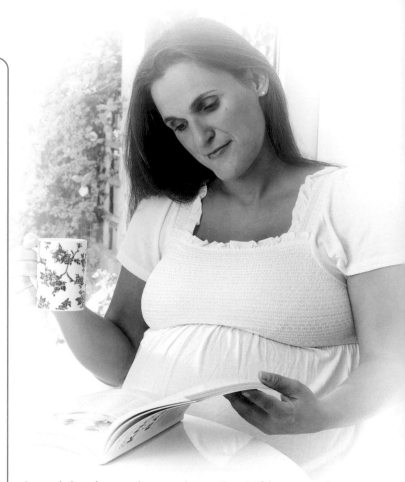

Lemon balm, ginger and peppermint are three 'safe' pregnancy teas, but drink no more than 2 or 3 cups of these a day.

physical deformities and mental retardation. I'm also more likely to miscarry.

A single unit of alcohol would be 85 ml of wine (a small glass is equal to 125 ml or 1½ units), ½ pint ordinary-strength lager, ale or beer (some continental varieties are stronger than formerly), a 25-ml shot of spirits or a 50-ml aperitif. An alcopop usually contains 1½ units. Many drinks, including wine, are served in larger than normal glasses.

Caffeine
Consuming too much caffeine reduces the absorption of nutrients and can result in low baby weight or miscarriage. In addition to tea and coffee, caffeine is found also in hot chocolate, colas, energy drinks and chocolate bars. I should limit my intake to less than 200 mg a day – 1–2 small coffees a day – and drink caffeinated tea and coffee half an hour after eating. I need to be aware that drinks sold in coffee bars are usually larger than those prepared at home and subsequently have larger amounts of caffeine.

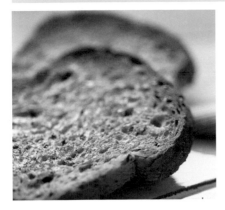

BREAKFASTS

Main Dishes
Fromage frais with chopped dried apricots
Wholegrain cereal with milk
Muesli with chopped dates and milk
Fortified breakfast cereal with milk
Bran flakes with milk
Porridge oats with maple syrup
Crusty bread roll with preserves
Boiled eggs
Scrambled egg with bagel
Grilled bacon with tomatoes and mushrooms
Pancakes or waffles
Wholemeal toast with yeast extract
Toasted fruit bun
Toasted muffin or bagel with jam or cheese

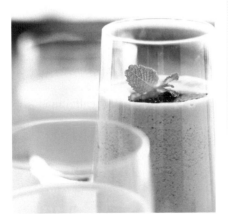

Accompaniments
Fruit juice or smoothie
Fruit salad
Melon half
Yogurt

LUNCHES

Main Dishes
Large baked potato with baked beans or low-fat cheese topping
Sandwich: chicken, ham, roast beef, canned salmon or cheese
Mushroom, ham or cheese omelette
Cheese and biscuits with a salad

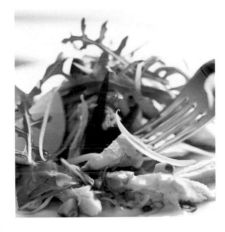

Salads: chef's, Niçoise, pasta, or lentil and rice
Hummus and pitta bread
Pasta with vegetables
Vegetable soup with crusty roll
Grilled sardines on toast with tomatoes
Vegetable pizza
Baked beans on toast
Frittata or vegetable quiche
Potato pancakes with apple sauce

Accompaniments
Fresh fruit or fruit salad
Vegetable juice
Cereal bar
Hard cheese and crackers

DINNERS

Main Dishes
Grilled chicken, turkey or fish fillet
Pasta mixed with salmon or topped with a meat- or cheese-based sauce
Chicken, beef or lamb casserole
Pan-fried beef or lamb steak
Grilled lamb or pork chop
Roast chicken, lamb, pork or beef
Steamed or grilled salmon steak
Roasted cod or haddock
Thai-style green chicken curry
Beef burger
Stir-fried lean pork, chicken or tofu and vegetables
Fish cakes
Pork or chicken brochettes
Macaroni and cheese
Mushroom risotto
Vegetable gratin
Crêpes stuffed with stir-fried vegetables, chicken or turkey

Accompaniments
Green vegetables or salad
Rice or noodles
Boiled or mashed potatoes
Baked sweet potato
Yogurt or sorbet
Stewed or grilled fruit

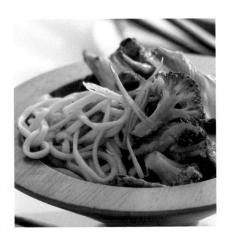

ESSENTIAL NUTRIENTS

Most of the vitamins and minerals I need I will get by eating healthily but my caregiver will prescribe folic acid and vitamin D, and possibly a multi-vitamin. If the iron level in my blood becomes low, I may be advised to take iron supplements.

Folic acid (folate)

Generally taken as a 400 mcg supplement, this B vitamin reduces the risk of my baby developing spina bifida and other neural tube defects. Many of the foods in my diet – green leafy vegetables, bananas, brown rice and fortified breads and cereals– are also rich in folate, the naturally occurring form.

Iron

Essential for the manufature of blood cells, I need to include lean red meat, green vegetables, and pulses in my diet as iron supplements can cause constipation. Vitamin C can help my body to absorb iron so I should have some citrus fruit or juice at the same meal. Coffee and tea may reduce the absorption of iron – another reason to cut down on these (see also page 50).

VEGETARIAN OR VEGAN MUM

Being pregnant may present some challenges but doing the following will ensure my baby and I thrive:

- For protein, I will eat dairy products or fortified soya-based foods such as tofu, tempeh or miso. I will also use beans, nuts and seeds, grains and lentils in my meals. These foods all contain large amounts of protein as well as iron, vitamin B and fibre.
- To get enough vitamin B_{12}, I can eat foods such as tempeh, vegetarian cheeses and spreads, and soya milk or take B_{12} supplements along with folic acid.
- For the 15 mg of iron needed daily, I need to increase my intake of legumes, dark green leafy vegetables and dried fruit and to take them with orange juice.

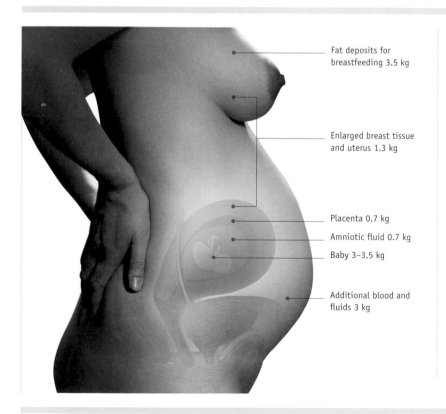

Fat deposits for breastfeeding 3.5 kg

Enlarged breast tissue and uterus 1.3 kg

Placenta 0.7 kg

Amniotic fluid 0.7 kg

Baby 3–3.5 kg

Additional blood and fluids 3 kg

WEIGHT GAIN

As I'm of normal weight with a BMI (body mass index) within the 18.6–24.9 range, I'm expecting to gain about 11.5–16 kg – most in the last trimester. I am expecting the weight to be distributed as shown opposite. If I was thinner, however, with a BMI of 18.5 or lower, I would have to put on more weight (about 13–18 kg is recommended) and if I was heavier with a BMI of 25–29.9, I should put on no more than 11 kg. Women who are overweight during pregnancy produce larger-than-average babies who go on to become overweight children with the potential to suffer life-threatening illnesses as adults.

Calcium

This mineral is needed for the healthy development of many parts of my baby's body including her bones and teeth, muscles, nerves and heart. The richest sources are dairy products, such as milk and yogurt (especially low-fat versions), but leafy green vegetables, fish with edible bones (like sardines), soya products, tahini and almonds also contain good amounts. To absorb calcium, I need vitamin D, which I get from a 10 mcg supplement as well as being out in the sun.

Vitamin D

Adequate vitamin D is important to maintain the bones and today many women are deficient. I've been prescribed a 10 mcg supplement.

CALORIES

Pregnancy is not the time to diet nor do I need to eat for two. As long as I'm not overweight, I will probably need to increase my calorie intake in the later months. The amount of calories I need depends on my activity level. Like most women, I need around 2,000 per day, increasing by 200 calories a day in the last three months and 200 more once I start breastfeeding.

EXPECTING TWINS

Regardless of pre-pregnancy weight, women pregnant with twins need to gain between 16–20 kg. Some of this – say 2.5 kg – should be in the first trimester, with a weight gain of 0.7 kg a week after this.

Women expecting triplets may need to gain a total of around 23 kg or about 0.7 kg per week.

It is not just additional calories that women with multiple pregnancies require. To support the additional increases in blood volume, uterus size, etc., as well as the development of two or more babies, there is a particular additional requirement for calcium, essential fatty acids and iron. It is important, therefore that the diet contains a good mix of nutrient-rich foods and an all-round antenatal supplement of 15 mg zinc, 2 mg copper, 250 mg calcium, 2 mg vitamin B6, 300 mcg folic acid, 50 mg vitamin C, 5 mcg vitamin D and 30 mg iron.

If I do nothing else I will ...

ENSURE FOOD SAFETY

By following basic food hygiene I will be able to avoid food-borne illnesses, which can harm my baby and me. I must:

✓ **Always wash my hands with soap and water** before handling food, particularly raw meat, after I have been to the toilet, handled rubbish or touched pets. I must wear gloves when gardening and when moving any animal waste (try to avoid).

✓ **Keep my kitchen and food serving area really clean.** I should bleach cloths and work surfaces regularly, wash tea towels daily and not use them as hand towels.

✓ **Transfer food to the fridge** as soon as possible after shopping; I mustn't leave it in a warm place such as the office or car.

✓ **Store foods at the right temperature.** My fridge needs to be below 5°C (41°F). The most perishable foods such as cooked meats, soft cheeses, salad leaves, ready meals and desserts need to be kept the coolest.

✓ **Wrap raw meats or fish,** which may drip onto other foods, or place them in containers in the coldest part of the fridge.

✓ **Store eggs in the fridge.**

✓ **Check use by and best before dates** on foods. I must throw out foods that are date-expired and not be tempted to buy reduced-cost, short-life products at the supermarket.

✓ **Have separate chopping boards.** I will keep one board for raw meat and fish and another for cooked foods to prevent cross contamination.

✓ **Ensure that meat and poultry is cooked through.** They need to reach 70°C (158°F) internally, which I can check with a meat probe. Another indication is when the juices run clear when I insert a sharp knife into the centre of the meat.

My exercise programme

I've always done some form of exercise and there's every reason to continue now that I'm pregnant. Exercising helps improve my posture and movement, increases my energy levels and releases endorphins, making me feel happier and less anxious. And, like my pregnancy yoga class, it's also a great way to meet other pregnant women and share experiences.

Of course, I mentioned to my caregiver that I was planning to exercise, in case there were any medical reasons not to, and was advised on suitable activities as well as the importance of warming up and cooling down at each session.

I was told not to start a new regime in the first trimester and to gradually build up to between 30–60 minutes per day. However, I'm an experienced exerciser and can keep to my present level but need to monitor my sessions so I don't overdo things. The second trimester is the best time for exercises; there's less danger of affecting the baby and many complaints have settled down. During the third trimester, my growing belly will affect my centre of gravity and I'll probably

feel quite tired and not much like exercising, so walking may be the best thing to do.

RECOMMENDED ACTIVITIES

While some things are off the menu (see opposite page), there are still a lot of things a pregnant woman can do – either alone, with a partner or in a class.

• Walking and swimming are so safe they can be done throughout pregnancy. Swimming keeps your body supported so is easy on the joints but the pool water should never be too hot.

• Yoga and t'ai chi are low impact exercises and not only keep you in shape but can help you to relax. It's best to take classes designed for pregnant women (or make sure that the instructor knows your condition), because some poses are not suitable.

• Gym equipment such as tread mills, stationary bikes, stair climbers and weight machines (not free weights) can be used as long as care is taken to breathe correctly and not to strain joints or use the equipment on a high setting.

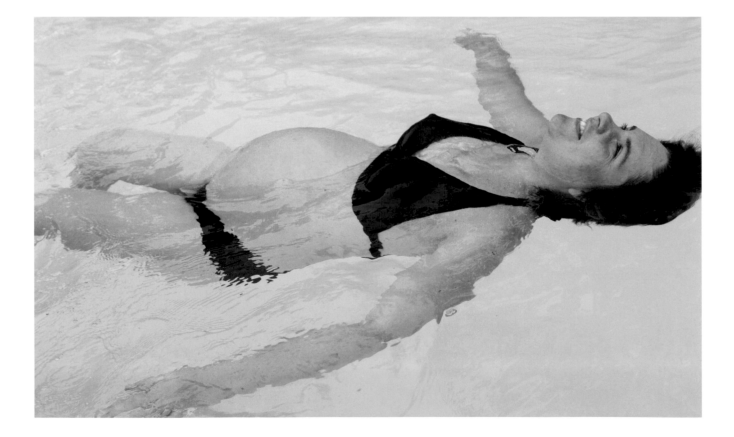

Off the menu ✕

The following sports/activities are either not suitable for pregnant women – particularly those new to the exercise – or need to be done under supervision. Also, I must avoid any exercise in which I have to lie flat on my back, as this position can reduce blood flow to the heart.

✗ **High-intensity aerobics.** This form of aerobics put unnecessary stress on the joints and in later pregnancy it is difficult to keep your balance during the exercises.

✗ **Downhill or water skiing and horse riding.** These can involve falls, which could prove very dangerous to baby.

✗ **Running,** unless you are an experienced runner. It can put you at risk of knee and hip injuries and can leave you dehydrated.

✗ **Weight training using free weights.** Unless done under guidance, there are a number of potential risks. Firstly, it's always possible that a weight can drop on your tummy; secondly, heavy weights can cause injury to the joints and thirdly, incorrect breathing can lead you to your bearing down and increasing abdominal pressure, which can reduce blood flow, increase blood pressure and place stress on the heart.

✗ **Roller blading and snow boarding.** The danger of falling is inherent in these sports.

✗ **Team and vigorous racket sports** such as volleyball or squash. As well as a risk of falls, joint stress and being hit in the stomach commonly occur.

✗ **Scuba diving;** gas bubbles could form in the baby's bloodstream.

• Low impact aerobics. A programme of strengthening and toning exercises working all the major muscles is a great way to keep in shape.
• Pelvic floor exercises (see page 56) can help make the birth easier and prevent complications later on.

WARMING UP AND COOLING DOWN

I know it's important to stretch my muscles before and after exercising to reduce cramps. My warm ups take around 10 minutes and I begin with a low-intensity rhythmic activity such as walking on the spot or stationary cycling, followed by slow, controlled stretches. I start slowly and then build up to moderately larger or faster movements.

I spend 5–10 minutes cooling down. Basically, while standing or sitting, I gently stretch each of the muscle groups in my feet, legs and arms.

If I do nothing else I will ... ✓

EXERCISE SAFELY
It's important when pregnant that I do the following:

✓ **Wear comfortable, loose clothing** in layers that can be removed as body temperature rises and to stop exercising when I feel too hot.

✓ **Drink plenty of water.**

✓ **Have regular sessions** – between 30–60 minutes at least three times a week – and warm up before and cool down afterwards.

✓ **Take care when I stretch.** I need to take things easy and not overstretch; nor should I spend time on my back after my fourth month.

✓ **Stop immediately** if I feel any pain or experience bleeding, palpitations, faintness or headache.

✗ **Not exercise in hot, humid conditions.**

PELVIC FLOOR EXERCISES

These exercises strengthen the muscles that control urination (the ones I use to break the flow of urine) and pregnancy can cause them to become slack. It's important, therefore, that I keep them in shape, because if they are toned it can prevent some of the discomfort of late pregnancy, including urine leakage and haemorrhoids.

Kegel exercises

So called because they were developed by Dr Arnold Kegel, these exercises can be done discreetly just about anytime, whether I'm driving in my car, sitting at my desk, travelling in a lift or relaxing on the sofa. Aside from the pelvic muscles, nothing else need move and it's important not to hold your breath.

The simplest way for me to tone these muscles is to imagine my pelvic floor as a lift: I contract my muscles, tightening them as I do when stopping urine, on the 'way up' – a little more each 'floor' – and holding them for at least 5 seconds. Then, I gradually release the muscles 'on the way down'. I repeat this about 4–5 times in a row.

Once this method is perfected, it's possible to gain greater control over each of the muscle bands surrounding the different openings.

The way to do this is to first identify the muscles surrounding the anus or opening of the bowel and then to squeeze these muscles tightly before releasing them slowly, then do the same for the vaginal muscles and finally the bladder muscles.

It's important, however, that I don't interrupt my urine stream on a regular basis. Doing Kegel exercises with a full bladder or while emptying the bladder can actually weaken the muscles, as well as lead to incomplete emptying of the bladder, which increases the risk of a urinary tract infection.

I try to aim for at least three sets of 10 repetitions a day – building up to hold each band of muscles for one minute – fitting in a set every time I do a routine task, such as checking email, commuting to work, preparing meals or watching television.

PELVIC FLOOR MUSCLES

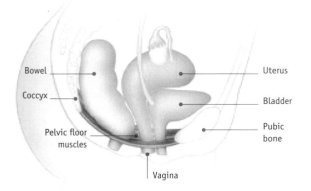

Bowel

Coccyx

Pelvic floor muscles

Uterus

Bladder

Pubic bone

Vagina

The muscles supporting the pelvic organs form a divided sling. Fastening at the coccyx and pubic bone, they surround the openings to the bowel, vagina and bladder.

Some women find it easier to make contact with their pelvic floor muscles by adopting an all-fours or kneeling position

Relaxation

Being able to relax will reduce stress, relieving anxiety, which tends to 'scatter' my thoughts and can release physical tension, which can be distracting when it causes discomfort or pain. Both are important for my health and that of my baby. I also want to use relaxation techniques during labour, when they may allow my body to function naturally and me to conserve energy.

The easiest way for me to relax is to be in a quiet place where I will not be disturbed. I turn off the phone, make sure I'm warm enough and lie or sit comfortably with my eyes closed and practise some breathing exercises (see below). However, sometimes I like to be massaged by my partner (see page 58).

BREATHING EXERCISES

To release tension in my body, I inhale slowly and then hold my breath for a count of five. Then I exhale slowly and repeat the procedure three times.

I also can relieve specific areas of tension by focusing on each body part, tightening and then letting go. For example, with my shoulders, I breathe in and push them down, breathe out and release them. I work through each part beginning at either my head or toes.

When relaxing in a quiet room isn't an option, I can adapt the above technique by thinking 'relax', pushing my shoulders down, and as I breathe out with a long sigh, letting all the tension from my head to my toes flow out with it.

Another technique is to take three deep breaths, and with each slow exhalation feel the tension flow out on the breath as my shoulders drop and belly softens.

MEDITATION

Concentrating on a single word, image or activity, enables me to withdraw from sensory input, forget the past or future and disregard all outside activity. The result is that my mind and body become calmed and re-energised. Meditating twice a day for 15–20 minutes is the most effective way to reap the rewards.

I find the best way to achieve mental stillness is through the repetition of a simple word, phrase or sound (mantra), which blocks the intrusion of other words and thoughts. I repeat my mantra (sometimes the word "relax") not just when I'm trying to meditate but also while doing housework, going for a walk or waiting in the doctor's surgery.

Some people prefer affirmations, which are phrases that have a meaning ('I love and cherish my perfect baby'), which is more important than the sound. Still others use a visual tool such as a lit candle or an imaginary scene that makes them feel relaxed, such as being on a beach.

It is important to establish a pattern by meditating at the same time every day: if I miss my usual slot it can be difficult to find another during the day. Convenient times are first thing in the morning (before getting involved in the day's activities), and early evening (but not just before bedtime when I can become too energised to sleep). Also, I don't eat or drink caffeinated drinks for an hour beforehand, as these can interfere with my mood. Meditation is most rewarding when I feel alert and rested.

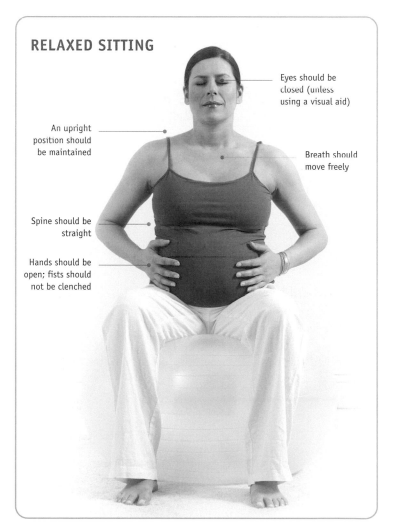

RELAXED SITTING

Eyes should be closed (unless using a visual aid)

An upright position should be maintained

Breath should move freely

Spine should be straight

Hands should be open; fists should not be clenched

Pregnancy massage

Massage is one of those age-old techniques that are particularly appreciated during pregnancy. Like most mothers-to-be, I rub my belly frequently as a way of keeping in touch with my baby, but massage can have other benefits. Throughout my pregnancy, my partner can use it to help relieve my various aches and pains and to connect with me and our baby. When I'm in labour, I will use abdominal and back massage for pain relief and comfort, as it should help to relax me and enable me to work with my contractions. I find it easy to massage myself if I need to relieve aching muscles.

USING OILS

In pregnancy, use only natural oils, as the body absorbs a percentage of everything put on the skin. Use a vegetable, olive or sunflower oil. Alternatively, use a beeswax-based product such as the Tui waxes from New Zealand; with a wax, there is no risk of spillage.

ABDOMINAL MASSAGE

This can be done on your own or with your partner; sitting, standing, lying on your side or on top of a ball; done through clothes or with belly exposed, with or without oil, and is enjoyable throughout pregnancy and in early labour. In pregnancy, you can use it to communicate with your baby. In labour, it can help you to breathe deeper, which can take your mind off the pain. It may also help to reassure your baby. Use gentle pressure throughout.

Vary the position by passing both hands from the front, along the hips, to the back and then moving from the back, passing along the hips, to the front.

Body position needs to be comfortable

Hand on lower back is kept still to give additional support

Use a ball to take the strain away from your arms and cover with a soft cloth

Massage in a clockwise direction to follow movement of the intestines

Wrists and hands should be relaxed

Be wary of using essential oils as these are powerful, medicinal oils that can overstimulate the body. If you want to use aromatherapy oils for your massages, first ask a qualified aromatherapist specialising in birth work to recommend oils that will be safe for you to use.

Pour your oil into a small bottle and make sure that it is within reaching distance, so that you can replenish your oil easily as you massage. When ready to begin, pour a small amount into your palm then rub your palms together to spread and warm the oil. Make sure you reapply when your hands feel dry or they stop gliding smoothly over your skin. Remeber to never pour any remaining oil back into the bottle, as it may now be contaminated.

PERINEAL MASSAGE

You can use this technique daily, from around 34 weeks, to stretch the tissue around your vagina and perineum in preparation for the birth.

- Always wash your hands before and after.
- Use a hand-held mirror to locate your vaginal opening, perineum and urethra.
- Sit or lean back comfortably, with a towel under your hips.
- Using a non-petroleum lubricant, such as K-Y jelly, coat your thumbs and perineal area. Place your thumbs 3–4 cm inside your vagina.
- Press gently down and to the sides. Stretch until you feel a slight tingling sensation. Hold this pressure for about 2 minutes.
- Maintaining the pressure, gently massage back and forth over the lower half of your vagina for 3–4 minutes. Take care to avoid your urethra because of the risk of urinary tract infection.

KEEPING IN TOUCH WITH MY BABY

Sitting down and rubbing my belly is a great way to spend some time relaxing with my baby and to enjoy just being with her. To help me focus, I place my hands on my lower abdomen and concentrate on my breathing. With each out breath, as my hands are drawn in by the movement of my abdominal muscles, I feel as if I am gently hugging my baby. I try to be aware of her position and feel for her spine, arms and legs. Sometimes I feel her move. As I breathe in, I imagine that I am creating more space for her.

Abdominal massage is a great way to get a baby ready for birth and to make me feel comfortable with letting her move out into the world. Shortly before my due date, I'll try and visualise my baby's head gradually going deeper down into my pelvis as she engages in preparation for birth. If she is not in such a good position, I will try visualising how she might be able to get into a better position and encourage her to move.

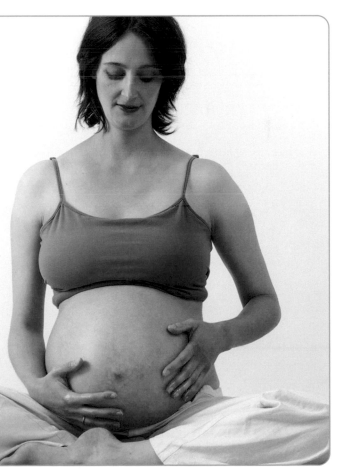

Avoiding potential hazards

Danger lurks in and around the home, outdoors and at work. In order to protect myself and my baby from proven risks as well as some that aren't yet proven, I need to be aware of the following hazards.

FOOD-BORNE INFECTIONS

Certain foods, as well as preparation techinques, can result in harmful organisms damaging my baby while in the uterus as well as making me dangerously ill.

Listeriosis

Caused by a bacterium (listeria monocytogenes) commonly found in the soil, a severe infection could lead to miscarriage, preterm labour, stillbirth or newborn meningitis. Listeria may be found in unpasteurised soft and blue-veined cheeses such as Brie and Camembert; unpasteurised sheep and goat's milk; ready-prepared coleslaw, pâtés and hot dogs; cooked food chilled for reheating and undercooked poultry.

Salmonellosis

Found in eggs and poultry, salmonella bacteria can cause food poisoning, which, if severe, needs immediate medical attention during pregnancy. I must take care to cook all eggs and poultry thoroughly and be wary when dining out or buying cooked foods from stalls and markets.

Toxoplasmosis

This serious infection, caused by the organism toxoplasma gondii, could lead to brain damage or blindness in my baby. It is especially risky during my last trimester. Found in soil, raw and undercooked meat and poultry, and in animal faeces (outdoor cats in particular), I must make certain that all my meat and poultry is cooked thoroughly, especially when dining out. I must also wash my hands thoroughly – before preparing or eating food, before serving fruits and vegetables and after touching pets. I have to wear gloves whilst gardening and avoid cat litter trays.

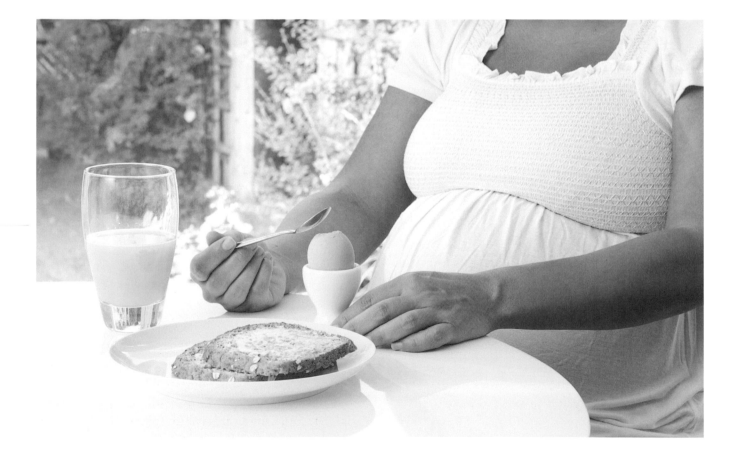

AROUND THE HOUSE

Cleaning and other products used in the home, paints and even personal care products can contain chemicals that are dangerous to a developing fetus. Pets, particularly cats, can spread toxoplasmosis. I must also take steps to ensure that my home has good air quality by checking for damp and mould, and installing carbon monoxide monitors.

Household products

I need to avoid highly toxic products such as oven cleaner or those with strong fumes. Any room that I'm cleaning should be well ventilated and I should take breaks often to ensure that I get fresh air. It's best that I avoid painting, particularly in the last months of pregnancy as some paints may contain lead or mercury, but if I have to, I need to keep the room ventilated and to use water-based paints.

The occasional use of insecticides isn't a risk, but I must avoid prolonged contact because long-term exposure to pesticides has been linked to birth defects. Instead, I need to use environmentally friendly, non-chemical products, which are completely safe.

Pets

Having pets in the household is generally safe as long as they are in good health and regularly wormed, but cats may carry a risk for toxoplasmosis. I try not to change my cat's litter box, but if it is unavoidable, I wear gloves and wash my hands immediately after.

Personal care

Environmental toxins, which could be dangerous to my body or baby, are found in many cosmetics and hair and skin care products – even those labelled 'green' or 'natural'. The main culprits are phthalates, which are hormone disrupting but are easily absorbed through the skin. The most frequently used phthalate in cosmetics, DBP, is also the most potentially harmful, capable of affecting a baby boy's reproductive system. It is found in skin lotions, perfume, night creams, sunscreens, mascara and deodorants. Parabens, the most widely used synthetic preservatives, are found in skin creams, face masks, foundations and deodorants. Traces of these chemicals have even been found in breast tissue, making it likely they can be transferred in breast milk.

I must therefore read all labels very carefully and stick to manufacturers known for producing products safe for pregnancy.

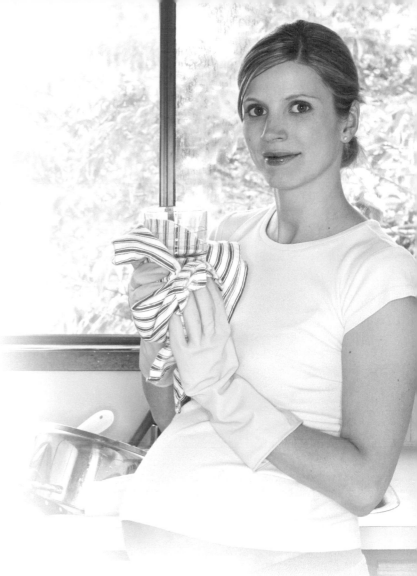

OUT AND ABOUT

Pollution is all around and hard to avoid, but anything that raises body temperature I need to avoid.

Pollution

Though city life is not known to be harmful to unborn babies, it is best that I minimise time spent in highly polluted areas to prevent any ill effects that may occur.

Jacuzzis, saunas and steam rooms

These are out of bounds because they will raise my body temperature above 38.9°C (102.2°F) for more than 10 minutes, which can harm my baby by causing neural tube defects such as spina bifida or miscarriage.

WORK-RELATED

Most jobs are safe while I'm pregnant, save for high-risk or physically demanding roles. Equipment such as computers or mobile phones are also safe and do not emit dangerous levels of radiation. However, I may have to adapt or ask for assistance for some routine roles.

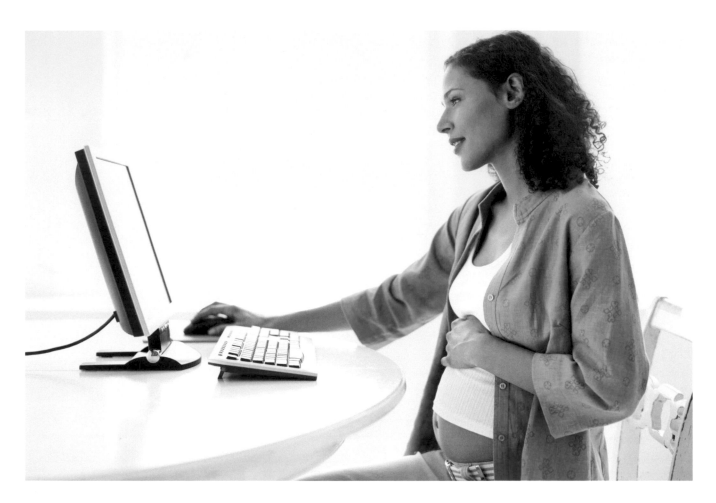

I must make sure I sit correctly while at my computer if I want to prevent backache, and use wrist supports and proper equipment to prevent carpal tunnel syndrome. Anyone working in a laboratory where contact with chemicals, biological agents, drugs or pesticides is unavoidable, should seek professional advice as to safety measures to take, the same goes for hairdressing salons. Workers in kitchens should ask to be moved to the safest station. In any event, I will speak to my supervisor or health and safety officer to ensure that my working environment is safe and proper precautions are being made to reduce stress.

DRUGS

Whether bought over the counter or prescribed by your doctor, medications can have serious side effects. Recreational drugs should always be avoided.

Prescription medications

Few medicines have been established as safe to use while pregnant, so I always discuss the pros and cons with my doctor if ever I'm prescribed medication, including over-the-counter painkillers. And, having

decided its safe and necessary to take, if I later feel uncomfortable about taking it – maybe because there's an unexpected side effect, I ask my doctor for advice before continuing.

If I was already on medication, say for a chronic condition or illness, such as diabetes or high blood pressure, I would make sure to dicuss my medication with my doctor or obstetrician in case a change in treatment is needed or the dosage needs to be adjusted. For short-term illnesses like colds, I ask my pharmacist what treatment is best, since most over-the-counter medicine isn't advisable when pregnant.

Recreational drugs

Whether legal or illegal, recreational drugs can be harmful for my baby. I need to stop drinking or greatly limit alcohol and caffeine.

I avoid all illegal drugs because they can harm the baby and me. They can increase the chances of delivering a premature or low-weight baby as well as cause behavioural or developmental problems. In addition to the above, use of marijuana can result in miscarriage or ectopic pregnancy. Cocaine can increase the chances of birth defects, seizures, developmental problems, neurological problems and SIDS. It can also cause a pregnant mother to have a stroke, heart attack or very high blood pressure. Narcotics and opiates, when not taken under medical supervision, can cause fetal growth problems, fetal death, preterm delivery and small head size. Having a narcotic addiction could harm my baby after birth, causing complications or death from withdrawal.

Amphetamines can lead to a decreased appetite, which can affect fetal growth and promote problems and defects, such as fetal stroke and death. Along with this, drugs can lead to higher rates of maternal malnourishment and sexually transmitted infections.

SMOKING
Even passive smoking is very dangerous, as it could result in low birth weight and developmental disorders.

If I do nothing else I will ...

PROTECT MYSELF AND MY BABY
I need to be proactive about safety so should:

✓ **Become alert to hazards** in my home environment and while out and about.

✓ **Wash my hands frequently,** particularly after handling animals and raw meats and poultry.

✓ **Keep my desk drawer topped up with healthy snacks** such as dried fruit, nuts and cereal bars.

✓ **Take frequent breaks** from working in front of my computer screen, I'll get up and move around.

✓ **Make sure my work station is properly set up.** My chair should be height adjustable with a back rest. I should use a wrist support and foot stool.

✗ **Not use strong-smelling products** of all types and check labels for problematic ingredients.

✗ **Not take medications,** even over the counter, without first checking with my caregiver.

✗ **Not smoke** nor let my partner do so. I'll avoid areas and places where people are smoking.

Smoking can impact negatively on pregnancy, resulting in preterm delivery, miscarriage, placenta praevia, placental abruption and preterm rupture of the membranes. It may also lead to sudden infant death syndrome (SIDS). My baby's heath will also be affected if my partner smokes, as secondary smoke is responsible for respiratory problems and SIDS.

It's not recommended to take nicotine substitutions and anti-smoking medications while pregnant.

TRAVEL-RELATED
Being away from home means most of all that I'll be away from my caregiver. I therefore need to ensure that I eat and drink safely, am properly immunised, have appropriate medications, insect repellents and sun screen on hand and travel in comfort. I've been advised not to travel where malaria is common. The best time to travel will be between about 18–24 weeks, when the risk of miscarriage or premature labour is low.

Safe food and drink
Particularly in underdeveloped countries, I need to be careful of what I eat and drink. I need to choose restaurants that look hygienic, and make sure I know what I'm eating. I need to be wary of food bought from stalls and markets, where dishes, and meats in particular, may be only semi-cooked. I should only eat fruit with a peel. To ensure I get plenty of safe water, I will only drink bottled water and avoid drinks containing ice. I will use bottled water also when brushing my teeth. If I still get diarrhoea, which can lead to dehydration, weakness, fainting, preterm labour, and reduced blood flow to my baby, I'll need to drink plenty of fluids and seek medical advice.

CAR AND PLANE TRIPS
On long car trips, I'll try and stop every couple of hours to get out and walk around a bit. Of course, I'll be wearing my seat belt with shoulder strap at all times, which keep me safe and won't hurt the baby, even if I'm involved in an accident.

I won't be flying after 35 weeks, and I'll make sure to regularly stretch my legs. Walking around keeps my circulation going and helps to prevent deep vein thrombosis (DVT). I'll sip water frequently as air travel can be dehydrating. If possible, I'll try and book an aisle seat, so I don't have to worry about disturbing my neighbour when I need to use the toilet for the umpteenth time.

Avoiding pregnancy complications

Like most women, I expect my pregnancy to be uneventful healthwise. However, there are a few conditions that can either develop as a result of pregnancy or be negatively affected by it. My antenatal care should pick up any signs of these conditions, but I also need to be aware of the symptoms and to take all preventative measures.

ANAEMIA

Many pregnant women develop some degree of anaemia – a lack of circulating blood cells – and in mild cases it doesn't cause problems. Even if I developed it, my baby shouldn't be lacking in iron since my body diverts its mineral resources to her.

There are a number of reasons why a pregnant woman can develop anaemia. Most commonly, she suffers from dilutional anaemia; the increased amount of blood circulating around her body, which is needed to support her baby (as much as 50 per cent more than usual), contains proportionally fewer red blood cells than required to the amount of serum.

Another common reason is iron deficiency, which can arise when a woman lacks sufficient iron to produce sufficient red blood cells for her and her baby. Most women don't have enough stored iron and it's difficult to ingest sufficient amounts.

Less commonly, anaemia can be caused by folic acid deficiency (the B vitamin needed to produce red blood cells), blood loss, chronic illness or as a result of hereditary haemoglobin abnormalities (which can be dangerous to the health of mother and baby).

To avoid anaemia, it is very important that I eat lots of iron-rich foods – molasses, red meat, kidney beans, spinach, fish, chicken and pork. To increase iron absorption, I need vitamin C, so citrus fruits and green leafy vegetables should also form part of my diet.

Symptoms
- Fatigue, loss of energy.
- Pallor.
- Decreased ability to fight illness.
- Dizziness, fainting, shortness of breath.

Treatment
If I'm found to be anaemic, I'll probably be prescribed an iron supplement, which I should take with a glass of orange, tomato or vegetable juice. In the unusual situation that I'd be unable to absorb adequate iron, injections of iron preparations may be given. Folic acid or vitamin B_{12} supplements may also be needed. In severe cases, blood transfusions may be required, especially if labour and delivery are imminent.

DEEP VEIN THROMBOSIS (DVT)

Because pregnancy makes your blood clot more easily as a way of preventing too much blood loss during childbirth, around one in 1,000 pregnant women develops a DVT at some point during her pregnancy. This occurs when a blood clot blocks a vein in one of the legs – usually the calf vein or a vein in the upper leg or groin area.

Being overweight, inactive and dehydrated are some of the precipitating factors, so I will aim to keep my weight under control, take moderate exercise and keep hydrated.

There's a similar but harmless condition known as superficial thrombophlebitis, whereby the small surface veins in the lower legs become red and sore, especially if one is overweight. In this case, using a soothing cream and wearing support tights will help.

Symptoms
- Pain, tenderness and swelling of the calf, upper leg or groin.
- Swollen area feels warm.

Treatment
If I think I might have a DVT, I need to go straight to hospital, because if left untreated the clot can travel to my lungs causing a pulmonary embolus, which can be life threatening. A blood test is available to confirm the diagnosis. A Doppler ultrasound scan (see page 26) can quickly tell if a DVT is present. Treatment usually consists of blood-thinning injections or medication.

GESTATIONAL DIABETES

During pregnancy, the placenta produces a hormone, human placental lactogen, which acts against insulin, so some women's bodies fail to make enough insulin to cope with their increased blood sugar levels and their babies can become very large. Delivery often has to occur no later than 40 weeks gestation.

During my antenatal visits, my blood sugar levels will be tested and if sugar is present in my urine, I'll probably just have to watch my diet.

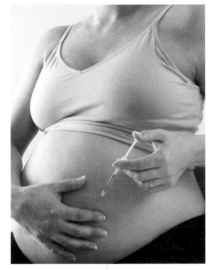

Symptoms
• Excessive thirst.
• Excessive urination.
• Fatigue.

Treatment
If I'm diagnosed with gestational diabetes, treatment may consist of my eating a relatively sugar-free diet. However, if this is insufficient to control the sugar, I may need to start having at least twice-daily insulin.

PRE-ECLAMPSIA, ECLAMPSIA AND HELLP SYNDRONE

Having high blood pressure can result in a number of serious conditions. Pre-eclampsia is characterised by high blood pressure, protein in the urine and leg and foot swelling. It affects 8–10 per cent of pregnancies (85 per cent of which are first-time pregnancies). Pre-eclampsia can develop into eclampsia, a life-threatening condition in which an expectant woman may suffer seizures. HELLP syndrome – H is for haemolysis (the breaking down of red blood cells); EL for elevated liver enzymes; and LP for low platelet count – is a unique variant of pre-eclampsia.

My blood pressure will be checked at my antenatal appointments – so it's important I don't miss any of these – and I can help to keep it down by avoiding stress, cutting down on salty and fatty foods, eating more calcium-rich foods, fruit and vegetables, and drinking plenty of water. It's vital that I immediately report any of the following symptoms to my doctor.

Symptoms
• Sudden, excessive lower leg swelling or excessive weight gain
• Persistent headaches.
• Blurred vision, flashing lights or spots before the eyes.
• Abdominal pain on right side of the body, just below ribcage.

Treatment
Birth is the only cure, though the two more serious conditions – eclampsia and HELLP syndrome – may require drug treatment as well. If I suffer badly from pre-eclampsia or am close to my due date, my delivery will be induced. If it arises early in my pregnancy or is mild, I may be prescribed blood-pressure medication, low-dose aspirin and possibly calcium.

CARPAL TUNNEL SYNDROME

The tendons and nerves that run to the fingers are located in a 'tunnel' in front of the wrist. If the hand and fingers swell in pregnancy, this carpal tunnel swells, too, putting pressure on a nerve. This pressure results in the sensation of pins and needles spreading down into all the fingers except the little finger. The symptoms of carpal tunnel syndrome tend to be worse at night, but usually ease during the day as the joints are used and become suppler. This condition generally disappears following delivery. I can help prevent this

PREGNANCY-INDUCED HYPERTENSION

Also known as PIH, this complicates 10–15 per cent of all pregnancies, and is defined as a BP greater than 140/90. It normally develops after 20 weeks, and becomes more common the nearer the delivery date. It is more common in first pregnancies. While mild high blood pressure is unlikely to be problematic, severe high blood pressure may lead to kidney failure or stroke. The major risk is to the 1 in 4 women with PIH who go on to develop pre-eclampsia.

happening by using a wrist support when working at the computer and keeping my hands elevated when sitting down.

Symptoms
• Pain in the wrist.
• Pins and needles extending from wrist down into hand.
• Stiffness of fingers and joints of hand.

Treatment
If I feel this pain in my wrists, sleeping with my hands raised on a pillow can prevent fluid from building up. When I wake up, I should make sure I drop my hands over the side of the bed and give them a vigorous shake to help disperse fluid and ease any stiffness. Wearing splints on the wrists also can help.

SYMPHYSIS PUBIS DYSFUNCTION (SPD)
Three bones – one at the back and two at the front – held together by ligaments make up the pelvic girdle. The bones meet to form three 'fixed' joints, one at the front, called the symphysis pubis, and one at each side of the base of the spine. The pregnancy hormone, relaxin, loosens all the pelvic ligaments to allow the baby easier passage at birth. However, these ligaments can loosen too much, making the pelvis move, especially when weight is put on it. The weight of the baby makes this worse and sometimes the symphysis pubis joint actually separates slightly and the result is mild-to-severe pain in the pubic area.

This condition can develop at any time from the first trimester onwards.

It's important that I safeguard this area to prevent the bones separating by remaining mobile most of the time and being careful when lifting and to perform activities correctly.

Symptoms
• Pain, usually in the pubis and/or the lower back, but can be in the groin, inner thighs, hips and buttocks.
• Pain is made worse when weight is on one leg.
• A sensation of the pelvis separating.
• Difficulty when walking.

Treatment
Untreatable during pregnancy as it's due to the effect of hormones, it should improve after delivery. Great care needs to be taken not to make SPD worse. If I should get this condition, I need to avoid putting weight on one leg as much as possible, so I should sit down to get dressed, get into the car by putting my buttocks on the seat first, and then lifting my legs into the car and keeping my knees together when turning over in bed. I shouldn't do breaststroke when swimming. If the pain is severe, I will ask about painkillers and whether I can see a physiotherapist, who may advise a pelvic support belt.

3 RARE CONDITIONS
Obstetric cholestasis, a liver condition, is most likely to affect Asian women. Its main symptom is intense itching (and consequent sleep deprivation), which is a result of a build-up of bile salts in the bloodstream. It can cause a pregnant woman to go into labour early, so there is a small risk of the baby dying before birth. The only treatment is vitamin K supplements.

An ectopic pregnancy is one that develops outside the uterus, normally in a fallopian tube. It can mimic a miscarriage (see page 67), because the symptoms and signs can be very similar – abdominal pain and vaginal bleeding, though normally bleeding is light. Any severe abdominal pain that may also be accompanied by shoulder or rectal pain must be investigated right away and surgery or a drug called Methotrexate will be used to remove the ectopic pregnancy.

Hyperemesis gravidarum, a severe form of morning sickness, affects approximately 1 in 200 women in early pregnancy. If a woman vomits excessively, hospital admission is usually necessary so that she can be rehydrated by intravenous drip. If left untreated, hyperemesis gravidarum can result in low levels of potassium in the bloodstream and prevent proper functioning of the liver.

Miscarriage

Losing a baby early in a pregnancy is very common – about 1 in 5 pregnancies ends before the end of the first trimester. Miscarriage is usually nature's way of dealing with pregnancies where the baby has chromosomal abnormalities incompatible with life, but infections, uncontrolled diabetes, thyroid problems, uterine abnormalities, or certain maternal antibodies may also be the cause.

Between 12–24 weeks, miscarriage is much less common and may be the result of an infection or an abnormality of the uterus, such as an incompetent cervix – one that opens under pressure of the growing uterus and baby – or in the placenta. If an incompetent cervix is diagnosed, a procedure known as a cervical cerclage will be carried out (see below).

After 24 weeks' gestation, the loss of a pregnancy is known as a stillbirth.

No matter what the reason, you will feel devastated if you lose a much-longed-for pregnancy. It is natural to feel grieved, sad and depressed even if your caregiver explains that the baby wasn't 'quite right'. It doesn't help matters that hospitals often treat the situation as routine, which can be very distressing. It is, however, important not to feel guilty that somehow you were to blame; this is a natural process and not a situation that you have caused. The happy fact is you have an excellent chance of a becoming pregnant again. That being said, a small number of women experience repeated miscarriages, and these need to be explored and treated to ensure a successful future conception.

There is no reason to wait before trying to conceive again. Taking folic acid and eating a well-balanced, nutritious diet will be helpful.

DIAGNOSING A MISCARRIAGE

Signs of a threatened miscarriage include vaginal bleeding, accompanied by lower backache or cramping abdominal pains, similar to period cramps, which may be constant or occur intermittently. Once the uterine contents have been expelled, the bleeding and pain subside and an ultrasound scan will show that the uterus is completely empty.

Where the uterus doesn't completely expel all of the pregnancy, a minor procedure under anaesthetic is generally done to clean out the uterus. Known as an ERPC (evacuation of retained products of conception),

it involves dilating the cervix and scraping tissue away from the lining of the uterus.

Occasionally, a miscarriage occurs without any symptoms or with very minor signs such as a small amount of brownish vaginal discharge. In this type of miscarriage, an ultrasound scan will detect that either there is an empty sac inside the uterus (the fetus has never formed) or that the fetal heart has stopped beating (the fetus died at a very early stage).

CERVICAL INCOMPETENCE

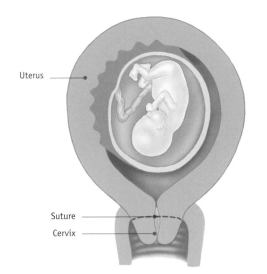

Uterus

Suture

Cervix

A cervix that opens can be 'repaired' by stitching closed the opening. The procedure is performed through the vagina under local anaesthetic or an epidural. The stitches are usually removed a few weeks before the estimated date of delivery; in some cases they remain in place until labour has begun.

Recognising medical emergencies

Most pregnancies run smoothly but occasionally something untoward occurs. I should contact my caregiver if I have any of the following symptoms or if I fall over or have an accident. However, in situations where I just don't feel well or something doesn't seem quite right, I shouldn't hesitate to get in touch.

CHILLS AND FEVER

I should consult my doctor the same day I have a fever over 37.8°C (100°F) even without having any other symptoms. If my fever is over 38.9°C (102°F), or I have other symptoms such as a sore throat or shortness of breath or cough, I need immediate treatment, as I may an infection that requires antibiotics and rest. If the fever remains high for a prolonged length of time, my baby's development could be hindered.

EXCESSIVE VOMITING AND/OR DIARRHOEA

If I can't keep anything down there's a risk of dehydration, while excessive diarrhoea depletes my bodily fluids, which is dangerous. If I have vomiting that is accompanied by fever, or the diarrhoea contains blood or mucus, I must call my doctor immediately.

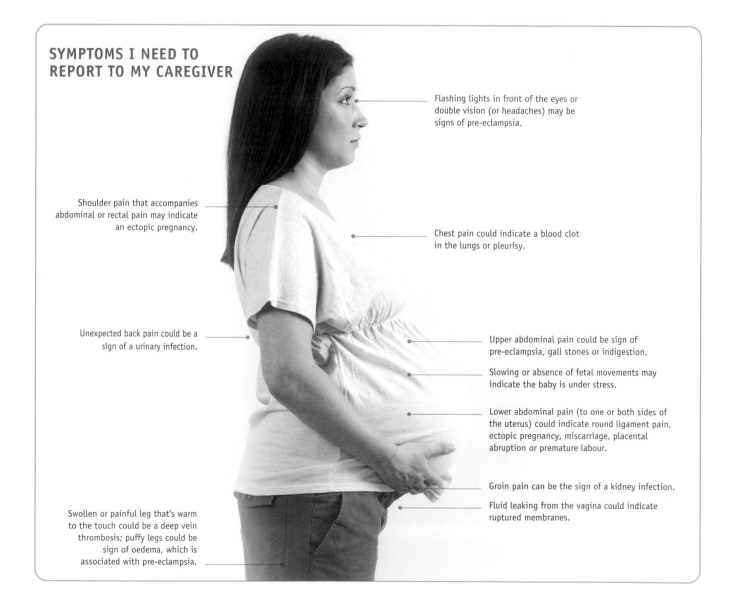

SYMPTOMS I NEED TO REPORT TO MY CAREGIVER

Flashing lights in front of the eyes or double vision (or headaches) may be signs of pre-eclampsia.

Shoulder pain that accompanies abdominal or rectal pain may indicate an ectopic pregnancy.

Chest pain could indicate a blood clot in the lungs or pleurisy.

Unexpected back pain could be a sign of a urinary infection.

Upper abdominal pain could be sign of pre-eclampsia, gall stones or indigestion.

Slowing or absence of fetal movements may indicate the baby is under stress.

Lower abdominal pain (to one or both sides of the uterus) could indicate round ligament pain, ectopic pregnancy, miscarriage, placental abruption or premature labour.

Groin pain can be the sign of a kidney infection.

Fluid leaking from the vagina could indicate ruptured membranes.

Swollen or painful leg that's warm to the touch could be a deep vein thrombosis; puffy legs could be sign of oedema, which is associated with pre-eclampsia.

ITCHING ALL OVER

This may be a sign of obstetric cholestasis (see page 66) especially if my skin looks yellow and my urine is a dark colour (signs of jaundice). Close monitoring of the baby will be necessary. In some cases, an early delivery may be needed.

PAINFUL OR BURNING URINATION, WITH FEVER, CHILLS AND BACKACHE

These are associated with a urinary tract infection, a condition that should be treated with antibiotics.

SEIZURES

A seizure may be the result of eclampsia (see page 65) and is a medical emergency. The administration of oxygen and drugs will be necessary to prevent any further seizures occurring. If I should suffer a seizure, I must call the emergency services without delay as in order for me to receive proper treatment, it will be necessary to deliver my baby right away

MEDICAL EMERGENCIES

Placenta praevia. When the placenta covers the cervix, it is less well attached to the uterine wall and is more likely to bleed from one or more of the huge number of blood vessels that cross the placental surface. Although it can be heavy, the bleeding often stops of its own accord. However, sometimes a blood transfusion is required. Rest in hospital from 34 weeks is required so that treatment can be given quickly in case of a bleed.

Placental abruption occurs when the placenta separates or shears away from the wall of the uterus. The amount of bleeding experienced is variable but can be heavy with clots.

Uterine rupture. Very occasionally, a tear occurs in the uterus during pregnancy or labour, usually due to weakness in the uterine wall caused by a scar from a previous caesarean or a previously repaired uterine rupture. An immediate caesarean is usually required, followed by surgical repair of the uterus.

BLEEDING IN PREGNANCY

Bleeding can occur for many reasons (see miscarriage, page 67). If I have bleeding that is accompanied by cramping lower abdominal pain and/or backache over several hours or any bleeding that occurs after 24 weeks of pregnancy, I must report this to my doctor. Painless vaginal bleeding may be the result of the following situations, which generally should not be cause for concern.

Implantation bleed may occur about 10 days after conception. A small amount of vaginal bleeding occurs for 24–48 hours as the fertilised egg implants itself into the wall of the uterus.

Hormonal bleeding. Around 4 and 8 weeks of pregnancy, there may be light period-like bleeding at about the time that a period would have occurred.

Cervical ectropion. During early pregnancy, particularly after sexual intercourse, cells on the inner lining of the cervix, which extend onto its surface, become inflamed and result in light spotting.

Marginal placental bleed. If one of the small blood vessels at the edge of the placenta ruptures, this can result in some light bleeding.

IMPORTANT PHONE NUMBERS

Emergency services: 999

Doctor:

Midwife:

Hospital:

Ambulance/Taxi:

Partner or friend:

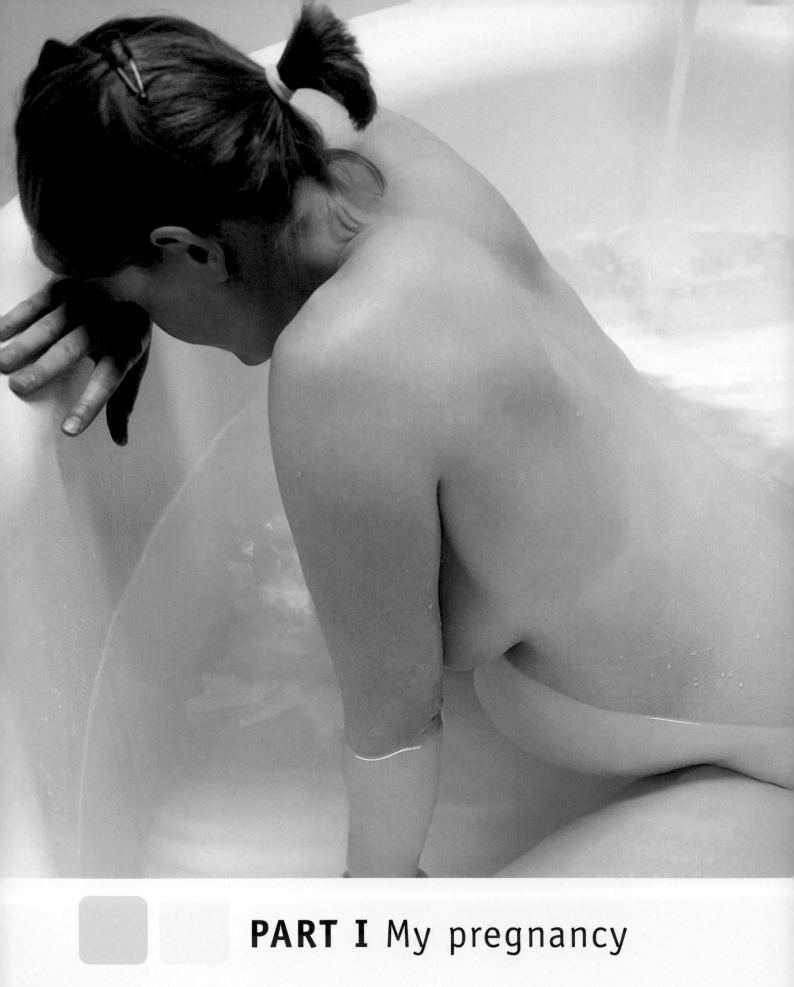

PART I My pregnancy

Choices in childbirth

Where and how to give birth needs careful consideration. How my pregnancy proceeds and many other factors will determine whether a birth centre or hospital is a necessity or if I might attempt birth at home. I also need to decide on the level of intervention and my preferred method or methods of pain relief. Once I've made my choices, noting them down on a birth plan will be vital when it comes time to giving birth – though I still have to be prepared for the unexpected.

Where to give birth?

Deciding where to have my baby is a big decision and one that will depend on my circumstances and caregivers. A hospital is the safest option should things not go as planned, but if my pregnancy proceeds normally, a midwife-led unit may be a good choice. A home birth may be harder to arrange and is generally not recommended for first-time mothers; I'd need to find a midwife or GP who would be prepared to deliver my baby at home.

HOSPITAL

The vast majority of women in the UK (97 per cent) have their babies in hospital. A hospital birth offers instant access to potentially life-saving technology, which can be very reassuring, and employs specialists who can deal with any complications – performing a caesarean or taking care of any problems with the baby. All the forms of partial or total pain relief are on offer. On the other hand, a hospital birth often entails medical interventions such as induction, fetal monitoring and episiotomies (see page 75), which may be unwanted. A better choice, if I decide to have as little intervention as possible, is to opt for midwife-led care in a hospital unit. These units aim to provide care in a home-like setting – relaxed décor with subdued lighting – and focus on natural birth with access to birthing pools.

Before I make my choice, I will visit all the local maternity units and ask advice from my GP, midwife and friends who have recently had babies. I'll also use the checklist, opposite, to enquire about the services on offer. I would want to choose a hospital near home, so that I don't have to travel too far for my delivery and antenatal visits.

HOME

Giving birth in familiar surroundings, with my partner and maybe other family members present, is another option if I want as little medical intervention during the birth as possible. However, I understand that a shortage of midwives can make this difficult to achieve. I would need to talk to my GP as the person responsible for organising my maternity care. A home birth would be overseen by midwives who have a GP or hospital obstetrician as a back-up should complications arise. In case of any problems at the birth, I would be transferred to hospital.

IMPORTANT QUESTIONS TO ASK

Answers to the following questions will give you an idea of what to expect – and whether this is the right place for you to give birth. You also should find out the centre's induction/caesarean rates and how long you will be in hospital

	YES	NO
Can I move around during labour?	☐	☐
Can I choose the position I give birth in?	☐	☐
Is fetal monitoring used continuously?	☐	☐
Will my waters be broken manually at a certain stage of labour?	☐	☐
Can I eat and drink during labour?	☐	☐
Is there a birthing pool and midwives experienced in water births?	☐	☐
Is there a 24-hour epidural service?	☐	☐
Will medical students/student midwives be involved with the birth?	☐	☐
Is there a limit to the number of people I can have in the birthing room?	☐	☐
Can my partner visit me outside visiting hours?	☐	☐
Will I get help with breastfeeding if I need it?	☐	☐
Are there security measures in place?	☐	☐
Are newborns identified so that they don't get mixed up?	☐	☐

Interventions and procedures

When considering the type of delivery I want, I may decide to avoid certain procedures as long as my baby and I are not at risk. Finding out as much as possible about what the various procedures involve will help me to make a decision. I need to be prepared, however, if the occasion demands, to allow my caregiver a role in judging if an intervention is needed. My doctor or midwife should discuss all procedures with me thoroughly beforehand. I should be told the reasons, method and potential risks and consequences for accepting or refusing the offer so that I can give 'informed consent'.

INDUCTION

Left to nature, I, like most women, will go into labour and deliver my baby within 2 weeks either side of my due date. If, however, at any time it's considered better for my baby to be born than remain inside the uterus, or if my health or my baby's is deemed at risk should the pregnancy continue, labour can be started artificially by a hormone drip or membrane sweeping (manual stimulation of the cervix).

Even if labour is not induced, my caregiver may help progress labour by giving me syntocinon (a synthetic form of oxytocin), which will result in artificially induced contractions that are often stronger and more frequent than natural contractions. These can lead to abnormal fetal heart readings, so were I to receive syntocinon, I'd be attached to a fetal monitor to see how baby is tolerating the contractions.

FETAL MONITORING

This device may be used to check my baby's progress during labour. Electrodes, which are hooked up to a machine that displays or prints out readings of baby's heartbeat and my contractions, will be placed on my abdomen. If I have a low-risk pregnancy and birth, I may be checked with a fetal monitor intermittently, or my baby's progress may be measured with a Doppler (a hand-held ultrasound device).

Some hospitals monitor women continuously, which has been shown to lead to an increase in Caesarean sections, which are often unnecessary, due to the readings being misinterpreted.

If my carers need a more detailed picture of baby's condition, they may want to use internal monitoring –

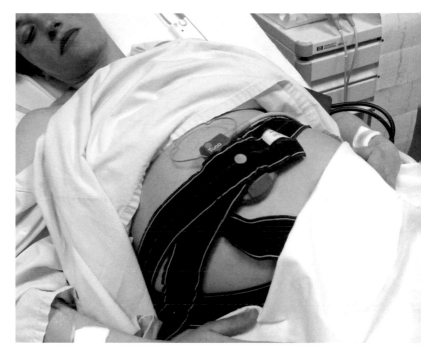

passing an electrode through my vagina and attaching it to my baby's scalp to measure her heartbeat.

EPISIOTOMY

A small cut may be made in my perineum (the skin between the vagina and anus) in order to enlarge the vaginal opening when my baby's head is about to be born. Nowadays this is usually only done to shorten the pushing stage of birth because of fetal distress or if a mother has a medical problem such as a heart condition and cannot cope with a long labour. It also

INCISION TYPES

Baby's head

Midline   Mediolateral

may be recommended to protect the delicate skull of a premature infant or to provide more space for the delivery of a breech or very large baby.

If I'm lucky, the skill and patience of an experienced midwife will stretch the area and allow my baby to be born with minimal or no tears and no need for an episiotomy.

FORCEPS AND VENTOUSE

In certain situations, medical instruments may be used to ease a baby out of the birth canal. Forceps (metal instruments resembling salad tongs or spoons) may be used if a mother can't push effectively or if a baby has to be born quickly. They also can be used to turn a baby into a different position and reduce the chances of trauma to him or her.

A ventouse or vacuum extractor works in a similar way to forceps, but instead of metal tongs, a soft suction cup is placed on the baby's head. As the mother pushes, suction helps to pull the baby out. Vacuum extractors can be used higher up the birth canal than forceps and cause less damage to the perineum.

PLANNED CAESAREAN

If I have a particular medical condition or there is an issue with my baby (see box page 108) that is detected sufficiently early, the baby may have to be delivered by caesarean section and this decision will be made well before the birth. However, during labour, it may become apparent that a caesarean will be necessary and in that situation, an unplanned or emergency procedure will be performed. While some women might prefer to have a caesarean birth to avoid the discomfort of labour, it is not recommended nor acceptable practice. Although surgical techniques have improved vastly in recent years, there are still much greater risks associated with caesareans than with vaginal births. In addition, the recovery period can be considerably longer, and a caesarean may make subsequent vaginal births more difficult.

While caesareans can be a safer means of birth for some babies, there are effects on the baby that may need to be overcome. Sometimes caesarean babies can retain fluid in their lungs – this is normally squeezed out in the birth canal. The newborn also may be drowsy from medication given to the mother.

A caesarean must be done in hospital as only an obstetrician or a surgeon can perform it. Under a general or regional anaesthetic, an incision is made in the lower part of the mother's abdomen and then

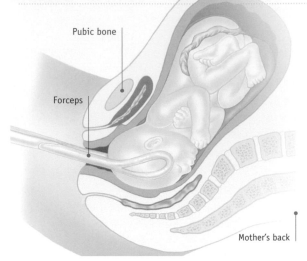

Pubic bone

Forceps

Mother's back

another one is made into the uterus and the baby is lifted out of the incision. The surgeon will then remove the placenta before the uterus and the abdominal wall are closed with stitches. Usually. the partner is allowed to be present and the mother will be handed her baby once he or she is born.

EXTERNAL VERSION

Breech babies – those presenting bottom first – are usually delivered by caesarean section. Some obstetricians, however, perform a manoeuvre, known as external version, in order to try and get the baby to turn head downwards so a vaginal delivery is possible. This is done around 37–38 weeks of pregnancy, when there is still sufficient amniotic fluid to allow for a small amount of movement, and involves manipulating the mother's abdomen. It is not without risks, however, which the obstetrician should make clear. Success rates vary from 50–70 per cent. Some women have found that assuming a breech tilt position – lying on the back with the knees flexed and the buttocks raised on pillows so that the pelvis is higher than the stomach or kneeling down on the floor with the buttocks raised as high as possible while the head rests on folded arms – for a minimum of 10 minutes twice a day can help a breech baby to turn naturally.

Pain relief in labour

Like all women, I will make use of one or more pain-relieving strategies during labour. Since I don't know how I will feel when the time comes, it's important that I remain flexible about what I will want.

DRUG-FREE METHODS

These include relaxation and breathing techniques, hot and cold compresses, massage, changes of position, visualisation and immersion in a birthing pool. Certain alternative therapies such as acupuncture, reflexology and hypnosis work for some women but require the support of a medical practitioner, while TENS (transcutaneous electrical nerve stimulation) machines may block the transmission of pain signals in early labour.

GAS AND AIR

Entonox (50% nitrous oxide, 50% oxygen) is a rapid-acting pain reliever, which you inhale via a mask from a

Many women in labour find having some of their pressure points stimulated can help to ease pain. Pressing into the hollow of the shoulder or between the first two toes may relax tension.

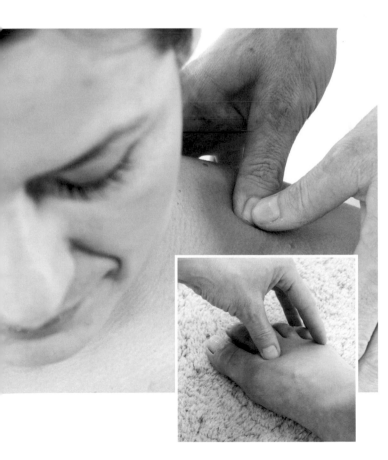

cylinder on a mobile support. It will take the edge off pain, and can be used as and when needed. It does not cross the placenta so cannot harm the baby. It can, however, cause nausea and lightheadedness.

PAIN MEDICATIONS

Among the standard medical therapies are analgaesics, which relieve pain, anaesthetics, which block sensations, and tranquillisers, which calm you. Local anaesthetics are commonly used for epidural insertion and pudendal blocks, and can be given at the time of birth and for episiotomies.

Analgaesics

These are injected into a muscle or given intravenously; pethidine is the one most commonly used. While it can be particularly helpful when early labour is prolonged and uncomfortable, allowing me to rest and taking the edge off strong sensations, it can make me feel sick, unsteady and sleepy. If given close to delivery, it can make baby drowsy and slow to feed and interact.

Regional anaesthetics

An epidural blocks most pain sensations in the abdomen, although pressure can still be felt. An anaesthetist places a small needle into the epidural space, in the lower part of the back, through which a very tiny, sterile tube is threaded and left in place when the needle is removed. Narcotic and local anaesthetics can be injected or pumped through the tube to take away or block pain. A pump provides a continuous low dose of the drugs. Side effects of epidurals can include difficulty urinating, lowered blood pressure and backache. Baby will be continuously monitored by an electronic fetal monitor.

A pudendal block numbs only the perineal area, so there is less pain, but contractions can still be felt. It is given at the time of delivery, by a needle inserted through the vagina usually with a forceps delivery or vacuum extraction and its effect can last through an episiotomy and subsequent stitching.

Tranquillisers

These are muscle relaxants, which can relieve tension. They are usually given with a narcotic to maximise the effect of a small dose of narcotic.

Childbirth classes and birth partner

As a first-time mum-to-be, there are lots of things to learn about pregnancy, labour and taking care of a baby, so I'm planning on signing up to a childbirth class to discover more about these things. I'm hoping that the instructors and other women attendees will able to answer all the questions I either forget to ask my caregivers or don't have time to ask. Also, they should be better able to prepare me physically and emotionally for the experience of birth and provide demonstrations and practice sessions for specific coping mechanisms.

I'm hoping that meeting in a group will be very supportive and that I'll make new friends who share a common interest in babies and children. A class should also be good for my partner, too, so that he can understand his role in the birth and become involved in the pregnancy and childbirth preparations.

CHOOSING THE RIGHT CLASS

I'm going to ask my doctor, midwife, friends and family for recommendations about the classes available in my area. Many private childbirth teachers approach the subject from a specific angle or philosophy, so it's important that I find a teacher who shares my views on childbirth, although it's also important to learn about different approaches to labour and birth so that I can make informed choices.

Childbirth classes usually begin at around 28–32 weeks and are held weekly – most often in the evenings and at weekends. All will cover what happens during labour and birth, when to call your caregiver, relaxation and breathing techniques, medical pain relief, caesareans and care of a newborn.

Health service classes are usually offered by hospitals, healthcare centres and doctors' surgeries. They are run by midwives or health visitors, sometimes with input from a doctor if there is something medical on the agenda. They are free, but are often conducted in large groups, possibly making it harder to make friends with other prospective parents.

Private childbirth classes are usually held in someone's home, or a community setting of some sort, and are run by a teacher trained by the organisation (such as the National Childcare Trust parenting charity (NCT), Lamaze International, Active Birth or Bradley Certification). The person offering the classes may not be a health professional. Some instructors will allow

you to sit in on a session so that you can decide if it's right for you. An ideal class size is around 5–7 couples – large enough to enable good discussion but small enough for everyone to get individual attention during sessions.

BIRTH PARTNER

Like most women, I will look to my partner to be present at the birth and to help me cope with labour. A supportive partner can help to shorten labour, decrease the need for interventions, decrease the risk of an unplanned caesarean and improve the outcome for my baby. However, should my partner not be available or feel uneasy about any aspect – he must be able to focus on my needs – I could hire professional labour support known as a doula, or ask a relative or friend.

Whoever is going to be there, he or she needs to be aware of the preferences expressed in my birth plan (see page 77) and should supply the needed support. I also plan to involve my partner in breathing and relaxation techniques so he is well practised by the time of delivery.

If I do nothing else I will ...

LET MY BIRTH PARTNER HELP ME

A birth partner can be invaluable in the delivery room. Some of the things I expect my partner to do are:

✓ **Offer emotional support.**

✓ **Ensure my privacy.**

✓ **Help me** with breathing and relaxation techniques.

✓ **Assist me** with changing my position.

✓ **Give massage or compresses** if requested.

✓ **Encourage me** to eat, drink and rest.

✓ **Keep me** cool (or warm) and comfortable.

BIRTH PARTNERS

I would like the following people to be at the birth

- [ ] Partner
- [ ] Friend
- [ ] Relative
- [ ] Doula
- [ ] Other children*

PHOTOGRAPHY

- [ ] I wish to have my birth photographed/videoed.

INDUCTION

- [ ] I would prefer not to be induced.
- [ ] I would consider induction for medical reasons only.
- [ ] I would prefer to be induced to control the time/date of my delivery.

LABOUR

- [ ] I want to be able to walk around and be out of bed if possible.
- [ ] I would like to drink fluids and/or eat lightly throughout the first stage.
- [ ] If available, I would like to use a birthing pool.
- [ ] I would like to keep the number of vaginal examinations to a minimum.
- [ ] I would like to view the birth using a mirror.

MONITORING

- [ ] I do not wish to have continuous fetal monitoring unless my baby is distressed.

PAIN MANAGEMENT

- [ ] I wish to have a natural birth and do not want pain medication offered to me during labour.
- [ ] I wish to have pain medication available but only given to me if I request it.
- [ ] I would like an epidural as early as possible.
- [ ] I would like an epidural later in labour.

EPISIOTOMY

- [ ] I would prefer not to have an episiotomy unless it is required for my baby's safety.
- [ ] I would prefer to have an episiotomy rather than risk a tear.

CAESAREAN

- [ ] If I need to have an emergency caesarean I would like my partner present at all times during the operation.
- [ ] I wish to have an epidural or spinal for anaesthesia.
- [ ] If I have to have a full anaesthetic, I wish my baby to be handed to (name of person) after the birth.

POST-BIRTH

- [ ] I would like to hold my baby immediately after the birth.
- [ ] I want to wait until the umbilical cord stops pulsing before it is cut.
- [ ] I would like my partner to cut the cord.
- [ ] I would prefer not to have routine syntocinon after the birth.
- [ ] I plan to breastfeed my baby.
- [ ] I wish to put my baby to the breast as soon after the birth as possible.

* Check with hospital about visiting policies.

PART I My pregnancy

Preparing for baby

As well as shopping for baby clothes and equipment and decorating and furnishing baby's room, I need to decide on whether to breast- or bottlefeed and what help I will need once she is born. I also need, along with my partner, to make the important decision about what she is to be named.

Shopping for my baby

Although a small baby doesn't need much in the way of equipment, having things ready at home will make the first hectic days of looking after her easier and will free up time and energy, which can be spent enjoying my baby. I'm glad I'm not having twins, but if I were, I'd need to double up on everything except the cot, as two babies can share initially.

Some of the equipment or supplies, such as for feeding, nappy changing and sleeping, will depend on my choice of method or bed. It's also not a good idea to buy too much, as I'm certain to receive gifts and maybe some second-hand items, so I'll use the list opposite to buy the essentials.

CLOTHES

I plan to choose clothes made of natural fibres (cotton and soft wools), which are colourfast and suitable for machine washing and drying. Easy-to-wear styles include vests with envelope-style necks (babies don't enjoy having things placed over their heads) and babygros fastened with poppers. I will wash all of baby's clothes, whether new or second hand, with a gentle detergent before use.

Baby clothes are generally sold according to age – newborn, 3 months, 6 months, etc., or in centimetre sizes starting at 50 cm. A big baby may not get any wear out of newborn size clothes, so if my baby's weight is projected to be 4.5 kg or more, I will want to start with a 3-month size. If my baby is very small or premature, there are special ranges.

FEEDING EQUIPMENT

This depends on whether I decide to breast- or bottlefeed (see page 83). For both, I will need small bottles, rings, teats and caps (two for breastfeeding to hold expressed milk, six for bottlefeeding), a bottle brush and a steriliser (with tablets depending on the type). For breastfeeding, I also will need a battery-operated breast pump to express milk and some breast pads – washable or disposable.

NAPPY CHANGING

With fabric nappies, I will also need plastic pants, nappy liners and safety pins (unless they are self fastening). 'Eco' nappies and coverings are now widely available. Additionally, I will buy two buckets – one for

THE LAYETTE AND ESSENTIAL EQUIPMEN

Indoor clothes

- [ ] 4 T-shirts or vests
- [ ] 2 pairs socks or booties
- [ ] 2 nightdresses or sleep suits
- [ ] 4 babygros
- [ ] 2 shawls
- [ ] 2 bibs

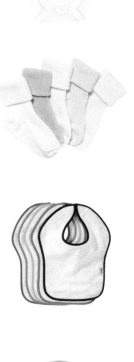

Outdoor clothes

- [ ] 1 hat (fabric and type depends on season)
- [ ] 3 cardigans
- [ ] 1 pram suit (for cold weather)
- [ ] 1 pair mittens

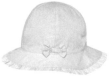

Changing supplies

- [ ] 24 fabric nappies* or 70 newborn disposables
- [ ] Changing mat
- [ ] Baby wipes
- [ ] Bin or 2 pails*

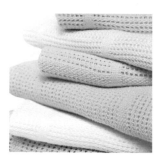

Bed and bath supplies

- ☐ Moses basket, cradle or cot (and mattress)*

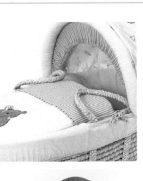

- ☐ 3 basket or cot sheets

- ☐ Baby bath

- ☐ 2–3 lightweight blankets

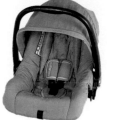

- ☐ 2 face cloths

- ☐ 2 hooded baby towels

- ☐ Baby hairbrush

Travel equipment

- ☐ Sling or carrier

- ☐ Infant car seat*

- ☐ Pram or pushchair*

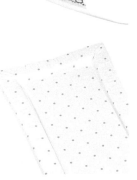

Feeding equipment

- ☐ 2–6 bottles*

- ☐ Steriliser

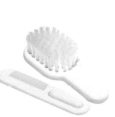

* See text for more information

---

soiled nappies and one for urine-soaked ones. If I use disposables, I will need nappy sacks and a covered rubbish bin (preferably pedal operated).

SLEEPING

A small baby can sleep in a portable Moses basket or a cradle or cot and there are different-sized sheets depending on my choice. I need to be aware that any cot or mattress I choose is safe (see pages 172–75).

CAR SEAT

I will need a car seat suitable for newborns to take my baby home from the hospital or birthing centre. Ideally, it should have a 5-point safety harness. It must be installed rearward facing and in a seat not fitted with an airbag. I need to install the seat before the birth as the set-up process may be tricky, time consuming and hard to manage once baby is here.

PRAM, PUSHCHAIR OR SLING

There's a vast choice of equipment for transporting my baby but I understand that only prams, flat-folding buggies and slings are suitable for newborns. An umbrella-folding pushchair is usually only suitable for babies from 3–6 months onwards.

Though prams are usually the most expensive, they are the most suitable for newborns. A baby can lie flat (which is recommended) and can be seen easily; many prams can transform into buggies or carry cots.

Flat-folding buggies are usually sturdy and if the seats are flat, padded and comfortable, they will be suitable for a newborn. Some have an adjustable handle height, which is handy as my partner is substantially taller than me. If possible, the seat should face inward; recent research seems to indicate that babies using outward-facing buggies may be losing out on acquiring social skills.

A baby sling or soft fabric carrier will enable me to hold baby close to my chest, and can be used indoors and out (see page 170). There are many different styles, but the important thing is that they don't interfere with baby's breathing. The item should carry a safety standards logo.

Preparing baby's room

I'm fortunate to have a separate room for my baby, although it would be possible to make space for her in part of another room. Initially, my concern is to ensure that all surfaces are easy to keep clean and that the furniture and storage areas are conveniently arranged. I need to make it easy on myself to get baby into and out of her cot, change nappies and dress her.

As my baby will probably use the same room throughout her childhood, I need to be sure that the decorations will grow with her. Plain, painted walls, which can be updated with borders, friezes and stencils, are the most flexible. The paint needs to be water based, with a washable or spongeable surface.

When placing the furniture, the cot needs to be against the wall, away from the window. It's important that from her cot my baby is not able to reach a window or curtain or blind cord or another piece of furniture, and that direct sunlight won't fall on her at any time.

ROOM ESSENTIALS

Besides the basic furnishings, there are some other items that will make it easier to care for my baby.

☐ **A comfortable rocking chair.** I will spend many hours feeding my baby, so I need to choose something with good support. I understand there are versions that recline as well as rock or glide and that have a matching foot support. The fabric needs to be spongeable or have a plastic covering.

☐ **Storage items.** I need different ones in which to keep clothing, nappies, toys and toiletries. Chests, crates, trolleys, stacking boxes or shelving are all possibilities.

☐ **A lamp.** One with a low intensity setting that can be used if I want to read while breastfeeding or expressing. The lamp should be able to function as a night light.

☐ **CD player or radio.** This will be soothing company at feeding times.

☐ **A clock.** This may be helpful for keeping track of how long I have been breastfeeding.

I either need to have a purpose-made changing table with space for storing nappies, wipes, nappy creams or ointments, etc. or to create a changing centre with a flat surface on which to lay the changing mat, with another piece of furniture to hold the necessary items. This, too, should be placed squarely against a wall and away from a window. The nappy bucket needs to be right next to the changing table.

As I will be breastfeeding, I need to set up an expressing centre and the nursery will be the most convenient. There needs to be a convenient place to store the pump, accessories and reading material.

My feeding choices

One of the most important decisions I have to make is whether to breastfeed or bottlefeed my baby. Although formula manufacturers claim they are able to produce a similar product, breast milk is the most natural and nutritious milk. It is also cheap and readily available and offers many health and medical benefits. Natural hormonal changes within the body ensure that breastfeeding becomes emotionally satisfying to both participants.

Some women, however, may have problems with breastfeeding. They may have an antipathy to it or may be on medication or have a condition, which isn't compatible with breastfeeding.

The most important, thing, however, is to decide on a feeding method that makes me feel comfortable and ensures baby can be healthy and happy, too. Deciding how to feed is a very personal matter and I want to spend some time understanding the benefits and drawbacks of each method in order to make an informed decision. One thing I need to bear in mind, however, is that it's harder to take up breastfeeding once a baby has started on a bottle, so I may not have another chance if I don't try it from early on. Even if I'm unsure about whether I will continue, I should aim at least to try breastfeeding (unless advised otherwise by my doctor or obstetrician). I understand that many women who don't do so sometimes later wish they had done.

BREASTFEEDING

Women and babies were designed to breastfeed, regardless of the size or shape of the woman's breasts, though if nipples are flat or inverted, a little help may be needed in learning to position baby. Most women manage it very successfully within a few weeks of the birth, though some with the help of a breastfeeding counsellor. Breast milk is most beneficial to a baby during the early weeks because it helps build up

immunity. But it is also possible to breastfeed long term and even if I go back to work. I can breastfeed when at home and leave expressed milk for baby's caregiver to give while I'm away.

BOTTLEFEEDING

Ready-prepared formula and modern sterilising equipment has made bottlefeeding less time consuming and easier to manage. All baby formulas are carefully produced under government guidelines to ensure that they replicate human milk as closely as possible and contain the correct amounts of fat, protein and vitamins that a baby needs. However, these artificial milks don't contain the protective antibodies of breast milk and in preparing and giving bottles, unless I strictly follow the recommended guidelines, I am more likely to introduce disease-causing bacteria.

Choosing a name

Coming up with a name for baby is another important decision I have to make. Until I find out the gender, I need to have both a girl's and boy's name in mind. As well as the most popular recent names shown here, I could refer to the many name books available, which usually contain the derivation and meaning of each name. Unlike some families, in ours there's no custom or tradition for naming children, such as naming a baby after a deceased relative or a boy after his father.

I'm not sure whether my partner and I will quickly agree on a name or names or whether it will be a long, drawn-out process. Compromise may be necessary.

A good method for choosing names is for each of us to make a list of our desired names for our baby, with our most favoured names highest on the list. Any names to which one of us objects would be removed from both lists. Then, if there are names that appear in both lists, we could choose the one that has the highest 'rating'. Another idea would be to make a list of favourite names and attach it to the fridge or a notice board so that we can look at the names frequently and get a good feeling for each one.

We also think we should be flexible about the name, changing our minds about the one chosen if, once our

If I do nothing else I will ... ✓

GIVE THOUGHT TO CHOOSING A NAME
Whatever name I choose, my baby is going to have to live with it for a lifetime. Therefore, I need to:

✓ **Pay attention to how the name sounds.** Does the forename go well with our family name?

✓ **Choose any middle name carefully.** What will the initials spell?

✓ **Consider whether current fads** and fashions are a good idea. In future, would names like Star, Suri, Brooklyn, Paris, Pixie, etc., be inappropriate?

✓ **Find out the derivation and meaning.** I can either buy a baby names book or look on the internet.

✓ **Try to think of possible nicknames.** Charles could become Charlie, Chuck or Chas but Fatima might be shortened to Fatty!

✓ **Think about others with the same name.** Maybe there is someone I like very much with the name or alternatively someone I don't.

✗ **Avoid difficult names.** Those that are easy to misspell or hard to pronounce.

DAD'S TOP 5 NAME CHOICES

	GIRLS	BOYS
1 Name:		
Meaning:		
2 Name:		
Meaning:		
3 Name:		
Meaning:		
4 Name:		
Meaning:		
5 Name:		
Meaning:		

baby is born, we decide that a different name seems to suit him or her better.

Unless we both consent, other relatives – the future grandparents, for example – should not get a vote, though we may consider their preferences in making our choice. Like some other prospective parents, we plan not to divulge the name until after the birth; hopefully, if any of our close relatives thinks our chosen name or names are inappropriate, our beautiful new baby can help to appease him or her.

MUM'S TOP 5 NAME CHOICES

		GIRLS	BOYS
1	Name:		
	Meaning:		
2	Name:		
	Meaning:		
3	Name:		
	Meaning:		
4	Name:		
	Meaning:		
5	Name:		
	Meaning:		

POPULAR NAMES

GIRLS	BOYS
Olivia	Jack
Ruby	Harry
Emily	Alfie
Grace	Oliver
Lily	Thomas
Jessica	Daniel
Amelia	Joshua
Chloe	Charlie
Isabella	Mohammed
Emma	George
Lucy	Lewis
Isabelle	Dylan
Megan	William
Ella	Samuel
Evie	Ethan
Charlotte	Ben
Hannah	Jacob
Ava	Joseph
Holly	Luke
Alexa	Ryan
Ashlee	Liam
Sophia	Max
Zoe	Tyler
Brooke	Callum
Chloe	Alexander
Faith	Finn
Laura	James

Childcare choices

Getting help with my baby at home – at least for the first few weeks after the birth – will probably make a huge difference to me. Also important is to find a GP that will look after my baby. If I decide to return to work then I'll have to arrange for more permanent childcare. I need to make sure that the people I choose are the right ones.

HELP AT HOME AND WITH BABY

Once I get home I'll want to get to know my baby and adjust to my new role in a relaxed atmosphere. It will be good, therefore, to have someone to help with household chores and cooking. If the birth is difficult or lengthy, I may also be tired and in need of plenty of rest. Ideally, my partner will be able to take paternal leave for some time or a close relative could help out. Alternatively, I could begin by employing a nanny or mother's help (see opposite page).

LONGER-TERM CHILDCARE SOLUTIONS

Once my baby is older and I'm thinking about returning to full- or part-time work, I'll need to arrange some more permanent form of childcare. It'll be a lot easier returning to a working life if I feel happy and confident about this. I'll ask my health visitor, family and friends for recommendations, and get a list of registered childminders from my local authority. The most important factor is to ensure the safety and wellbeing of my baby. I must always double-check licences, training certificates and references and investigate thoroughly any facility that I am considering using. My options are:

Shared parental care at home

This is the ideal option; one of us stays at home to look after our baby, or we both work different hours so that the care can be shared.

Family

Having my mother or other relative look after baby can be an excellent solution, as baby will be provided with continuity of care. However, if we disagree over baby's care, this could lead to long-term problems. Not every grandmother wants to spend her retirement years looking after a young baby and I have to be certain even if she is willing, that she is physically able.

CHILD-FRIENDLY PRACTICE

In order to find a GP who has a special interest in paediatrics, I need to ask my health visitor, midwife, friends and relatives for their recommendations. I can then either telephone and/or visit the surgery to find out answers to the following questions.

- What is the type of practice? Is it solo or group? (It may be better to choose a group practice where there'll always be someone on call.)
- Are there dedicated baby clinics?
- What are the surgery hours, typical waiting times and on-call group policies?
- How are after-hours calls handled?
- What happens in emergencies?
- Is the waiting area welcoming and clean, and are there plenty of toys and books to keep young children entertained?
- Are the reception staff welcoming and friendly, and how do they interact with children?

Once I'm happy with the answers to the above, I'll need to make an appointment to meet the GP and to find out what he or she thinks about issues about which I have an interest such as:

- Breastfeeding.
- Supplementation.
- Newborn jaundice.
- Circumcision.
- Antibiotic use.
- Immunisation.

If I do nothing else I will ...

HAVE DAD HELP WITH BABY

There are lots of things dad (or another helper) can do. He can:

✓ **Change nappies.**

✓ **Feed baby** or bring baby to me for feeding.

✓ **Get up** in the night to tend to baby.

✓ **Help with housework and chores.**

✓ **Do the food shopping,** replacing essential items as necessary.

✓ **Cook meals** and clean up afterwards.

✓ **Comfort our crying baby.**

✓ **Deal with visitors,** allowing me as much privacy and relaxation time as possible.

Nanny

Dedicated in-home care will be expensive, but if I'm planning to have another child fairly soon, and I have the room, it will become more economical. There's no doubt that one-on-one care during my baby's first year of life will be very beneficial, but that depends on my finding a reliable, experienced nanny who's in tune with my baby's physical and emotional needs.

Mother's help

Hiring someone who lives in and can help not only with my baby but can perform other useful functions such as running errands, cooking and assisting with the household chores may be an option. However, mother's helps are not available full time and many are learning English, so there may be communication problems.

Childminder

I could look for someone licensed to offer childcare in her home, possibly someone already looking after her own or other children. This arrangement will provide playmates and a family environment for my child, and has the advantage of her having the same caregiver long term and being in a small group. A negative is that she will be more likely to come down with colds and other illnesses from contact with the other children.

Nursery

This could be an option when my child is older (not all nurseries take babies under the age of 12 months). The important thing is to find one that is of a high standard and is recommended by people I trust. Obviously, it also needs to be affordable and be open convenient hours. Again, my baby will be able to benefit from interacting with others and from the facilities the nursery should offer – play equipment, water table, etc. – but there will be a greater risk of illness as well .

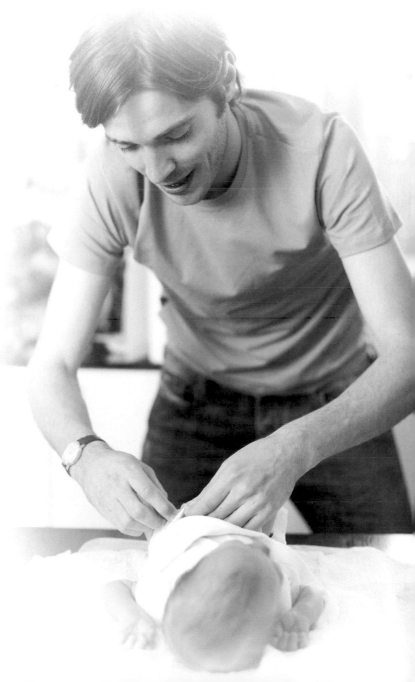

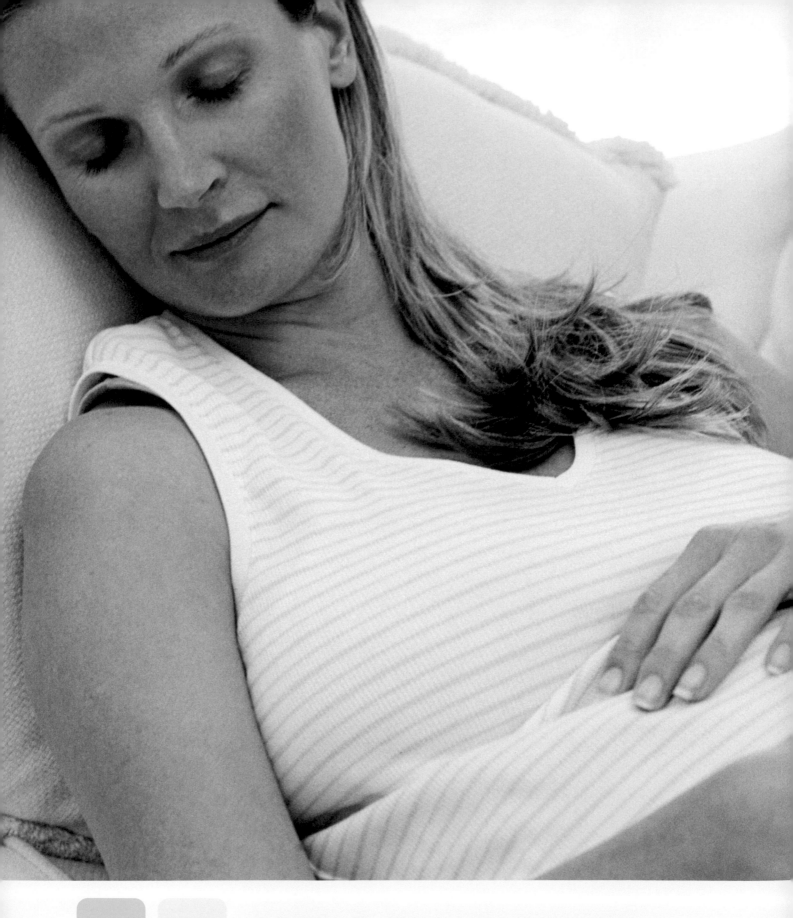

PART I My pregnancy

Preparing for the birth

Now that I've reached the last weeks of the last trimester I know that my baby will be born soon. I want to be able to recognise labour when it begins and to have prepared myself for the experience. In these last weeks, however, it becomes increasingly uncomfortable for me to go about my daily routine and all the effects associated with an enlarged tummy and around an extra 9–13 kg or so take their toll.

Easing late pregnancy complaints

During these last weeks of pregnancy, I am find it increasingly hard to get comfortable as baby grows, takes up more and more space in my adomen and assumes her delivery position (see page 91).

SWOLLEN FEET AND LEGS

At the end of a day or if I've been standing or sitting a lot or if it's hot, I've noticed that my feet and legs (and sometimes by hands and fingers) swell and feel spongey. Known as oedema, this is due to excess fluid circulating throughout my body.

I can help to ease the condition by avoiding standing for long periods, sitting or lying down with my legs elevated, wearing comfortable shoes or slippers and drinking at least 8–10 glasses of liquids a day

ABDOMINAL STRETCHING

Frequently I feel an uncomfortable burning sensation over my taut tummy. Sometimes called hot spots, these are superficial pains irritated by tight or heavy clothing.

To prevent these pains occurring, I must stop wearing tights and stick to loose clothing. Applying an ice pack can relieve the burning and wearing an abdominal support also may help. Performing my pelvic exercises regularly and strenghtening my

If I do nothing else I will ...

LOOK AFTER MYSELF

I may need to make adjustments to my normal habits because of changes like increased fat deposits and a faster metabolism. I will:

✓ **Wear light, loose clothing** because I may feel hotter than normal.

✓ **Get as much sleep as possible,** as it is difficult to get a good night's sleep with having to go to the toilet frequently. I will supplement my nightly sleep with naps.

✓ **Drink plenty of fluids** so that I can relieve swelling feet and legs. I must keep my body hydrated.

✓ **Take a break** whenever I can, making sure I put my feet up for 10–15 minutes, 3 times a day.

✓ **Increase my intake of protein.** Eating plenty of milk, eggs, meat and fish can improve my stamina.

ABDOMINAL TIGHTENER

I do this lying on my side, but it can also be done while sitting or standing. I place my hands behind my head and slowly curl my body towards my knees, contracting my abdominal muscles and breathing out. Then I relax for about 30 seconds and repeat. I do this as many times as I can without becoming tired.

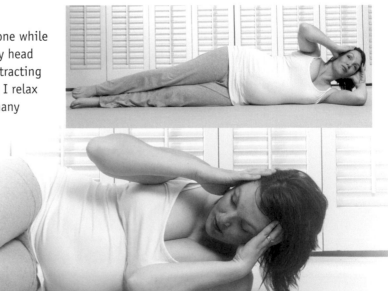

abdominal muscles (see opposite page) can help improve my posture and relieve pain.

INDIGESTION

One of the most common discomforts of late pregnancy, this is caused by my growing baby putting pressure on my abdomen, causing a reflux of wind and gastric juices into my oesophagus. It is exacerbated by hormones having relaxed the sphincter between my stomach and oesophagus.

I can help to ease this by avoiding large meals, not eating close to bedtime, and sleeping with extra pillows to prevent acid from rising up. Antacids containing calcium carbonate aren't generally effective as they cause an increase in stomach acidity.

PREGNANCY SUPPORT

Worn occasionally, an abdominal support designed for pregnancy can help relieve pain in the abdomen, back and legs. This is especially helpful if your abdominal muscles are stretched by a twin pregnancy or large baby.

BABY'S POSITION

Before about 32 weeks, when my baby is still relatively small, she has room to change positions frequently. After this, like most babies, she will settle into her preferred position. It's important that I know what this is, since this profoundly affects the birth. My caregiver can ascertain baby's position by palpating or gently pressing my belly.

Head down

The best position for my baby to be in for birth is head down with her spine facing away from my back. In this position, the narrower part of her head comes down the birth canal first. This is known as the anterior position and more than 95 per cent of babies adopt it. If, however, she is lying head down but with her back against mine (posterior position), a wider part of her head is presenting and it may be more difficult for her to move down the birth canal and the birth can be more painful.

Breech

If, like 4 per cent of babies, my baby is lying with his head up and his bottom facing down (see opposite), my doctor may not want to deliver him vaginally because there are small, but significant, risks to a vaginal birth of a breech baby, especially for first babies.

Transverse

If baby is lying across my uterus with neither his head nor bottom in my pelvis (see bottom, opposite), like around 1 per cent of babies, it will not be possible to deliver him except by caesarean section.

Changing his position

External version (see page 74) and visualisation (see page 94) may help my baby turn naturally into the anterior position.

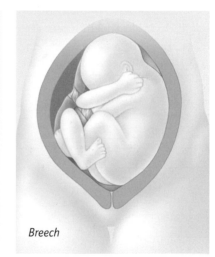

Breech

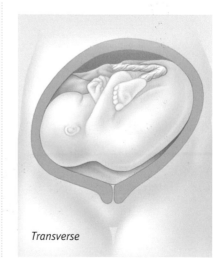

Transverse

My labour preparation

As my due date approaches, there are things I need to do to prepare myself for the birth. I need to be in shape both physically and emotionally, and to take it easy whenever I can, which will promote both. I also need to work on some of the techniques and positions I might use to help make the birth easier and less painful.

PHYSICAL PREPARATION

Certain exercises and positions (see box, below) can help prepare my body for labour, and I need to add them to my regular routine from about 28 weeks of pregnancy. It also helps, at around the same time, if I start building up the intensity of my pelvic floor exercises (see page 56). I now need to hold each squeeze for a count of 10, and repeat 4–6 times, at least 3 times a day. Changing the speed of the pull ups will lead to greater flexibility and control, so I can either count quickly to 10 or 20, alternately contracting and relaxing my pelvic floor for each number, or do it slowly, contracting for a slow count of 4, waiting for a

PRIMING THE BODY

Stretched muscles will make it much easier for my baby to pass through my pelvis and sitting tailor fashion can help improve pelvic flexibility. Pelvic rocks can ease backache and modified squats can strengthen the thigh muscles and encourage my baby to descend properly. into the pelvis.

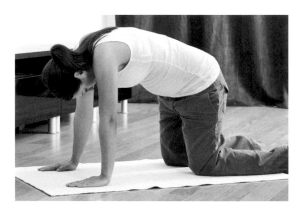

Sitting with feet touching and knees spread produces a stretch that needs to be held for a count of 12 and repeated daily. In time, as I get more flexible, I'll be able to remove the pillows and push my knees closer to the floor.

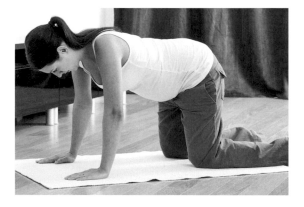

Pelvic rocks involve assuming an all-fours position. I must round my back and shoulders, drop my head and briefly tighten my abdomen and buttocks. I hold this position momentarily before gradually releasing. I repeat this 10 times twice daily.

count of 10 and then slowly releasing the muscles for another count of 4.

EMOTIONAL PREPARATION

Sometimes I feel thrilled knowing my baby will arrive soon and other times totally unprepared for labour, birth and motherhood. I've been told all these mood swings are entirely natural, as is feeling a little down during the last weeks of pregnancy. It's not unusual to feel that baby has taken over completely.

I know that fantasies and fears very often rise to the surface in late pregnancy, so it's important that I discuss anything untoward with my midwife or bring it up at antenatal class. Focusing on the positive, through

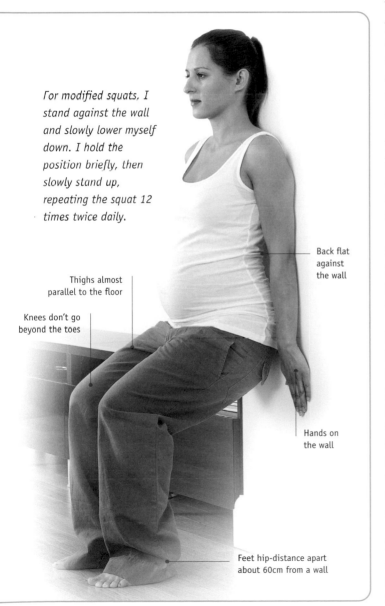

For modified squats, I stand against the wall and slowly lower myself down. I hold the position briefly, then slowly stand up, repeating the squat 12 times twice daily.

Back flat against the wall

Thighs almost parallel to the floor

Knees don't go beyond the toes

Hands on the wall

Feet hip-distance apart about 60cm from a wall

meditation and visualisation, can also help as can treating myself to a baby-shopping spree or lunch out.

If I'm planning a hospital birth, a tour of the delivery suite where I'll give birth can help, while deciding on how to get to the hospital will make me more confident about transport arrangements. My partner and I should map out the easiest route and try it out, bearing in mind that we may need a different route during rush hours. We should know which entrance we need and where to park. I also plan, as backup, to ask a friend to be prepared to take me and to have the number of a reliable taxi service handy.

Worries and anxieties can affect a birth in a very direct physical way. Being unprepared for the pain of normal contractions can be frightening and can disrupt breathing, which can increase tension – and therefore pain – in the muscles, and may even decrease the flow of oxytocin, the hormone that causes the uterus to contract. It is therefore important that I learn as much as I can about labour and what my body is up to; once I realise that these sensations are totally normal, I may be able to view my contractions as 'work' and not 'pain'.

Another way my mind can help my body to 'work' is by focusing on a goal – in this case the arrival of my baby. Distracting myself may help me to cope with any distressing body sensation. There are all sorts of mental distraction techniques I can practise and later use, including breathing, massage, meditation or visualising.

Finally, relaxed muscles will make it much easier for my uterus to do its work and to stretch as baby passes through the pelvis. Therefore, I need to practise the positions (see box) and use those activities, such as massage or meditation, which can help me relax.

Breathing

Breathing correctly is an important component of successful labour; muscles deprived of oxygen can be painful and insufficient oxygen going to the uterus and placenta can lead to baby becoming distressed. As well as the patterned breathing taught in antenatal class, slow breathing in early labour helps to promote relaxation. Sufficient oxygen will get to my baby if I take deep, relaxing breaths at the beginning and end of contractions. It's important I don't breathe too quickly or hold my breath for prolonged periods.

Panting or deep blowing can be helpful in later labour if I need to slow down pushing at the time of actual delivery of my baby's head. Breathing out will stop my lungs from expanding and pushing down on my uterus when pushing isn't appropriate.

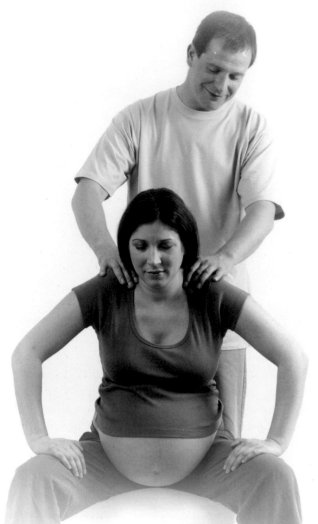

Massage
Having my muscles kneaded or stroked can help to release muscle tension and promote relaxation. Between contractions, massage can provide a pleasant tactile sensation to help to lift my spirits and during contractions it can help to take my mind off the pain.

Meditation and visualisation
Meditation and visualisation both use a device – meditation a word, sound or phrase and visualisation an image – which either helps to slow down breathing or relaxes tense muscles. By concentrating hard on the sound of the meditation or the image in visualisation, my mind will be distracted from pain.

Water
Whether at home or in hospital, spending part of my labour in warm water will help my muscles to relax, which can speed up the birth process. Some women even give birth in the water, but opinion is divided as to whether this is sufficiently safe. Most water births tend to be carried out by midwives in midwife units or in the home (pools can be rented), but some hospitals provide birth pools for use in labour.

LABOUR POSITIONS
In addition to mental strategies to ward off pain, it's important that I find and experiment with comfortable positions – with or without my birth partner.

During labour, different positions may be needed at different times. Some may be better at relieving backache or promoting rest, others may aid baby's progress through the curvature of the lower abdomen and pelvis. Recommended positions include sitting on a chair facing the chair back or kneeling forward on a pile of cushions, leaning over my birth partner or having him or her support me in a squat or getting down on hands and knees. Other positions can be achieved more simply by lying down with plenty of pillow support for my head, bump and thighs or using a birthing stool.

For birth, an upright position is best. This enlists the aid of gravity to help to push baby out. I may want to stick to one position or, again, try out a few.

Sitting backwards facing the back of a chair with my bottom off the end can take pressure off my sacrum.

Leaning over my birth partner can help baby rotate if she is facing backwards in the birth canal. I kneel down and rest my arms on my partner so he supports me as I bear down.

Squatting encourages baby to descend rapidly and may widen the pelvis by as much as 2 cm. I don't have to put as much effort into bearing down, but it can be a tiring position to hold for any length of time. Having my birth partner support me from behind or using a birthing stool can help.

Assuming an all-fours position can help to relieve backache and rotate a backward-facing baby. It may be useful to slow down baby's descent if she is coming too fast. If I have backache, I'll try rocking my hips from side to side while in this position.

Recognising labour

Beginning some weeks before my due date, my body will undergo certain changes that precede the start of real labour. Some of these are a result of my baby assuming her final position for birth. The exact cause of the onset of labour remains unknown. The most widely held theory is that my baby produces substances that result in a change in pregnancy hormones. But I will know that I'm in labour when I experience regular contractions, which will cause my cervix to dilate. Prior to that, there will be a few other signs that mean labour is imminent.

ENGAGEMENT

Between 2–4 weeks before labour starts, my baby's head will descend lower into my pelvis. Known as engagement, there are some related benefits and minor discomforts to my baby's head being lower down. While I'll have more space to breathe, any heartburn symptoms should ease and I'll not feel uncomfortably full after a meal, I will also pass water and bowel movements more frequently, have aches in my pubic bones and back, sharp twinges in my pelvis and swollen legs and feet. Pelvic rocks (see page 92) and

HOW THE HEAD ENGAGES

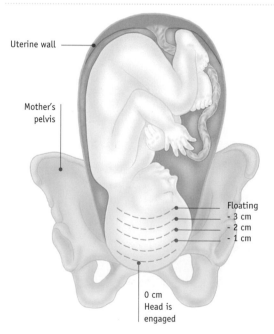

Uterine wall

Mother's pelvis

Floating
- 3 cm
- 2 cm
- 1 cm

0 cm
Head is engaged

⚕ **EXPERTS ADVISE**

Suspicious vaginal discharge
Although increased vaginal secretions are likely as labour approaches, a healthy discharge will be colourless or tinged pink. A yellow, green, brown or frothy discharge may signal an infection or the leakage of amniotic fluid containing meconium (a baby's first bowel movement and often a signal of distress), so you should report it immediately to your caregiver.

lying on my left side can help to relieve some of this pelvic pressure.

NESTING INSTINCT
During this last month, I find I have a sudden desire to empty drawers, clear out cupboards and scrub the house from top to bottom. This is an inbuilt maternal urge to prepare the home for the imminent arrival of baby. While I want to make the most of this burst of energy, I have to take care not to overdo it.

MUCUS PLUG AND BLOODSTAINED SHOW
As my cervix softens, shortens and begins to dilate, the mucus plug that has sealed the cervix for most of my pregnancy will be dislodged. This is called a bloodstained show – or sometimes just a 'show' – and usually appears as a small amount of bright red or brownish mucus. A show may also appear as a heavier discharge or it may simply be unnoticeable. Though a show can be a sign that labour's imminent, it can occur as much as 6 weeks before the birth. However, if I have a show, I need to contact my midwife for advice.

RUPTURE OF MEMBRANES
The amniotic sac containing the fluid around my baby usually will rupture – known as the 'waters breaking' – at some point during labour. Occasionally, however, it may rupture before contractions begin in earnest. Most women go into labour within 24 hours of their waters breaking, as the rupture causes the release of prostaglandins, contraction-stimulating substances.

Sometimes a woman may have been having contractions before her waters break but has not been aware of them. Once the waters break, contractions can intensify, as the baby's presenting part (the part that will be born first) now presses directly onto the dilating cervix.

If my waters break at home, I need to note the time they break and the consistency (fluid containing meconium would be dangerous), and notify my midwife. Amniotic fluid is usually clear and odourless, and once the bag of waters has ruptured at term, it will go on leaking until delivery (urine or vaginal secretions may leak from time to time). If the waters break before my due date or before baby is engaged or if baby was high in my pelvis at my last examination, my midwife may recommend that I go into the hospital to be assessed before contractions start.

Once my waters break it's important that I not put anything into my vagina as there is a possible risk of infection. Showers are preferable to baths until active labour has begun and my baby has been assessed by my midwife. If I become aware of something pulsing in my vagina after my waters break, this may be a prolapsed cord, so I need to call the hospital right away.

CONTRACTIONS

Well before true labour begins, Braxton Hicks contractions can occur, which stretch the lower part of the uterus so that baby's head engages and the cervix thins and softens. In the run-up to labour, these practice contractions can intensify, producing a tightening or 'balling up' sensation in the abdomen. Lying down usually helps to ease any discomfort. These early contractions are sometimes, therefore, called 'false' labour, because they occur only intermittently as they prepare the uterus for true, progressive labour.

At some point, any brief, irregular contractions will be replaced by ones that have a rhythmic pattern and longer length. These contractions progressively contract the upper uterus while stretching the lower part and opening or dilating the cervix. By this mechanism, the powerful upper uterine muscles push the baby through the stretchable lower uterus.

Sometimes contractions are strongly felt in the back. If I experience back pain every 5 minutes, I need to call my midwife and go to the hospital.

TRUE OR FALSE LABOUR?
Contractions are the one sure way I'll be able to tell if I'm in labour or not. This chart can help me assess whether my contractions are the real thing or are 'practice' ones known as Braxton Hicks contractions.

TRUE LABOUR

✓ Contractions have a regular pattern – coming every 5 minutes.

✓ Contractions become progressively stronger.

✓ Contractions don't abate when walking or resting.

✓ Contractions may be accompanied by a show.

✓ Progressive cervical dilatation.

FALSE LABOUR

✗ Contractions are irregular – coming every 3 minutes, and then every 5–10 minutes.

✗ Contractions don't intensify with time.

✗ Contractions may recede with changes in activity or position.

✗ Contractions usually not accompanied by increased mucus or bloodstained show.

✗ No significant cervical change is detectable.

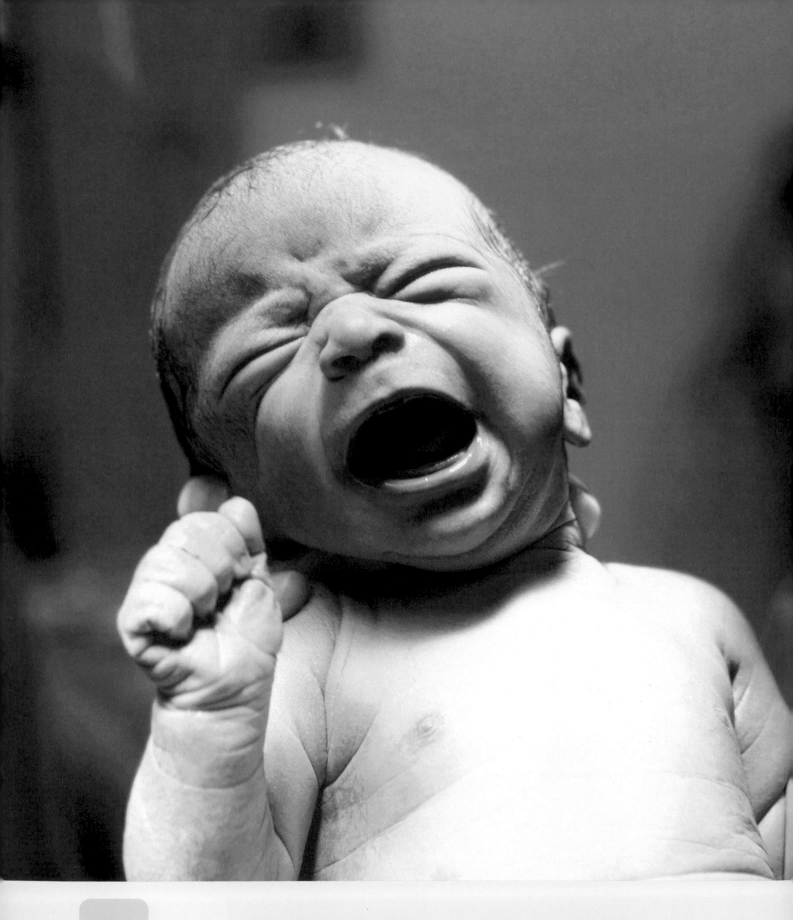

PART I My pregnancy

My labour
and birth
experience

It's time to head for the hospital and deliver my baby. My bag is packed and I'm experiencing contractions or it's the day agreed for a planned caesarean. Although most births are uncomplicated, situations could arise that will necessitate unforeseen procedures. Knowing that I'll be meeting my baby soon will fortify me when the going gets tough.

Going to hospital

Only 5 per cent of women actually deliver on their due date; the majority give birth a little late. In any event, in a first pregnancy, it is common for a baby to be overdue – on average, 8 days past the due date. A pregnancy is only considered officially overdue after 42 weeks. If I do go beyond my due date, I'll try and use the extra days (or weeks!) for crucial extra resting time before the birth. If I go to the hospital and am told I'm in false labour, I'll try not to be embarrassed about asking my midwife to check me. I understand it can be easy to misinterpret the signs of labour, especially with a first pregnancy, and it's best if I err on the side of caution.

IS IT TIME?

The early part of labour – with symptoms including cramps, backache, increased urination, bowel movements and vaginal discharge, pelvic pressure and leg and hip cramps – can take hours. If I'm able to manage the discomfort, I'm planning to stay at home in familiar surroundings where there's plenty to do to distract myself. If the contractions first appear at night, I'll try to continue resting as much as possible. If I can't rest, I'll try to read, watch a DVD, do some tidying up or make final touches to baby's room – nothing too taxing. It's also important that I keep hydrated and eat light snacks – labour is hard work and my body needs energy in order to cope.

WHEN TO GO

I'll probably want to head for the hospital once I'm not able to ignore the discomfort. I've been advised to think about leaving when contractions are so intense that I'm unable to hold a conversation during one and if the contractions have been regular for over an hour – 5 minutes apart, each lasting 45–60 seconds. Intense contractions that are less than 3 minutes apart are often a signal that birth is very near.

I may also need to go if my waters break in the midst of regular contractions. However, if this occurs before regular 5-minute contractions are happening, I'll need to call my midwife or hospital for advice.

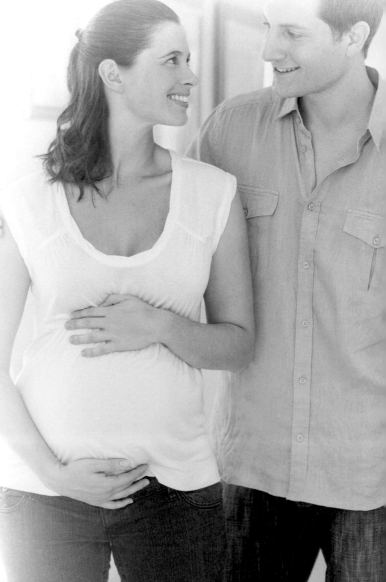

EXPERTS ADVISE

Going overdue

A small number of pregnancies outlive the placenta's ability to nourish a baby. Since this can cause problems, a number of checks after 40 weeks can help ensure that your baby is doing well. You should expect to count at least 10 movements over a period of 12 hours during the day for your kick-count sheet (see page 29). If you do not, or if your baby seems less active than normal, call your midwife or go to the hospital immediately. Medical procedures to check on your baby include fetal heart rate monitoring and a special ultrasound (a biophysical profile) that measures your baby's limb and lung movement, and the amount of amniotic fluid.

HOSPITAL ESSENTIALS BAG

- [ ] Mobile phone
- [ ] Money, particularly coins for parking or snacks
- [ ] Phone numbers of friends, relatives, maternity nurse, nappy service
- [ ] Camera or video equipment and extra batteries
- [ ] Magazines, books and other distractions
- [ ] Snacks for me and my birth partner
- [ ] Isotonic drinks
- [ ] Lotion or powder for massage
- [ ] Cold and warm packs for back relief
- [ ] Slippers and thick socks for cold feet
- [ ] Toothbrush, toothpaste and mouthwash
- [ ] Toiletries and make-up
- [ ] Hairbrush, clips and bands
- [ ] Pillow, if appropriate
- [ ] Dressing gown, nightgowns and underwear
- [ ] Maternity sanitary pads
- [ ] Breastfeeding supplies: nursing bra, breastfeeding pads, purified lanolin for nipples
- [ ] Changing bag and nappies for baby
- [ ] Baby clothes
- [ ] Birth announcement cards, address list and a pen
- [ ] Baby book for footprints and signatures

GOING HOME BAG*

- [ ] Loose outfit
- [ ] Comfortable shoes
- [ ] Bag for carrying home gifts and hospital supplies

Going home outfit for baby:
- [ ] Vest
- [ ] Nightgown or all-in-one suit
- [ ] Socks (optional)
- [ ] Hat
- [ ] Shawl

If weather is cold:
- [ ] Cardigan
- [ ] Warmer hat
- [ ] Warmer shawl
- [ ] Nappies and baby wipes
- [ ] Infant car seat

* Depending on how long you'll be in hospital – generally 24 hours with a first baby and 3–4 days after a caesarean, you may just need to take only one bag with you and ask your partner to bring the going-home bag later.

Giving birth

Childbirth is divided into three stages. During the first stage, known as labour, uterine contractions cause the cervix to fully dilate. In the second stage, my baby will pass out of the uterus, down the birth canal and be delivered into the outside world. The third stage is when the placenta is delivered. The entire process takes, on average, up to 18 hours for a first baby and up to 12 hours for later babies. Some labours, however, progress more slowly during the first stage and then speed up at the beginning of the second stage. Labour may slow down if a baby is in the wrong position, contractions are weak, the baby's head needs more moulding to fit through the birth canal or the pelvic tissues need more stretching.

LABOUR

Labour is often divided into three phases: early or latent labour, active or established labour and transition or hard labour. Many women experience these as distinct stages; other women may not notice such clear-cut differences.

Early or latent labour

Usually the longest though generally the easiest part, it is during this time that the cervix thins out and progressively dilates to 3–4 cm. At this stage, contractions are usually manageable, and I'm told I may be able to sleep through them.

Contractions last from 20–60 seconds and initially, they may be as far apart as 20 minutes, becoming increasingly stronger and closer over a 6–8 hour period. It is now that my mucus plug may become dislodged or my membranes rupture. I'm hoping to spend early labour at home.

If I first notice the contractions at night, I'll continue resting as much as possible. If I can't rest, I'll try to find

During second stage labour, it is common for a woman to focus in on herself and not feel sociable. It's important not to feel that labour is never going to end. If you are worried about how well things are progressing, ask your midwife or have your birth partner ask about anything that's bothering you.

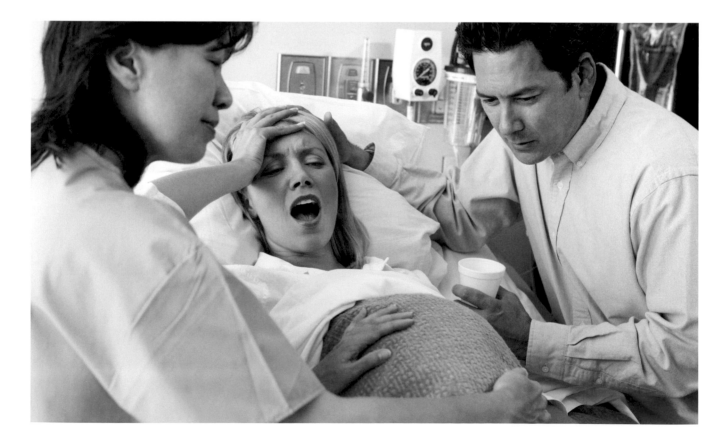

a distracting, but not taxing, activity. It's a good idea to eat light snacks during this early stage. While women used to be advised not to eat at all in labour in case they needed a general anaesthetic, in which case it was thought that they might breathe in food, studies have shown that this risk is very small. Eating light solids in labour can actually improve labour outcome – labour is hard work and the body needs energy in order to cope.

Symptoms in early labour may be similar to those of pre-labour – cramps, backache, increased urination, bowel movements and vaginal discharge, pelvic pressure, and leg and hip cramps. Many women also experience a burst of energy, but if I do so, I'll try to conserve this energy for later on.

Active labour

This is the time when the cervix begins to dilate rapidly – usually at a minimum of 1cm per hour. Contractions become stronger and noticeably more intense and last 45–60 seconds. From every 5–7 minutes, they occur every 2–3 minutes.

As my contractions become stronger and longer, I may need to work harder to relax through and between them. Moving around and changing position may relieve muscle tension. The sheer physical effort of labour can lead to increased breathing, heart rate, perspiration and even nausea, so it's important I drink plenty of isotonic drinks to guard against dehydration. I'll also try to concentrate on the fact that this phase is usually rapid and that every contraction is one nearer to my baby being born.

As contractions strengthen, there will be increased aches and tiredness. If they haven't done so already, my membranes may rupture.

Transitional labour

Lasting between around 1–2 hours, this is labour's most difficult and demanding period. It is now that the cervix fully dilates from 8–10 cm (see opposite). Contractions become very strong, lasting from 60–90 seconds and come every 2–3 minutes.

Because this phase is so intense, it can be accompanied by dramatic physical and emotional changes. As my baby is pushed into my pelvis, I may experience strong pressure in my lower back and/or perineum. I may have the urge to push or move my bowels and my legs may become shaky and weak. It's not unusual to suffer significant stress reactions such as perspiration, hyperventilation, shivering, nausea, vomiting and exhaustion. I may find every touch or

ACTIVE MANAGEMENT OF LABOUR
Many hospitals expect that labour proceeds within a certain time-frame and will help it along if it seems to be taking longer. Once labour is diagnosed – with regular painful contractions, dilation (opening up) of the cervix and, sometimes, ruptured membranes – women are expected to deliver within about 12 hours. Frequent vaginal examinations are used to check that the cervix is dilating at a rate of 0.5– 1 cm per hour. If labour appears to be slowing down, the membranes will be ruptured artificially (see page 73) and a dose of syntocinon will be given. Women giving birth in hospitals that actively manage labour generally have shorter first labours and a lower chance of having an unplanned caesarean.

labour aid unacceptable and may reject my birth partner's help. Like many women, I may lose all inhibitions, and may verbalise my distress uncharacteristically by shouting and swearing. It's important, therefore, that I keep the goal in sight. The

THE CERVIX DILATING IN CM

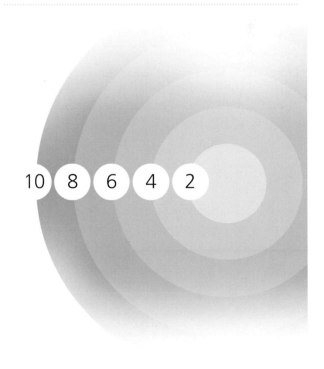

10 8 6 4 2

pushing stage will come soon and my discomfort will be much more controllable. Stronger contractions will bring this phase to an end faster.

I mustn't be afraid to express myself – making it clear what helps and what doesn't. I'll also try to relax; it's the key to conserving strength and the best way to help my contractions to accomplish their goal.

DELIVERY

The second stage of labour usually takes an hour, but can take as little as 10 minutes or as much as 3 hours. It may be significantly lengthened if anaesthesia has been given. Contractions still last for 60–90 seconds but may come every 2–4 minutes. My position can influence their pattern – staying upright can intensify contractions; reclining and knee-chest positions may slow them down.

I know that I'll have an overwhelming urge to push, but it's important to wait until my midwife says that it's okay. There will be huge pressure on my rectum, and a tingling, burning feeling as my baby's head appears at the entrance to my vagina. I'm hoping that the excitement of thinking I'll be meeting baby at last will help me cope with any exhaustion or pain.

Time to push

Once I'm given the go-ahead to push, bearing down when the urge occurs will bring satisfying relief from pent-up sensations. As long as the second stage isn't too fast and my perineum stretches gradually, this can be a time of pressure, not pain. Often the extreme pressure of the baby's tight fit and the subsequent compression of nerves produces a form of anaesthesia. For many women, this nerve compression can block the sensation of perineal tears, surgical incisions and repairs. My body will tell me when it's time to push (if not, the midwife will do so). As my baby presses on my pelvic floor muscles, receptors trigger an urge to bear down. This urge to push can feel like having a bowel movement, because the pressure of baby on my rectum stimulates the same receptors as does a bowel movement.

Usually the urge to push occurs 2–4 times within the course of a contraction, or as one long, continuous urge. If my pushing doesn't produce results – maybe because my cervix is not fully dilated – I'll try lying on my left-hand side or going on all fours for a few contractions. Sometimes 'blowing' breathing can help: this is breathing as if blowing out a candle, and it prevents me from holding my breath, which would

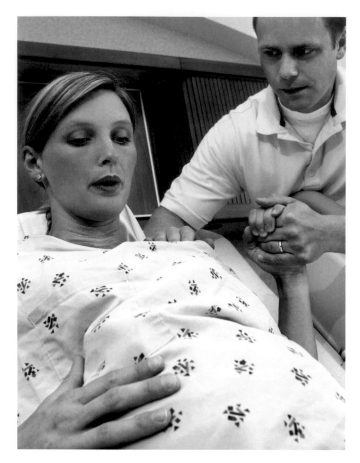

When pushing, I need to take a deep breath, relax my pelvic muscles, and bear down with my abdominal muscles. The length of the push isn't as important as timing with the contraction. Shorter pushes – for about 5–6 seconds – are usually fine and allow more oxygen to enter my bloodstream.

result in downward cervical pressure. Moving to a knee-chest position can reduce the pressure on the cervix and pelvic muscles, decreasing the urge to push.

My baby's coming...

With each contraction, my baby's head becomes increasingly visible at the vaginal opening. Once her head stops slipping back and remains at the opening, this is called crowning.

In just a brief period of time, my perineum will thin from approximately 5 cm thick to less than 1 cm. This is totally natural, and the distension reverses within minutes after the birth. I may feel this distension as strong pressure, possibly with some mild stinging as my baby's head – or buttocks if she's breech – stretches the vaginal opening. If it looks as if I'm going to tear badly, it is now that I may be offered an episiotomy.

As my baby starts to emerge, I will try to manage slow, controlled pushing; this will allow my perineum to stretch gradually, helping to prevent tears. My midwife will tell me whether or not to push.

Cutting the cord

Once my baby is born, her umbilical cord will usually be clamped in two places and cut in between. My partner has indicated that he would like to cut the cord and I've checked that the hospital permits this. It's not vital to clamp and cut the cord immediately, but it enables the hospital staff to check my baby, if necessary, and permits more freedom of movement with baby.

THE THIRD STAGE

This is when the placenta is delivered. Generally, this is relatively automatic and requires little effort. As soon as my baby leaves my uterus, the uterus continues to contract, causing a massive decrease in volume, which usually shears the less flexible placenta from its walls. Further contractions push the placenta out.

Most hospitals actively manage this third stage to prevent heavy bleeding after delivery. Immediately after my baby is born, syntocinon or syntometrine will be injected into my thigh, which encourages the uterus to

stay contracted. My midwife will help the placenta to be expelled by gently pulling on the cord. I may be asked to bear down or push or the midwife may massage my uterus.

Once the placenta is out, it will be examined to check that fragments haven't broken off inside the uterus. Very occasionally, some of the placenta remains behind, which can result in bleeding. To remove any placental fragments, an obstetrician needs to feel inside the uterus and manually remove them. This usually takes place in the operating theatre under epidural for pain relief.

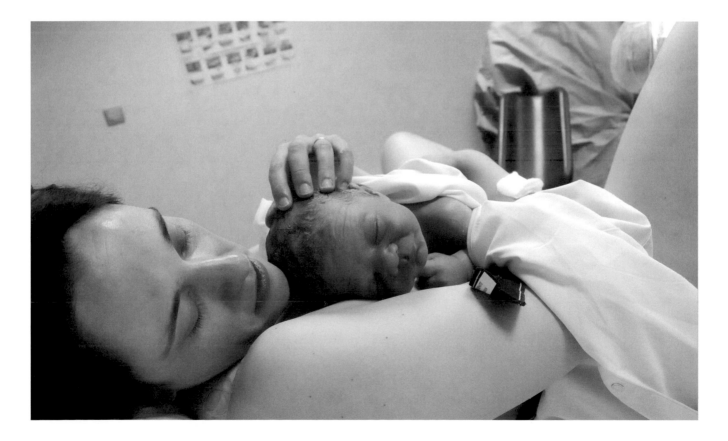

Special deliveries

Some births may become complicated by the number of babies or by a singleton's position and, occasionally, the problem only becomes apparent either during labour or while the baby is being born.

TWINS OR MORE

Although a caesarean section is generally recommended for twin pregnancies, many women give birth to twins vaginally without any problems. A twin birth tends to be faster than a singleton birth. However, extra care has to be taken with a multiple birth, so an anaesthetist will be standing by in case a caesarean is needed. The first baby may deliver vaginally without any problem, but the second baby may be positioned awkwardly and need assistance. The second baby should arrive 10–20 minutes after the first. If progress is slow, syntocinon may be given to speed up delivery, or the baby helped out with forceps. The placenta or placentas may follow soon after, or an injection may be given to speed up their delivery. Women who are expecting triplets or more will have them delivered by caesarean.

BREECH

Breech babies are positioned so that their legs or bottoms are closest to the cervix. In a frank breech, the thighs are up against the chest and the feet by the ears. In a flexed breech, the thighs are pressed against the chest, but the calves rest against the back of the thigh with feet just above the bottom. A footling breech is similar to the above, but the hips are not flexed so much and the feet lie below the bottom.

Breech positions can make delivery difficult because the baby's head is the largest part of her body and it could get trapped if the body slips through a partly dilated cervix. Vaginal delivery is possible with a frank breech but normally breech babies need to be delivered by caesarean section to avoid trauma to baby or mother.

POSTERIOR PRESENTING

A baby who descends into the birth canal with her head down and her back towards her mother's spine is referred to as occiput posterior (OP). Posterior babies may be harder to deliver as they present a slightly larger head diameter when passing through the narrow birth canal; such labours may take longer or involve greater back pain. Not infrequently, however, the baby turns in mid-labour or during the pushing stage. If a baby doesn't turn spontaneously, the midwife may be able to encourage her to rotate by strengthening the contractions with a syntocinon IV.

FORCEPS OR VACUUM EXTRACTION

If a baby has entered the birth canal at an awkward angle or is in distress, or if the mother has a medical

FRANK BREECH

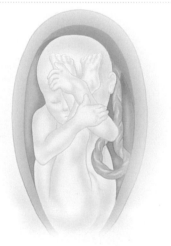

POSTERIOR

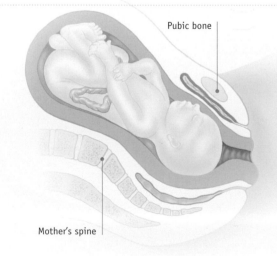

Pubic bone

Mother's spine

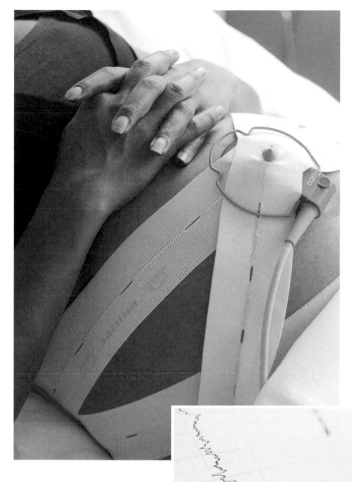

CORD PROBLEMS

Sometimes, the umbilical cord becomes knotted or tangled in the uterus, even wrapping around the baby's neck. This can reduce the baby's blood supply. Rarely, the baby's umbilical cord can fall into the birth canal ahead of the baby's head or other parts of the baby's body. It's vital that any cord problems are resolved quickly.

A knotted cord or prolapsed cord may be suspected where there is a decrease in fetal activity. If a cord is thought to knotted, which can cut off the blood and oxygen supply to the baby, immediate delivery, usually by caesarean, is necessary.

Prolapse is more likely to happen if a woman has too much amniotic fluid (polyhydramnios), if the baby is breech or in a transverse lie, during delivery of the second baby of twins or if the membranes rupture, either naturally or during a vaginal examination, before the baby descends into the pelvis.

If the cord is still pulsating and can be seen or felt in the vagina, the midwife or consultant will support the part of the baby delivering first to take pressure off the cord. To assist with this, you may be asked to get on your knees and bend forward. The midwife will keep a hand in the vagina until the baby is delivered the fastest way possible, usually by emergency caesarean section or possibly with forceps or vacuum extractor.

condition such as heart disease or is too exhausted or over-medicated to push effectively, forceps or a vacuum extractor will be used to help the baby out and shorten the second stage. If speed is an issue, forceps is the preferred option; 10–15 per cent of vaginal deliveries need forceps or vacuum extraction.

If forceps need to be used, a local anaesthetic or pain medication will be given to numb the area. If there is an epidural in place, this will be 'topped up' so that it is working well. Alternatively, a spinal anaesthetic may be suggested. The midwife will gently slide one side of the forceps at a time into the vagina until they fit around the sides of baby's head. The midwife will gently help to pull the baby out during contractions while you push.

If the midwife uses a ventouse, the rubber or plastic cup will be attached to the top of baby's head at the back. Suction is created by a pump, and the midwife will gently pull on the instrument to help the baby along while you push.

FETAL DISTRESS

This is a term used to describe any situation in which an unborn baby is thought to be in jeopardy – usually through decreased oxygen flow. The distress can be caused by a variety of problems including: maternal illness such as anaemia, hypertension, heart disease, low blood pressure, a placenta that is no longer functioning well or has separated prematurely from the uterus, umbilical cord compression or entanglement, fetal infection or malformation and prolonged or excessive contractions during labour.

Fetal distress is manifested by a change in or absence of fetal movements or changes to the fetal heartbeat.

Immediate delivery is usually recommended, generally by emergency caesarean particularly if vaginal delivery is not imminent. The mother may first be given medication to slow contractions, which will increase oxygen to the baby, and to dilate her blood vessels, which will improve blood flow to the baby.

Caesarean birth

Generally, caesarean deliveries are planned but occasionally, during a vaginal delivery, a baby may become distressed or at risk of trauma from the birth process or the mother develops a serious medical condition, such as pre-eclampsia (see page 65), which makes rapid delivery necessary.

WHAT HAPPENS IN A PLANNED CAESAREAN

If a caesarean has been decided on in advance, I'll be admitted to the hospital prior to the surgery and an intravenous drip (IV) will be started in my arm, to keep me hydrated and able to receive necessary medications.

Depending on my medical condition and the reason for the caesarean, I'll be given either a general or a regional anaesthetic. A general anaesthetic is an anaesthetic gas mixed with oxygen that is given through a tube in the throat via the mouth. I might require general anaesthesia if I have certain conditions such as back problems. It would put me to sleep so I wouldn't remember anything.

A regional anaesthetic will block pain from the waist down so that I'll be awake and alert and hopefully able to see and hold or touch my baby. I would like to meet the anaesthetist before the surgery so that I can discuss all the options. The night before my caesarean, I won't eat or drink anything, not even water, for at least 8 hours. This helps to avoid anaesthetic complications.

My partner is planning on being in the operating room. He'll be seated by my head and be under the direction of the staff.

Before surgery, a catheter (a small tube) will be placed in my bladder to drain urine during surgery, and for several hours following, and a small area of my lower abdomen, where the incision will be made, will be shaved. My abdomen will given an antiseptic wash and covered with sterile drapes.

The surgeon will make an incision in my lower abdomen and will push aside the muscles there. Then he or she will make another incision in the uterus. I'm told I may hear a whooshing noise as the amniotic fluid is sucked out.

My baby will then be lifted out through the incision; I'm told I might feel pressure and a tugging sensation. I may be able to see my baby right away or after she has been first assessed by another member of the team. My baby will be given a quick physical examination as well as some basic tests, including the Apgar score (see page 111). Once the surgeon has removed the placenta, my uterus and abdominal wall will be sewn closed with absorbable sutures and then my skin will closed with either sutures or staples. Once this is done, I should be reunited with my baby before we are taken to a recovery room where I will be able to hold, bond with and breastfeed my baby.

TYPES OF CAESAREAN

A planned caesarean will be done if:
- The baby is very large (estimated fetal weight greater than 4.5 kg where the mother has diabetes and greater than 5 kg otherwise).
- Placenta or vasa praevia (the placenta or umbilical cord lie over the cervix) is present.
- Fetal presentation is transverse lie or breech.
- Previous uterine surgery (removal of fibroids, caesarean section, etc.) was done.
- Twins, triplets or more babies are expected.
- Certain maternal medical conditions – heart and inflammatory bowel disease – are present.
- The woman wishes.

An unplanned but non-emergency caesarean will be done if:
- Labour stops progressing or progresses slowly because either the baby is thought to be too big to fit through the birth canal or the position of the baby's head makes vaginal delivery unlikely.
- Fetal monitoring suggests that the baby is not tolerating labour.
- Maternal medical conditions – pre-eclampsia, maternal heart disease, etc. – worsen.

An emergency caesarean will be carried out if:
- There is a prolonged drop in the baby's heart rate.
- Excessive bleeding occurs.
- The baby's umbilical cord or a fetal part prolapses or protrudes through the cervix.

WHAT HAPPENS DURING AN EMERGENCY CAESAREAN

The surgical process involved is much the same as a planned one, but the circumstances of an emergency procedure can make it more stressful. The staff may be rushed, my birth partner may not be allowed in the operating room and I may be given general anaesthesia. If the baby is in an awkward position or if it's necessary to work fast, a larger incision may be necessary.

PAIN RELIEF OPTIONS

Caesarean deliveries are safest for the mother and baby if they can be performed with regional anaesthesia – an epidural or spinal (see page 75). Less medicine is passed to the baby, the mother can be awake to greet her newborn, and family members can also be present.

Sometimes, however, general anaesthesia is necessary for the mother's or baby's safety. Because it takes effect more quickly, it may be necessary if, for instance, the baby is in distress.

Usually, general anaesthesia is a combination of IV medication and anaesthetic gas administration. During the surgical procedure, general anaesthesia usually requires the use of a respirator to protect the mother from developing serious pneumonia and from aspiration (inhaling food particles and stomach acid into her lungs).

ALTERNATIVE INCISIONS

During a Caesarean birth, the surgeon will make two separate incisions: one through the skin and abdominal wall and the other, beneath this, through the uterine wall. Most often, a surgeon will make a 'bikini' incision, so-called because it is made across the lower abdomen, just above the pubis. In rare circumstances – if the surgeon needs a large area in which to work or when the baby must be removed quickly – a vertical skin incision from the pubic area to the tummy button will be done.

The most common uterine incision is the low transverse (side-to-side) incision, which is made across the lower part of the uterus As this is the segment of the uterus that stretches rather than contracts, incisions made here have less risk of reopening or rupturing in future labours. Many women who have this incision have a vaginal birth the next time (VBAC). A disadvantage of this incision is that it takes longer to perform, so it may not be used in the case of emergency caesareans, where time is critical.

A vertical uterine incision allows more room to avoid birth trauma to mother and baby if the baby's in an awkward position, if it's a multiple pregnancy, or if the lower uterine segment isn't stretched enough to allow delivery through the transverse incision. If I require a vertical incision and it extends into the upper portion of my uterus, I will need to have a caesarean for future deliveries as there's a higher risk – greater than 2 per cent – of scar separation in future labours.

Checks on my baby

My baby will receive a considerable amount of medical care immediately after her birth and during her first few days to make sure that all is well. As I'm having my baby in hospital, she will probably be first checked by a paediatrician. If I were to have her at home, my GP would make this first assessment.

A FULL PHYSICAL EXAMINATION

At 1- and 5-minute intervals after her birth, hospital staff will perform the Apgar test (see page 111). This test was developed by Dr Virginia Apgar as a quick assessment of a newborn's health. The word 'Apgar' stands also for the signs that the doctors and nurses are looking at – appearance, pulse, grimace, activity and respiration. For each of these, my baby will be given a score of 0, 1 or 2. Babies rarely receive a total score of 10, but a score above 6 is usually fine. If my baby receives a low score, I shouldn't worry as it is not an indicator of her future health, it simply means she needs some medical help and close monitoring initially.

At some stage within her first few days, my baby's features, spine, anus, fingers and toes will be checked; she'll be weighed, and her head size and length may be measured. Her hips will be checked for proper movement and placement.

VITAMIN K INJECTION

At many hospitals, newborns receive an injection or drops of Vitamin K shortly after birth. This is because newborns often have low levels of this vitamin, which is necessary for normal blood clotting. An injecion at birth provides the most protection. However, breastfed babies may receive two oral doses in the first week of life and another oral dose at one month of age, while bottlefed babies may receive two doses of vitamin K in the first week of life. Formula milk contains higher doses of vitamin K than does breast milk.

HEEL PRICK TEST

At 5–8 days of age, my baby may have a blood sample taken from her heel. This blood can be used to check her thyroid function, as well as test for a rare metabolic

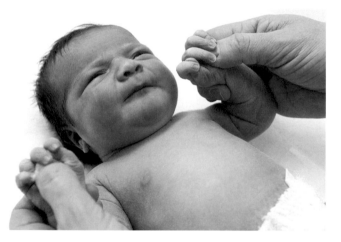

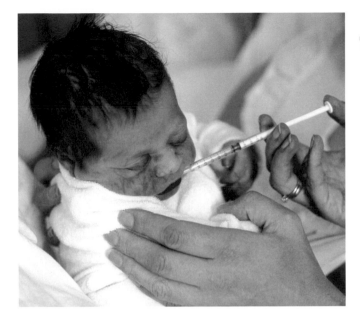

MONITOR BABY'S BODILY FUNCTIONS

As I'm with my baby all the time – and my doctor is not – I'm best placed to ensure that she thrives. I need to be aware of:

✓ **How much she takes** when feeding (grams of formula or one or both breasts).

✓ **How often she feeds.**

✓ **Frequency and appearance of her urine.**

✓ **Frequency and appearance of her stools.**

disorder called phenylketonuria. If there is a family history of any conditions, a test may be done for them. The tests offered vary among GPs and hospitals, so it's important I find out which ones my baby will be given.

HEPATITIS B VACCINE

Before being discharged from hospital, my baby would receive the Hepatitis B close family member was suffering from the disease. If given, the course is completed in three doses by the time baby is a year old. Some babies also have an immunoglobulin injection aftr birth to help prevent them being infected. This gives quicker protection against the disease.

WEIGHT

My baby will probably be weighed regularly in her first few days. It is normal if her weight drops at first; babies commonly lose up to 10 per cent of their birth weight in the first few days. She should begin to gain weight again by the time she's one week old.

HEARING

My baby will be screened for hearing problems a few days after birth. This involves placing earphones over her ears and analysing by computer whether the emitted sounds are picked up by the brain. Of course, I need to be aware of whether she responds to noises.

APGAR TEST

Sign	Points		
	0	1	2
Appearance	Pale or blue all over	Body pink, extremities blue	Pink all over
Pulse	Not detectable	Below 100	Over 100
Grimace (reflexes)	No response to stimulation	Grimace	Lusty cry, cough or sneeze
Activity (muscle tone)	Flaccid (no or weak activity)	Some movement of extremities	A lot of activity
Respiration	None	Slow, irregular	Good, crying

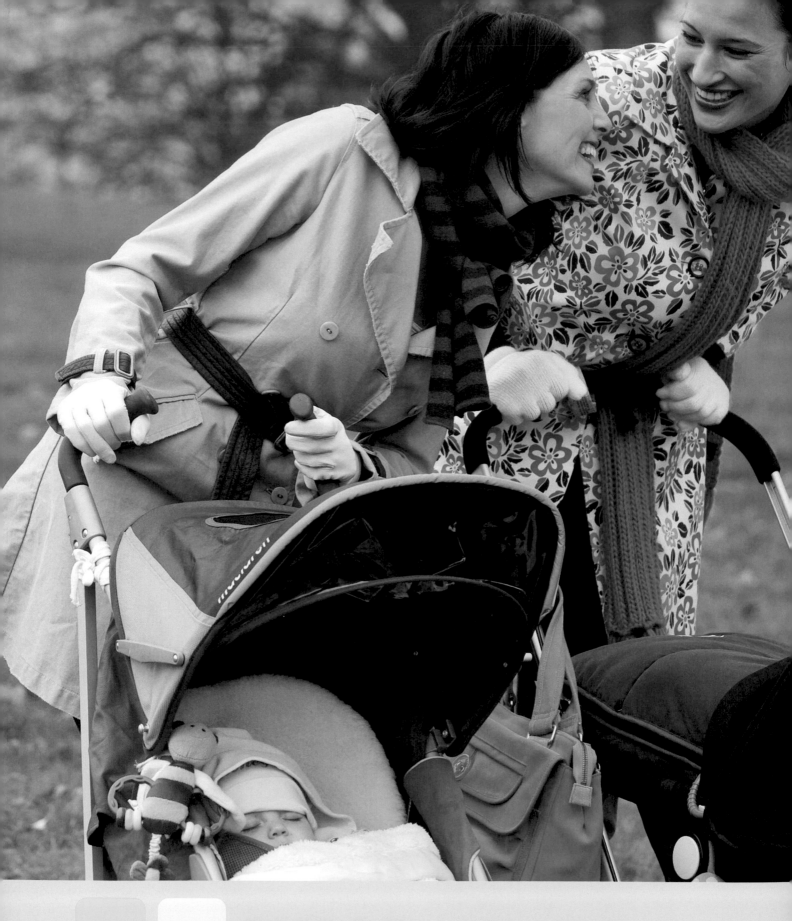

PART I My pregnancy

Getting back in shape

Recovering my pre-pregnancy figure should not be done in a rush. It took

nine months to acquire a new shape so I won't expect

it to take much less to revert to the way I was. Eating a good diet,

engaging in a safe, habitual fitness programme and monitoring my

emotions are all part of the process. I should also be on the look out for

problems that can arise as a result of the birth or breastfeeding.

My body after the birth

The sheer effort of giving birth has made every muscle in my body ache and my emotional responses are unpredictable. What disappoints me the most, however, is that although I've lost quite a lot of my belly, it is still distended and sagging. At my postnatal appointment, about 6 weeks after the birth, I'll be able to discuss my recovery with my caregiver, as well as contraception.

PHYSICAL CHANGES

Immediately after baby was born, I felt strong pains, similar to period pains, in my abdomen. Known as afterpains or postnatal uterine cramping, these are triggered by the release of oxytocin, the hormone that initiates birth contractions and contracts and shrinks the uterus to decrease bleeding afterwards. My uterus will shrink in size over the next six weeks or so, and will do so more rapidly as I'm breastfeeding, which involves the release of greater amounts of oxytocin.

Happily, the discomfort from postnatal contractions decreases each day. If necessary, I can take safe, pain-killing medications such as ibuprofen or paracetamol, even though I'm breastfeeding. Warm baths can be soothing, too.

Lochia

After the birth, blood, mucus and tissue exit from the uterus. Known as lochia, this discharge initially is heavy, dark red and thick and may contain large blood clots. It can be particularly heavy when getting out of bed and breastfeeding.

Lochia can last up to six weeks, but gradually the flow becomes less heavy and lighter in colour. Special maternity pads (extra-large sanitary towels), not tampons, should be used to absorb the discharge, and may need changing frequently. If the bleeding suddenly becomes heavier, turns bright red, contains unusually large clots or smells unpleasant, I must notify my GP immediately as this could be a sign of infection.

Soreness and swelling

My genital area is swollen, sore and stretched. With a long, difficult labour, tearing, stitches or an episiotomy, there will be a lot of pain and discomfort and the perineum (the area between the vagina and anus) may feel quite numb. It's important that I use as many of the self-help remedies (see opposite page) as possible.

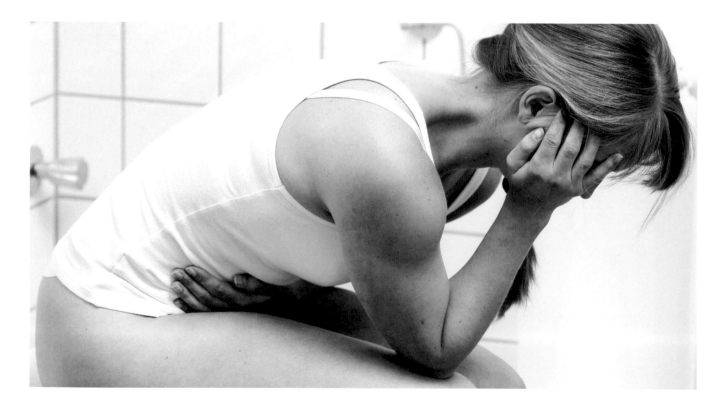

Elimination difficulties

Although it's essential that the bladder is emptied within 6–8 hours of delivery to avoid urinary tract infections and to prevent the bladder from becoming distended, which could cause a loss of muscle tone, I may, like some women, not feel the urge to go at all, or that I want to go but can't. Drinking plenty of fluids and getting up and walking about as soon after delivery as allowable will help to get my bladder working. After

If I do nothing else I will ...

EASE PERINEAL PAIN

Taking the following self-help measures will mean I recover more quickly. I should:

✓ **Start pelvic floor exercises** (see page 56), from early on. Not only will they reduce pain but they can help me to regain muscle tone and promote healing by increasing circulation in the area.

✓ **Drink plenty of fluids** to dilute my urine so that it doesn't burn as much, and empty my bladder regularly.

✓ **Put an ice pack** or pack of frozen peas, wrapped in a soft cloth, on my perineum for 5 minutes, every couple of hours during the first 24 hours to decrease swelling and relieve the discomfort.

✓ **Squat over the toilet** rather than sit down. I need to angle my bottom so urine misses the tender spot.

✓ **Keep a jug of cool water** in the bathroom so I can pour water between my legs as I urinate and when I have finished so that there is no urine left on my skin.

✓ **Sit in a sitz bath** (a bowl filled with warm water) or apply warm compresses for about 20 minutes 3 times a day.

✓ **Soak a maternity pad in witch hazel;** it will cool the area and prevent blood sticking to pubic hair.

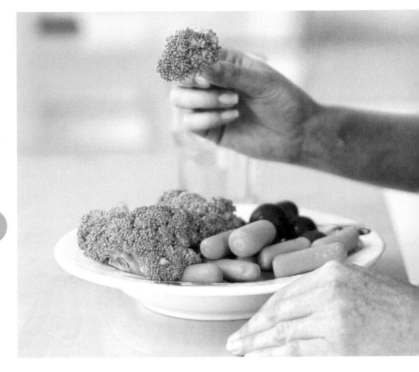

24 hours, it is expected that I will urinate frequently and copiously as the body fluids of pregnancy are expelled from my body.

As I've had stitches, I am somewhat concerned about possible discomfort and that a bowel movement could split them open. I've been told that although my first few bowel movements are likely to cause discomfort, my stitches won't be affected, and I should be back to normal within a few days. Eating fibre – whole grains and fresh fruit and vegetables – and

▼ EXPERTS ADVISE

Avoiding postnatal infection

It's vital to keep your genital area scrupulously clean. When you wash your perineal area or after you've been to the toilet, always wipe from the front towards the back to prevent the transfer of bacteria from your rectum to your urethra. Change your maternity pad every 4–6 hours, at least, to keep the area fresh and to check the amount of bleeding. Always wash your hands before and after you clean your perineal area and after changing a maternity pad.

drinking fluids will help to get my bowels moving again. Gentle exercise and pelvic-floor exercises will help to ease any discomfort. However, my GP may suggest stool softeners or a laxative if I become constipated.

Breast discomfort

The hormonal changes that prime my breasts for breastfeeding take place about 2–4 days after birth (this is also true if a woman decides not to breastfeed). Known as engorgement, my breasts become larger and firmer and may be painful as they prepare to provide milk. To feel more comfortable, it's essential that I wear a well-fitting, supportive bra, possibly 24 hours a day during the engorgement period. Before breastfeeding, I may find it helps to stand under a very warm shower or put warm compresses on my breasts. The moist heat will dilate the milk ducts and when baby sucks, the milk will flow more freely, and my breasts will be relieved of pressure. Engorgement usually lasts around 2–5 days.

If you're not going to breastfeed, try putting a cool compress on your breasts and take an analgaesic such as paracetamol or ibuprofen. Don't stimulate your breasts or try to express milk to relieve pressure, as this will only cause your body to produce more milk. Lack of stimulation by a sucking baby will gradually slow and then stop milk production.

Care of the breasts normally just involves washing with mild soap and rinsing well. If, however, my breasts become inflamed, extremely uncomfortable or my nipples crack (see page 122), I should see my doctor.

Skin and hair changes

Pregnancy-related skin pigmentation such as the linea nigra and chloasma (see page 33) should fade gradually, but some changes may never completely disappear. To prevent dark areas from getting darker, I need to avoid excessive sun exposure and use a good sunscreen at all times. Stretch marks will fade in time though never completely disappear.

For as much as 6 weeks post birth, sweating can seem excessive as my body gets rid of the extra fluids accumulated during pregnancy. Breastfeeding speeds up my metabolic rate and results in more sweating. It can help to drink plenty of fluids and wear natural fibres, such as cotton and wool, which allow my skin to breathe. If I have a temperature over 37°C, I need to talk to my GP, as I may have an infection.

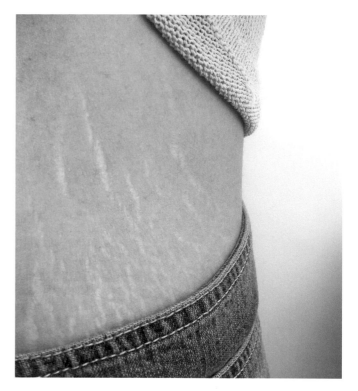

Pregnancy hormones, which stop the normal cycle of hair growth, plummet after birth and the result is hair loss, often on a massive scale. Within 6 months, however, hair should resume its normal pattern. To prevent exacerbating hair loss, I should wash hair only when necessary, using a mild shampoo and a nourishing conditioner, and avoid heated rollers, hair dryers or straighteners, which may cause damage. Until hair is back to normal, I should also avoid chemical-based hair treatments, such as perms or hair-relaxers.

Body shape and weight loss

On average, giving birth results in a 5 kg weight loss. My breasts seem huge because they are preparing to feed baby and my stomach sticks out due to fluid retention and a distended uterus. My skin is sagging because my skin is overstretched and I've lost muscle tone. Over time, my body will get closer to its pre-pregnancy shape if I eat a healthy, nutritious diet and exercise regularly.

Back pain

During pregnancy my back had to support the weight of a growing baby, as well as compensate for weaker abdominal muscles. The hormone, relaxin, loosened my ligaments and joints and shifted my centre of gravity leaving me with a tendency to lean back and push my tummy forwards. Giving birth can exacerbate back problems, especially if labour is long and exhausting. As I had an epidural, it is not unusual to feel pain in my lower back, where the anaesthetic was injected. Bending to pick baby up or put her down, or sitting for long hours breastfeeding can make matters worse. If my pain becomes severe, it should be investigated to rule out any more serious underlying condition such as a bruised, or even broken, coccyx.

Back pain can last for many months but it depends on individual circumstances. Gentle exercise that builds up the abdominal and back muscles can alleviate a lot of the discomfort, as can assuming proper posture: when standing, imagine that a wire is pulling your head towards the ceiling. Relax your shoulders so that your chest isn't too tight. Gently pull your tummy in and lengthen your spine. If you're sitting down for long periods, make sure that your lower back is always supported. Slowly roll your neck to the front and side to relieve tension in your shoulders.

Getting periods back

Periods will probably start within 4–6 weeks, though as I'm breastfeeding, periods may be irregular or not appear until I have stopped. The amount of menstrual flow for the first few cycles can range from light to quite heavy, but should soon settle down into a more consistent pattern after that. Ovulation begins again after the first period following childbirth, so having unprotected sex could result in another pregnancy. To prevent this, some form of contraception is needed as soon as I start having sex again. Breastfeeding mothers like me may be able to take a progesterone-only pill. Those who are not breastfeeding can start taking birth control pills about 2–3 weeks after the birth. Barrier contraception should not be used if stitches are present or until the cervix is completely healed.

EMOTIONAL CHANGES

More than half of all new mothers suffer from the baby blues – mood changes; vague sadness, feeling weepy, irritable, anxious and confused – which may occur a day or two after birth and last for about 10–14 days. Although the exact cause of baby blues is not known, rapid hormone shifts and sleep deprivation are common suspects, which is why I'm planning to nap whenever I can and try some relaxation techniques. Lack of sleep can be a big contributing factor; physical fatigue can reduce the amount of stress I can handle. I need to make sure I take advantage of the times that baby sleeps by sleeping then myself, and taking any help that is offered.

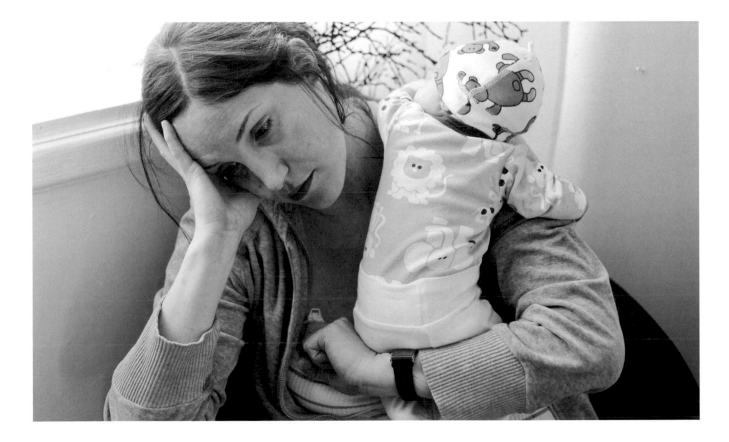

Eating and exercising after the birth

Although I would like to regain my pre-pregnancy figure as soon as possible, I realise that it's better to take things easy at first and not rush into dieting or exercising too strenuously. The key to regaining one's pre-pregnancy figure is to combine healthy eating with a strengthening and toning exercise regime.

A BALANCED DIET

Eating right means eating a diet similar to the one I ate during pregnancy (see page 48), which was rich in fresh foods and low in fats, oils and sugars. Unrefined carbohydrates, such as brown rice and wholegrain bread, cereals and pasta are high in essential nutrients and should provide the energy I need to look after baby. I do realise, however, that caring for baby may make it hard for me to eat the 3 meals necessary (see opposite), so keeping some healthy snacks to hand will be invaluable. The best are:
• Cashew nuts and almonds
• Pumpkin and sunflower seeds
• Fresh and dried fruit
• Wholewheat toast or fortified breakfast cereals
I also need to drink plenty of liquids – 6–10 250 ml-glasses a day. I need to make sure I keep a glass of water beside me when I'm breastfeeding and to take frequent sips. Alcohol will pass into my breast milk, altering its smell and possibly upsetting baby, so I'm limiting myself to a single small glass of wine, only drunk after feeding times. Caffeine drinks (see page 50), too, will affect baby as she is not able to eliminate caffeine easily, so it may accumulate in her system and she may become irritable and unable to sleep well. If I must have coffee or tea, I'll limit myself to one cup per day drinking it at least 2 hours before breastfeeding.

CUTTING BACK ON CALORIES

All new mums should try losing any excess weight slowly and sensibly; it's important not to be too strict with oneself too soon! Contrary to much received advice, breastfeeding does not require a greater intake of calories but you may want, like me, to wait until feeding is well established before attempting moderate weight loss. The important thing is to maintain energy levels and keep hydrated. Over a period of weeks, I plan to start cutting back gradually to my pre-pregnancy requirement of at least 1,800 calories a day.

MY DAILY DIET

The following meal suggestions include all the essential vitamins and minerals required for breastfeeding.

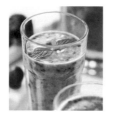

BREAKFAST

I start my day with a fortified breakfast cereal enriched with folic acid and iron, to which I add fresh or dried fruit and low-fat milk or yogurt. Or I may eat a slice of whole grain toast with jam or butter. Eggs – boiled, poached or scrambled – on wholewheat toast make a filling breakfast. I round my meal off with fruit juice or a smoothie.

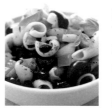

LUNCH

I often eat an open or closed sandwich using different types of bread, such as ciabatta or focaccia, topped with sliced cheese, ham or chicken. Or I make a pasta or couscous salad with chopped vegetables such as red peppers and broccoli florets sprinkled with some chopped nuts. A piece of fresh fruit is a good ending.

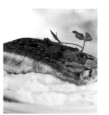

DINNER

I make a variety of dishes containing meat, fish or other protein (lentils and beans), combined with a carbohydrate and vegetables. Some of my favourites include pan-fried chicken or beef fillet with boiled potatoes and cooked spinach, grilled tuna with a baked potato and green salad or steamed tofu in spaghetti with sugar-snap peas and yellow peppers. Dessert choices include fruit with yogurt, meringue nests filled with apricots garnished with cream or rice pudding.

GETTING FIT AGAIN

This should be a gradual process. I can start simple exercises almost immediately (see below) as well as taking baby out for walks, but I can only start on an aerobic programme once lochia and any bleeding subsides and I get the go-ahead from my GP, after my first postnatal check-up. He or she should check that I don't have a condition known as diastasis recti, which is when the abdominal muscles separate during pregnancy. I will start with exercises that target the areas that have become particularly weakened over the past 9 months and need the most work to get back to the way they were. The 'hug technique' and modified sit-ups are good abdominal strengtheners.

I also need to practise contracting and releasing my pelvic floor muscles (see page 56) during everyday activities, such as doing washing.

- **Hug technique:** I need to lie on my back with my knees bent and arms crossed at the waist as I raise my head and shoulders off the floor.
- **Modified sit-ups:** Lying on my back on a firm surface (not my bed) while keeping my shoulders on the floor, I need to slowly raise just my head to look at the ceiling and then to lower it.
- **With baby:** With my knees bent and baby placed carefully on my abdomen, I should lie on the floor and grab my thighs on either side while slowly raising my head and shoulders. I need to keep my neck straight and my chin away from my chest.

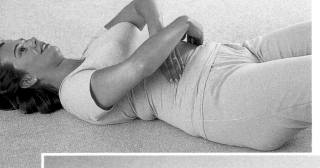

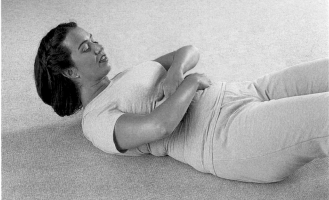

GRADUALLY REGAIN MY FITNESS

To ensure my safety I need to do the following :

✓ **Wear a good support bra.** Breastfeeding mums like myself should not wear a sports bra as this binds the breasts and may hinder lactation.

✓ **Exercise after I feed baby** or express milk so that my breasts aren't full. I should try not to do anything too strenuous because lactic acid – a by-product of exercise – can build up in my milk.

✓ **Spend 5–10 minutes warming-up and cooling-down** when performing aerobics or muscle-conditioning activities. Stretching and relaxation exercises should be part of the cool-down.

✓ **Start by exercising 3 times a week,** slowly increasing to a maximum of 5 times a week.

✓ **Begin with 15 minutes of activity** at my target heart rate then increase by 5 minutes every week. 40–60 minutes is my maximum target time for working out.

✓ **Exercise every other day** to allow my body to recover from the work-out, especially as I'm breastfeeding.

✓ **Sip water before, during and after activity.** If I don't replenish my fluids, I may suffer from dehydration and be unable to produce as much breast milk.

✓ **Get a qualified instructor** to design a safe weightlifting programme. I must use low weights (manageable for 2 sets of 12–15 reps).

✗ **Not exercise if I feel any pain, dizziness or faintness.** If it continues, I'll ring my GP immediately.

Recovering from a caesarean

Initially, dealing with the pain, getting mobile and taking care of my incision will be my main concerns. I've been told that it can take a year, or even longer, before I am back to my old levels of energy and fitness. In addition to pain from the abdominal incision and any side effects from anaesthesia, I will experience many of the same postpartum discomforts as a mother who has had a vaginal birth, such as uterine contractions and lochia (see page 114). The catheter collecting urine will be removed once I can walk to the bathroom, but the IV line will be kept in place until my intestines begin to work again – when I start to experience rumbling in my stomach and gas pains.

As I'm planning to breastfeed, I should start as soon as I feel able – in the recovery room, or perhaps an hour or two after surgery. Any pain relief medication that I received will have been checked to make sure it's suitable for use with breastfeeding. I may need to experiment with positions and supports in getting comfortable.

If I do nothing else I will ... ✓

ACT TO RELIEVE THE PAIN
Being pain-free means I will be able to move around more freely and hold and position my baby better. I need to do the following:

✓ **Ask for pain medication** before the pain becomes unbearable.

✓ **Wear a maternity belt** (over my bandages, if necessary) for support, which can relieve pain.

✓ **Get up and take short walks** as often as possible as soon as I can.

✓ **Change my position frequently** when resting.

✓ **Rock gently backwards and forwards** while sitting in a chair.

✓ **Wait before reintroducing solids** into my diet and avoid carbonated drinks.

EXPERTS ADVISE

Monitoring the incision
Although after the first 2–6 weeks there should only be minimal discomfort, it is a good idea not to lift anything heavy during this period or to drive during the first 4 weeks because of the risk of haemorrhage if in an accident. You may not feel like having sex for 6 weeks or so and positions that keep your partner's weight off, such as a side-by-side position, will be best. If the bleeding from the incision stops and then starts again, or if it soaks more than one dressing every hour or turns bright red, you should talk to your GP. However, if the area becomes painful, red or swollen, or there is an unusual discharge, you must seek immediate medical attention.

EXERCISES
During the course of my recovery and the next 6 months, it's important to exercise gradually – starting from a supine position, then sitting and standing. In time, I can exercise with my baby.

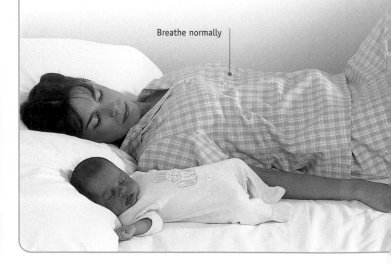

Assume the position then push the heel of the extended leg into the bed 4 times before changing to the other foot

Bend knee

Breathe normally

GETTING MOBILE AND COMFORTABLE

The surgery and anaesthesia can cause fluids to accumulate, which may lead to pneumonia, so movement is very important. Mobility improves lung function; when I breathe deeply, it boosts blood circulation, and this lowers the risk of blood clots, improves digestion and helps the bowels start working again. I need to be sitting up and getting out of bed as much as I can, as soon as I can. I'll probably have to experiment with different positions and use cushions and pillows in order to move a little more each day.

I should start to sit up and walk short distances within 6–8 hours. Once up, I should place my hands, a pillow, or a rolled-up towel against my abdomen for support. The more mobile I am, the easier moving will become and the more quickly I will recover.

TAKING CARE OF MY INCISION

The nursing staff will show me how to clean my incision and check for any redness or swelling. Initially, there will be some pink, watery drainage. If this discharge continues for more than 6 weeks, it may be a sign of an infection that needs medical care.

I've been told there may be a hard ridge along the line of the incision, which should gradually soften as time goes by. The area may be numb with some tightening around the scar, which, when I move around or pick things up, may be accompanied by a slight pulling sensation, around the two end points of the scar. If I experience any discomfort, a heated pad or a warm, moist towel placed against the area should help. As it heals, the incision may itch and become tender around the time of my period.

Showering or bathing is fine as long as I use mild, unscented soap when washing the incision site and dry the area thoroughly. I should wear loose clothing over the top during the day and leave the area open at night.

If I find it hard to get into a comfortable sleeping position, I can use pillows or cushions for support; I may also need them to protect the scar area when breastfeeding.

The scar will gradually fade as time goes by, but I'm told I need to keep it out of the sun for at least 6 months after the birth and that it can take up to a year to heal completely.

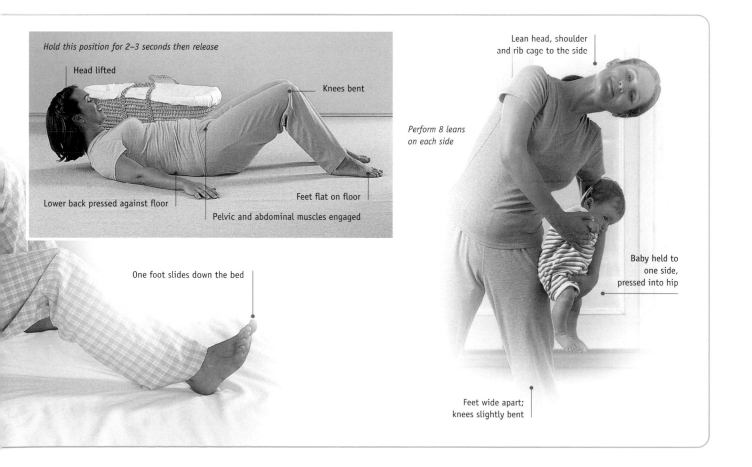

Hold this position for 2–3 seconds then release

Head lifted

Knees bent

Lower back pressed against floor

Feet flat on floor

Pelvic and abdominal muscles engaged

One foot slides down the bed

Lean head, shoulder and rib cage to the side

Perform 8 leans on each side

Baby held to one side, pressed into hip

Feet wide apart; knees slightly bent

Possible postnatal problems

Major problems after childbirth are normally rare. However, it's estimated that up to 8 per cent of all births will be followed by an infection and some breastfeeding mothers experience problems with their breasts.

POSTNATAL INFECTIONS

Most commonly, the lining of the uterus becomes infected, but infections can also occur in the cervix, vagina, vulva and perineum. Sometimes, bacteria invade the site of an episiotomy. Premature rupture of the membranes, prolonged labour, frequent internal examinations, internal fetal monitoring, an infection already present during pregnancy, diabetes and being overweight increase the likelihood of an infection occurring.

Symptoms
• Fever.
• Pain in the abdomen or perineum.
• Offensive vaginal discharge and odour.
• Inflammation, redness or swelling.

Treatment

My doctor will prescribe me a 2–7-day course of oral or intravenous antibiotics. I may be sent to hospital if further treatment is required. Once treated, any infections should clear up within 7–10 days. I can continue to breastfeed during most treatments.

If my stitches get infected, this can usually be resolved with careful hygiene and frequent baths. Occasionally, my stitches may come apart prematurely. I may require further stitches, but simple hygiene procedures are often sufficient for healing to occur.

BLOCKED MILK DUCTS AND MASTITIS

Producing excess milk or a baby not latching on properly, not emptying the breast or sleeping through and missing out on being fed, can lead to the milk ducts becoming blocked.

If bacteria find their way into a blocked milk duct – often through a cracked nipple (see opposite, top) – the milk within may become infected, resulting in inflammation of the duct or the condition mastitis.

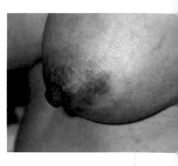

Symptoms
• Tenderness.
• Redness, with or without heat.
• Lumpiness, which reduces with massage or after feeding. or stays painful and inflamed.
• Fever, flu-like muscle aches.
• Nausea.

Treatment

If my duct is simply blocked, applying heat, such as a face cloth dipped in warm water and squeezed dry, to the affected area, along with massage before each of my breastfeeding sessions can help to relieve the problem. It also can help to feed frequently and use a breast pump at the end of a session if my breasts have not been completely emptied. Trying different positions at each feed and making sure my baby is latched on correctly (see page 149) are also important.

If the blocked ducts become infected, my doctor may prescribe antibiotics and analgaesics in addition to the measures given opposite. The medicines prescribed will be safe for me to use while breastfeeding, because an important part of the treatment is continued breastfeeding. If there is no improvement after 24 hours of taking antibiotics, I will ask my GP for advice, as there is a risk of an abscess.

CRACKED NIPPLES

While sensitive and sore nipples are very common during the first few days of breastfeeding, vigorous sucking, incorrect positioning and milk left on the nipple can cause the nipple to crack. Cracked nipples are very painful and may become infected.

Cracked nipples often get infected with the yeast candida albicans, resulting in thrush. Women who are prone to vaginal thrush yet have no problems with breastfeeding also can develop thrush on their breasts.

Symptoms
- Small cracks on the nipple, which may bleed.
- Sharp, piercing pain during feeding.
- Itchy, irritable, pink or red nipples.
- Tiny white spots on nipples.

Treatment
I should continue breastfeeding, making sure that my baby is latched on correctly (see page 149). I can use a breast pump to empty my breasts if they still feel full when baby has finished feeding. I must expose my nipples to the air for a short while after each breastfeeding session, and always wash my nipples with plain warm water – never soaps or disinfectants – and gently pat dry. Breast shields may also help.

If thrush is present, it can be passed from me to baby, so both of us may need to be treated, usually with an antifungal medication. Although it is likely to be painful, I should continue breastfeeding during any treatment.

URINARY INCONTINENCE
Physical changes that occur in the body during pregnancy – rather than weak pelvic floor muscles, as was previously thought – are now believed to cause urinary incontinence. A common problem after a vaginal delivery, urinary incontinence may last for a few weeks or months.

Stress incontinence (a type of urinary incontinence caused by laughing, coughing and straining), is very common, too, and can last up to a year after delivery. It usually improves over time.

Symptoms
- Leaking small amounts of urine.
- Feeling of fullness and an urgency to pass urine.
- Inability to control urine flow.

Treatment
Whatever the cause, I should do regular pelvic floor exercises (see page 56), performed as 8 repetitions at least 3 times per day. This is the best method of combating urinary incontinence. It may take a few weeks before any improvement my bladder control is noticed, but I will persevere for at least 3 months. I should wear sanitary pads or protective underwear to forestall leaks. In severe cases, I may require surgical procedures, several of which are available.

FAECAL INCONTINENCE
A forceps delivery, severe tearing or an episiotomy can damage nerves and muscles of the anal sphincter, the muscles responsible for opening and closing the bowel. This can lead to loss of control over bowel movements. The duration of faecal incontinence depends on how much damage has been done. Women who are affected can take from 6 weeks to 4 months and more to regain control of their bowels after childbirth.

Symptoms
- Involuntary bowel movements.
- Passing excessive wind.

Treatment
Anal plugs and incontinence pads are available for me to use in the short term. I can follow a high-fibre diet, too, which may also help, and I should avoid spicy and fatty foods and dairy products. Pelvic floor exercises (see page 56) can strengthen the muscles that control the opening to my bowel and increase blood flow to the perineum, which may help my recovery. If the incontinence doesn't improve with these exercises, it's important that I discuss the problem at my postnatal check. I have no need to feel embarrassed about it; it is far better to get the problem treated as soon as possible. My doctor may recommend bowel retraining and biofeedback techniques, as well as surgery.

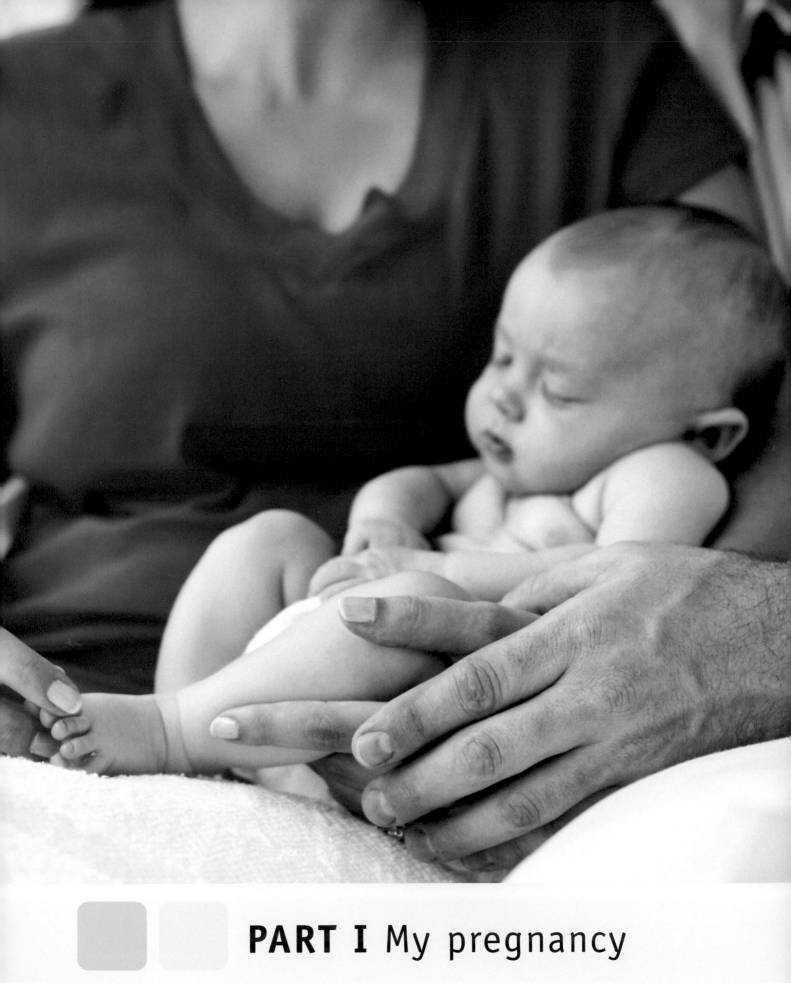

PART I My pregnancy

Becoming a parent

Throughout my pregnancy, I took care to protect baby as well as I could and made many decisions about her care and wellbeing. During these 9 months, when baby was carried safely inside me, my partner and I talked much about what she would be like and how family life might change once she arrived. Now, all our assumptions will be tested and baby's actual presence will have an effect we may not have anticipated. Whether we wll be successful as parents and whether our family life will be as harmonious as desired, depends a lot on whether we can find a consistent approach from early on.

Parenting choices

Having a baby means confronting all kinds of new experiences – some exhilarating, others daunting – and having to make many decisions on a daily basis. Of course, there will be times when I'm not sure what will be the best thing to do, but I'd like to think that I'll get it right most of the time.

Parenthood involves commitment. In the early months, particularly, my baby needs me to be there for her. No matter whether I'm tied up doing something else or feel exhausted, if my baby is hungry, tired, bored or sick, I must find the necessary strength to tend to her needs. However, this should result in a strong emotional attachment between us, which will make the tough times easier to bear.

In my new role, I am finding out I can do a lot more in a day than I previously thought, and that I possess hidden strength and determination, I'm also amazed by the depth of love and protectiveness I feel for my baby.

DIFFERENT APPROACHES

Like every parent, I want to be the best parent in the world, to get everything right, to not make any mistakes and to raise wonderful and loving children. However, these ideals are complicated by personality factors (mine, my partner's and baby's) as well as my other responsibilities at home and/or with work. Having an approach to parenthood should enable me to be consistent, which is important for baby. However, it's important that I not be dogmatic in my approach because baby's behaviour and development may require changes to meet her needs.

One popular system of classifying parents is according to the extent to which we are led by our children's internal emotional needs and demands or the extent to which we require our children to adapt their needs to an external structure and routine. Looked at from this way, parenting can be divided into three common types: child-orientated, schedule-based or flexible. Most professionals think that a flexible parenting style is the most effective as children thrive

Holding my clean, warm, satisfied-looking baby close to me makes all the hard work and effort worthwhile.

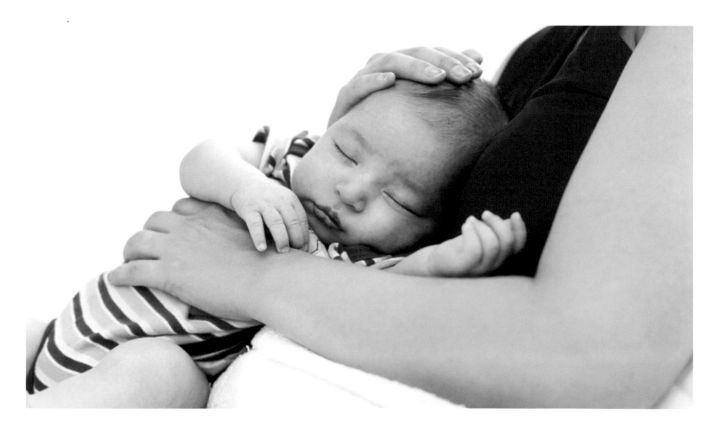

best in loving environments, in which there are clear guidelines for behaviour but the occasional relaxation of the 'rules'.

Child-orientated

Do I consider that the best way to raise my baby is by responding to her emotional and physical needs as they emerge? Will I, for example, immediately give comfort when baby cries, will I feed her immediately when she's hungry or will I play with her right away if she's bored? The advantage of this approach is that my baby's needs are satisfied instantly, which could mean she might never feel alone, isolated or ignored. On the negative side, she may grow up to expect the world to totally revolve around her and may miss out on opportunities to develop resilience and coping skills of her own.

Schedule-based

Do I believe that routine is good for baby and that I am the best person to decide that routine? Will I feed baby at strict intervals and put her to bed according to a predetermined schedule (whether or not she wants to feed or sleep at those times)?

On the plus side, this approach shows that I have very clear ideas of what to do with baby right from the start; baby will learn very quickly that her needs are not the only priority. On the negative side, she may resist the imposition of a fixed schedule that might not fit in with her changing emotional needs.

Flexible

Am I someone who recognises that routine matters to a growing child and that every child is an individual with her own particular blend of characteristics. Would I be willing, therefore, to change a feeding schedule, at least occasionally, to accommodate baby's desires and not insist on always putting her to bed at the same time?

This approach means I might be better able to match my child's stage of development and changing emotional needs. The downside is that baby can become confused if schedules and routines change constantly and I may never stick to anything long enough to know if I'm getting the best results.

A TRUE PARTNERSHIP

No matter which type of parent I want to be, in a two-parent family, it is vital that both parents agree on parenting style. While my partner and I don't have to be carbon copies of one another – I'm sure our child will benefit from our individual natures and personalities –

If I do nothing else I will ...

ESTABLISH MY APPROACH

Coming up with a parenting strategy may help me respond better to my baby's needs – even if I change my mind later. I should:

✓ **Weigh up all the alternatives carefully.**

✓ **Follow through with commitment.**

✓ **Be prepared to admit I've made a mistake.**

✗ **Not assume I am wrong.**

✗ **Not always go for the easy option.**

✗ **Not chop and change too quickly.**

it is in her best interests for there to be a broad consensus on the main parenting concerns such as discipline, behaviour, relationships and routine.

When differences in parenting attitudes and style arise between me and my partner – which is bound to happen in every family at times – we will try to resolve the disagreement privately, without our child having the opportunity to listen in. To increase our child's psychological wellbeing, her confidence in us as parents and her sense of emotional security, we need to present a united front to our child so that she sees both of us support each other.

SINGLE PARENTHOOD

Although single parents face many challenges – in terms of money, time and support, among other things, routine conflict with a partner over how to raise their child is not one of them. Of course, single parents have friends and relatives who may have differing opinions, but for most of the time, they make all the decisions on their own without anyone battling against them.

On the plus side, a single parent doesn't have to resolve disagreements over baby care with anyone else. She is the sole decision-maker. The downside, however, is that single parents need to have confidence in their judgements as a parent – and that's not always easy; everyone is bound to have self-doubts sometimes.

Managing early parenthood

Family life with a new baby takes a lot of getting used to. It was scary to suddenly realise that I was in total charge of a helpless being, completely dependent on me to feed, change, bathe, protect and love her and to be able to diagnose and find a solution to any problems she had. On top of that, my daily routine became completely unpredictable and I felt mentally and physically exhausted by the lack of sleep, the effort of learning new skills and the worries all new parents have. It took time to get on top of things, but I try to be patient and not let the occasional minor upset rock my confidence in my abilities.

HOUSEHOLD TASKS

Almost immediately, there was a change to the management of household tasks. I found it helpful to list the various tasks and agree with my partner which ones he would do and which would fall to me. There are, of course, some we share.

MAKING TIME FOR MYSELF

Although this seemed hard at first, there were plenty of free moments, once I knew how to make them. The most important thing was to establish a basic routine; I decided on set times to take baby out for a walk, give baths and put her down for naps and to bed, etc. While she was asleep or my partner was caring for her, I took time to rest myself, putting my feet up. I was also happy to accept offers of help from relatives – whether looking after baby or doing some shopping or chores.

SUCCESS WITH FEEDING

Although I've decided to breastfeed and have been able to do so effectively, some women who want to find that it doesn't 'work' for them or that it becomes a source of anxiety. In these cases, it's important to go with one's natural instincts. If a woman decides, for example, that she'd rather bottlefeed than breastfeed, it's important she not become concerned that bottlefeeding will have a detrimental effect on the emotional bond she has with her baby. She needs to bear in mind that what's important and manageable is the sensation of relaxation and comfort that she creates. Feeding isn't only about nourishing a baby physically, it's also about providing emotional nourishment.

If I do nothing else I will ...

MAKE THE MOST OF THE GRANDPARENTS
Although there may be the occasional disagreement, their help will be invaluable. I need to ensure I:

✓ **Am welcoming and encouraging when they offer help.** Some grandparents stay away from their grandchild, fearing that they'll be considered too dominant.

✓ **Involve them in baby's care.** If I think they're 'out of practice', I'll give them a simple task to start with, such as reading baby a story, or show them the way I change a nappy.

✓ **Ask for their advice.** There's bound to be something that I'm not sure about – or maybe there is a family history of something – so they should appreciate it when I ask for their opinion. Of course, I won't ask their advice about anything I feel strongly about.

✓ **Make them feel wanted.** I'll keep them informed about what baby is doing and, as she gets older, will tell them how fond she is of them and how we all look forward to their visits.

✓ **Give them notice when I need them to help out.** Grandparents can have pretty busy lives, so I can't expect them to baby-sit at a moment's notice. I'll also be sure to thank them for helping out when they do.

✓ **Let them know how I feel about certain things, like discipline.** If I think they are being too lenient, I need to discuss this with them and make my expectations clear.

In the first few months, many feeding problems – perhaps baby has trouble latching on or possets some milk during a feed – begin as very minor difficulties but if fuelled by parental anxiety and tension, may soon grow into major problems. If a mother becomes anxious, this can affect her baby and set up a vicious circle. In the above cases, once you're certain your baby doesn't have a health problem, it's a good idea to experiment with changing your feeding position or, if you're bottlefeeding, changing the teats.

If your baby feeds too slowly or feeds hurriedly then sleeps before finishing, step back and have an objective look at the whole process. Ask yourself the following:
• Do I look forward to feeding times?
• Do I enjoy holding my baby while I feed her?
• Does she look very settled and comfortable in my arms and when taking the breast or bottle?
• Does she seem satisfied when she's finished?
If the answer to any of these questions is 'no', then you need to create a relaxed atmosphere, which is useful for both breast- and bottlefeeding.

COPING WITH CRYING

I need to remind myself how delighted I was to hear baby cry moments after delivery – the signal that she had arrived safely – as now that she's home, her repeated cries can wear me down. It's important to bear in mind that crying is baby's main way of communicating and a sign of healthy development not a reflection that I'm doing something wrong. As time goes by, I'm getting better at figuring out what her cries mean so that I'm less stressed and frustrated about what to do to help her to settle. Like all babies, mine rarely cries just for the sake of it, so I always look for an explanation.

As well as trying to understand why my baby is crying, I need to ensure that I'm not tense and anxious when I pick her up, as she will sense the tension and another vicious circle can arise. If I do become tense, I try to take a short break, as a few minutes' respite is usually all that's needed to put me in a more positive frame of mind.

WHY IS BABY CRYING?

☐ Hungry; does she need feeding?

☐ Too hot or too cold; do her clothing, blankets or the room temperature need adjusting?

☐ Wet or dirty; maybe she's uncomfortable and needs her nappy changing?

☐ Bored and wants me to amuse her?

☐ Lonely and in need of some loving attention?

☐ Tired but needs gentle rocking to sleep?

☐ Distressed because there is loud noise or bright lights and needs holding in a quiet, darkened place?

☐ Ill and must be seen by the doctor?

SLEEPING NEEDS

According to research, a new baby will result in her parent(s) losing 400–750 hours of sleep in her first year. Up until her fifth month, 2 hours' sleep a night will be lost and this gradually falls to about 1 hour a night until the child is 2 years old. It certainly felt like that to me! I had to be philosophical and accept that lack of sleep is part of parenthood at this early stage in my baby's life. I found catnapping an effective way to recharge my batteries as well as sharing baby's care at night with my partner.

Of course I realise that my lack of sleep is due to baby's development. While a newborn may spend most of each day asleep, she will wake frequently to cry and be fed. She'll only sleep for a maximum of 4 hours at any one time. By 3 months of age, a baby will spend roughly 14–16 hours of her day asleep, although this is still spread evenly throughout the day and night. It's only later that she'll start to sleep more during the night and less during the day. The fact that I want her to sleep longer at night makes no difference to her!

Postnatal depression

While feeling down is very common after childbirth, true postnatal depression (PND) affects only about 10–20 per cent of mothers. Although there is no one known cause, fluctuating hormone levels and stress are contributing factors. Women who have had a caesarean, particularly an emergency caesarean, are particularly at risk. As having a caesarean birth is one of life's more difficult experiences, it can leave its mark resulting in feelings of low self-esteem, disappointment and failure.

Most commonly, PND begins in the first 6 weeks after birth and peaks at 10 weeks. Common symptoms include loss of interest in one's usual activities, difficulty concentrating or making decisions, fatigue, feelings of worthlessness or guilt, recurrent thoughts of death or suicide, significant weight gain or loss, changes in appetite or sleep and excessive anxiety about baby's health.

Contact your GP if you find that you:
• Get angry easily.
• Feel anxious about how your partner feels toward you and have low self-esteem.
• Have fears about your baby's health.
• Cry excessively.
• Are lethargic but can't sleep.
• Experience panic attacks and feelings of being overwhelmed.
• Have feelings of hate toward your baby and/or your partner.

Some new fathers also experience PND – but they are less likely to ask for help!

Although it may be difficult to talk about your feelings with your GP or health visitor, PND is an illness and requires treatment, usually with counselling and medication. If you're breastfeeding, it's important that any prescribed medications are suitable. If you feel uncomfortable about talking to your GP, or you are unsure whether you actually have depression, there are organisations that specialise in the condition. Do a search on the internet then call one of the helplines and talk to a counsellor.

If I do nothing else I will ...

PROTECT MY EMOTIONAL HEALTH
By taking the following steps, I'll be more likely to keep my spirits raised. I need to:

✓ **Make time for things that make me laugh,** such as watching my favourite comedies.

✓ **Ask for help with tasks or situations** that make me feel pressurised or cause anxiety.

✓ **Spend time relaxing.** If necessary, I may use meditation or visualisations to still my mind when I'm worried.

✓ **Pay attention to my appearance.** If I think I look good, I'm sure to feel better.

✓ **Get out and about.** Taking baby for a walk, or getting my partner to look after baby while I go out with a friend will get me away from domestic chores and is sure to be cheering.

✓ **Join a new mothers' support group** or a postnatal exercise class as a way to share experiences and help lift my spirits.

✓ **Let my partner know how I feel.** If he appreciates that sometimes things can get too much, he'll be better able to help out and give me the support I need.

✗ **Avoid sugar, chocolate and alcohol,** which can have a depressant effect. I need to eat plenty of healthy fresh foods.

Settling into family life

Caring for baby can be all-consuming, but it's important I do not lose sight of myself as an individual and that the relationship between my partner and me is maintained. Once the newborn period is over, I am keen to re-establish my own lifestyle, and I need to think about whether to return to work or pursue other interests. Probably the biggest decision I will make over the next few months is whether or not to return to work. I'm going to take my time thinking about this and move forwards in a way that suits me, my partner and my baby.

OPTING TO STAY AT HOME

If I decide to care for baby full time, I'm hoping this will provide me with all the satisfaction I used to get from my job, though I know that some women worry that by staying home they will somehow lose their individuality. If I start to feel like this, I will focus on the fact that the job I have now – that of bringing up baby – is equally, if not far more important, than my previous one. Many of my friends with babies tell me how enjoyable it is discovering things with their babies

and watching all the incredible changes they go through. And I'm planning to share my experiences with them and others.

OPTING TO GO BACK TO WORK

If I decide to return to work, I need to fix on a date and make the necessary arrangements for childcare – whether a nanny, childminder or nursery (see page 86).

I'm sure that when the time comes to return to work, it's inevitable that I will feel a bit sad or guilty, thinking about the precious times I could be spending with baby or wondering what will happen if she has an accident. If I'm returning to work it's because I either want or have to, so I'll try not to let such feelings get me down. I need to concentrate on the notion that I'll feel more independent and fulfilled while working, and that will make me a happier mother, which will benefit my baby. My working will provide her with a stable financial background.

I'm hoping that baby will develop a close bond with her caregiver, but this shouldn't affect the relationship she has with me. I will find time to spend alone with

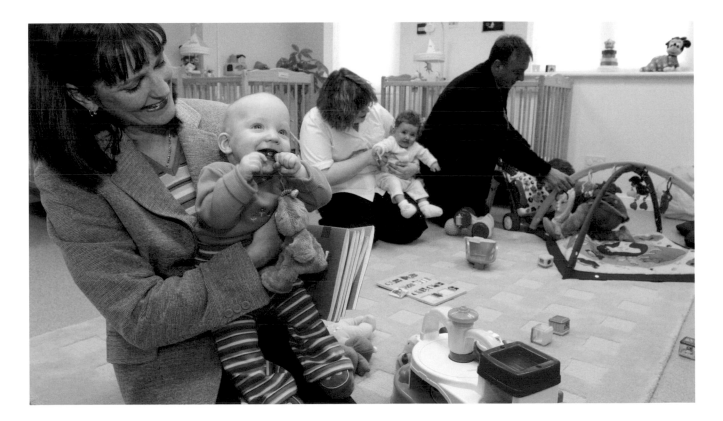

her and build this into my routine, and once I'm home in the evenings and at weekends, I can feed her, play with her and then put her to bed.

Returning to work is certain to be difficult at first. I'm sure to be tired and it'll take time to get used to juggling my workload and responsibilities at home.

BEING PART OF A COUPLE

Living with a baby affects each partner in different ways. Maybe one of us now will stay at home, whereas before both of us held down full-time jobs, or maybe my partner will resent the attention I'm giving to baby. Unexpressed, these concerns can create barriers between us. Honest communication is the best way to maintain a strong relationship, and for it to evolve as our family grows.

There are a number of things we need to do. Having a social life is one. We don't need to go out for the entire evening at first, but watching a movie or visiting some friends will provide a welcome break.

We also need to share ideas about parenting with one another, as well as any concerns. I will listen to my partner's hopes and fears, and make sure I voice my own. Even if he is passionate about baby, he may feel hurt and left out by the apparent switch in my affections – and I need to reassure him how important he is to both of us.

I need to resist the temptation to keep everything to myself. Initially, I felt as if I wanted to spend all of my time with baby and that I was better at caring for her than my partner could, but it soon became apparent that I could share baby's care without worrying about loss of control. I tried to bear in mind that baby was learning different things from each of us.

PUTTING SEX BACK ON THE MENU

Although my GP has advised waiting 6 weeks before having sex, doing so really depends on whether and when I feel ready. As my birth was relatively easy and I don't have much discomfort, I don't see any reason to wait that long. Other women, who've had a difficult birth and stitches, may prefer to wait longer than 6 weeks. When I do feel ready, I'll take it at my own pace, finding what feels good and what doesn't. If penetrative sex doesn't seem to be on the menu, then kissing and cuddling, massage, mutual masturbation and oral sex will be satisfying until I feel ready for penetration. I'm told it's a good idea to avoid the missionary position until I feel completely comfortable and pain-free, but making love in a position in which I can control my partner's depth of penetration – me on top or us lying side to side – ensures that if the pressure becomes

✚ **EXPERTS ADVISE**

Use lubrication
After the birth, when oestrogen and progesterone levels plummet, you may temporarily experience a loss of vaginal lubrication, as well as hot flushes and sweats. These may continue for some time. So, when you're ready for intercourse or want to try masturbation, use a water-based, vaginal lubricant. Don't use petroleum jelly, because this is oil-based and can lead to an infection.

uncomfortable, I can ease away. I also understand it's very common for sex drive to decrease after childbirth what with the exhaustion, lack of sleep and the massive adjustment that a new baby demands and that sex might not be as spontaneous as it was before.

Ovulation can start even though I'm breastfeeding and my periods haven't returned, so I need to use some form of contraception when I resume sex. Condoms are probably the best option at first. If I want to use other forms of contraception, I'll need to speak to my GP. An oestrogen-based pill won't be suitable as it can block milk production, but I understand it's usually safe to take the 'mini-pill', which contains only progesterone. If I want to have an IUD fitted or a replacement diaphragm prescribed, I'll need to wait until my cervix has recovered, which may take around 6 weeks.

KEEPING ON TOP OF THINGS

At first the reality of parenthood didn't always match up to my expectations; I found it more demanding than I'd anticipated and it was hard always being on call to respond to baby's needs. But having confidence in myself and my ideas made problems easier to overcome. I had doubts and made mistakes – everybody has moments of uncertainty and at times wishes that he or she had done something differently – but I try not to let these occasional moments affect my self-confidence. I tell myself that other parents have the same thoughts, too. I also find it a help sharing my ideas and feelings with my partner and close friends. Explaining my ideas to others helps me clarify my thoughts, even when my listener doesn't offer any advice. And when advice is given, I listen to what the other person says and discuss the matter further. I don't always change my mind in the end but I feel more confident about my decisions.

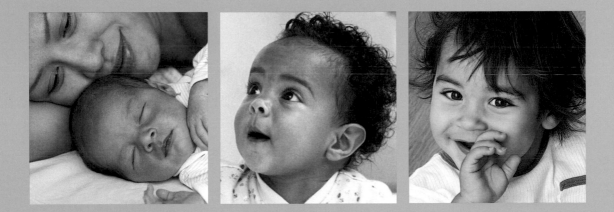

PART II My baby

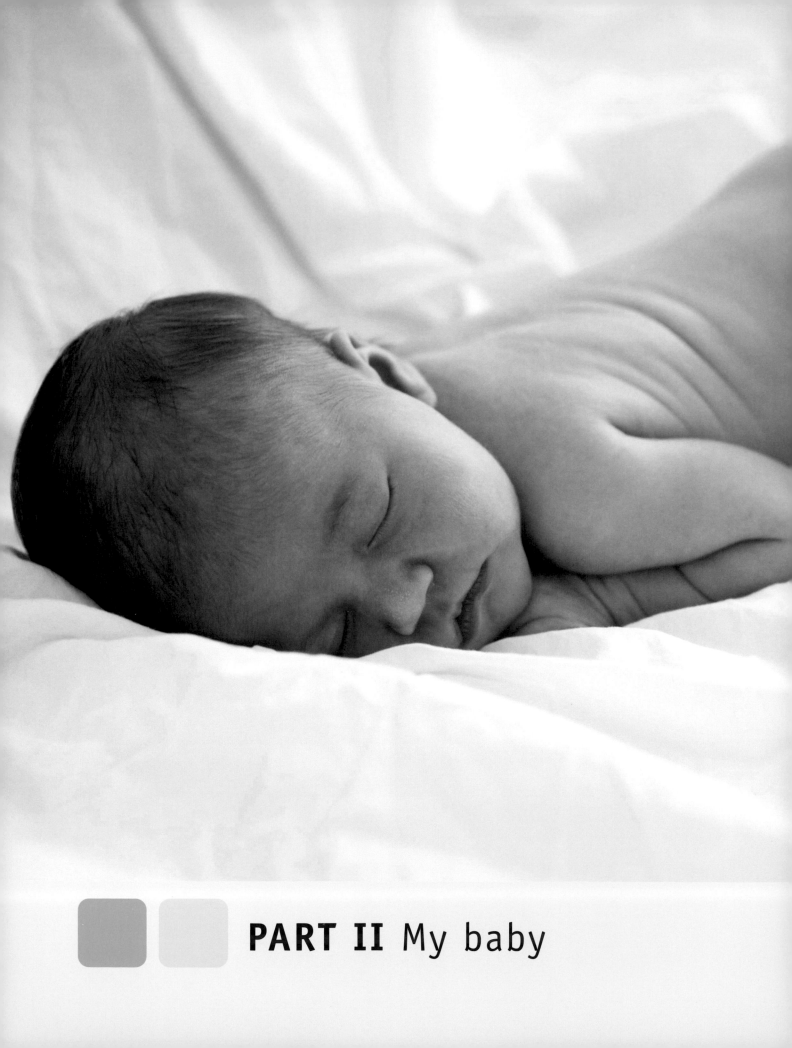

PART II My baby

My marvellous newborn

At last, after 9 months of anticipation, my baby is actually here. I'm simply amazed at how beautiful she is and that she is perfect in every way. I feel exceedingly lucky. Some babies, I know, need special care at birth or are born with problems. Fortunately, these babies, too, can, in most cases, be helped to live long, healthy and happy lives.

What my baby looks like

Once she was born, I couldn't believe how absolutely gorgeous my baby was! Not in a conventional sense, perhaps, but here she was, perfectly formed, the baby I had for months longed to know, and I felt utterly amazed when she was handed to me. If she had been born by caesarean, she would have had a more rounded head and less squashed face, since she wouldn't have had to go through the narrow pelvic canal, but otherwise, most newborns look pretty similar to my baby. A baby delivered with the help of forceps or ventouse or who had a scalp electrode attached prior to delivery may have bruising and swelling on her head.

THE UMBILICUS

My baby's tummy button may be an 'outie' or an 'innie'. If the umbilical cord was short or if a longer cord was twisted around her while she was in the womb, more tension would have been applied at the umbilicus and her tummy button will protrude. If very little cord tension was present before birth, the button will be recessed. If the amount of pull was in between, the tummy button will be at the level of the abdominal skin. Should my baby's umbilicus stick out, I'll not worry; many outies eventually sink and become innies.

The remnant, or stump, of the umbilical cord is still attached. It is yellowish-white and soft, with a clip applied at birth to the end. This prevents any of her blood from exiting her body via umbilical vessels. In another day or two, it will shrink, become dark in colour, and very hard and the clip will be removed.

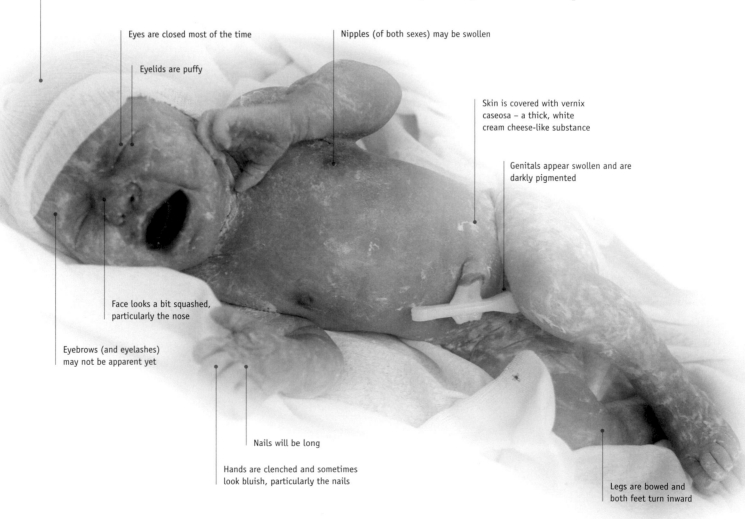

Head is elongated and swollen

Eyes are closed most of the time

Eyelids are puffy

Nipples (of both sexes) may be swollen

Skin is covered with vernix caseosa – a thick, white cream cheese-like substance

Genitals appear swollen and are darkly pigmented

Face looks a bit squashed, particularly the nose

Eyebrows (and eyelashes) may not be apparent yet

Nails will be long

Hands are clenched and sometimes look bluish, particularly the nails

Legs are bowed and both feet turn inward

BIRTHMARKS

Although my baby doesn't have any (yet), they are common to babies and come in several types.

HAEMANGIOMAS

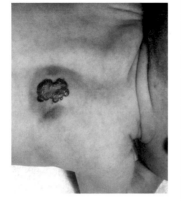

At birth these 'strawberry' marks are flat, well defined and often pale-purplish in colour. They are essentially a collection of many small blood vessels in a localised area, but may not be visible until the vessels begin to grow. As they grow (mostly up off the surface of the skin), they become larger, redder and raised. Haemangiomas continue to grow for the first 6–9 months of life, then slowly begin to shrink and lose their colour. The vast majority, even very large ones, are completely gone in a couple of years without treatment. Rarely, a large haemangioma becomes problematic due to its location near important structures (the eye, nose or mouth) or in areas that can be easily irritated (hand or nappy area) and these can be treated with cortisone injections or laser.

PIGMENTED SPOTS

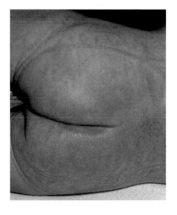

Commonly called 'Mongolian spots', these are large, flat and greyish-black areas of up to several centimetres across. Most commonly found over the lower back and upper buttocks in an enlongated shape, they also can be found in other areas such the back of the hands and upper back and shoulders. They are very common in black infants and those of Asian descent. Usually, these pigmented spots become much less noticeable with age.

NAEVI FLAMMEUS

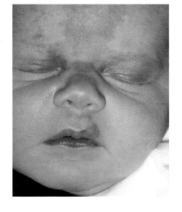

Flat and pinkish-red, these areas of skin are also made up of extra blood vessels but, unlike haemangiomas (see above), they are present at birth and don't grow. Common locations include the nape of the neck ('stork mark'), upper eyelids ('angel's kiss'), on the nose or just above it, and the forehead. These birthmarks will gradually lighten and usually disappear in time. However, when baby cries or strains to have a bowel movement, naevi flammeus will momentarily become redder.

NAEVI

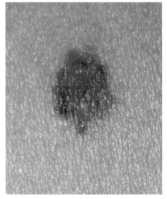

Thess are black birthmarks that may be flat or raised. Like haemangiomas, naevi (plural) also may not be present at birth but appear later on. Many are small and look like moles in older children and adults. Occasionally they are larger. While they don't get larger, they do not disappear.

What my baby can do

As well as taking her first breath, my baby also gave her first cry! Although crying is now well established, I've also been surprised by the number of other noises she makes – hiccups, sneezes and snorts. Some of her behaviour is reflexive – she reacts to certain stimuli in particular ways – but other things that she does seem to indicate that she is using her senses. Moreover, she seems to have a particular temperament.

REFLEXES

Some newborn reflexes exist to help my baby cope with the outside world, but others are a mystery! Breathing is one of the first reflexes to be apparent at birth. My baby's lungs didn't operate in the uterus but now she needs to take in vital oxygen.

Feeding is supported by a number of reflexes – rooting, sucking and swallowing. These ensure my baby turns towards a milk source (breast or bottle), latches on and takes in food.

Her eyes are protected by the pupillary and blink reflexes, which cause her pupils to constrict and her eyelids to close in response to bright lights.

Sudden noises or sensations elicit the Moro or startle reflex of splayed out limbs, which demonstrates she is alert to a potential danger nearby (see opposite).

If I hold my baby up so her feet touch a firm surface, she will demonstrate the stepping reflex, by appearing to walk and, if something is placed in her hand, she will grab it very tightly (the grasping or palmar reflex). These latter two reflexes quickly fade but may be a result of something learned in the womb

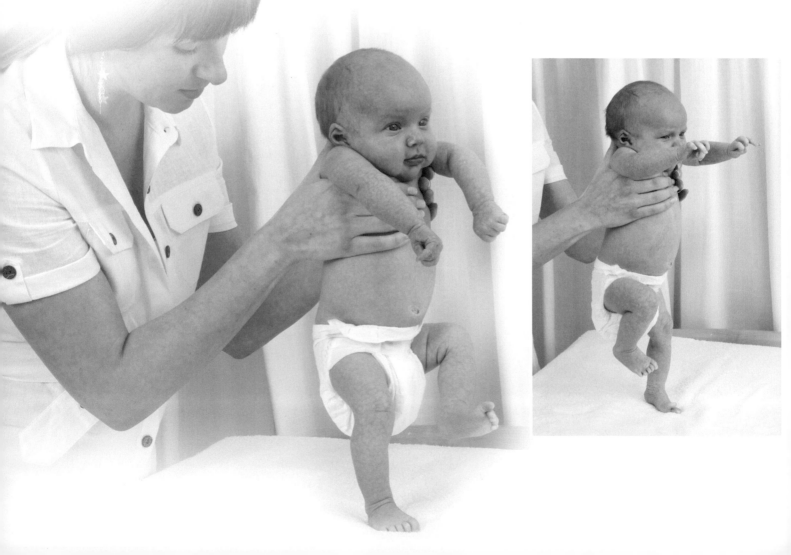

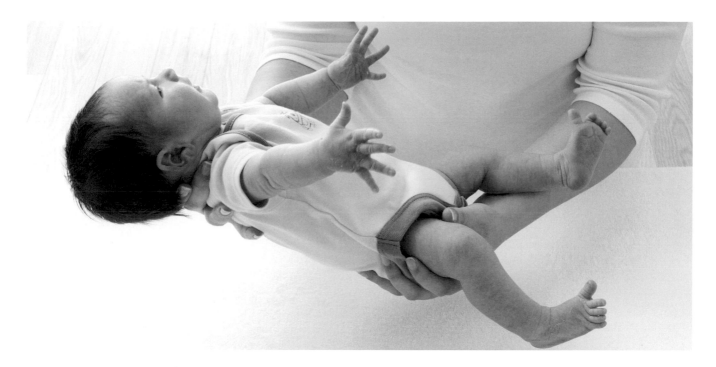

(grasping one's umbilical cord) or that may be important to later development (stepping when walking); nobody knows!

SENSORY AWARENESS

Right from birth, my baby can see me quite well, but focuses best at 20–25 cm away from something. Interestingly, this is the approximate distance between my eyes and baby's face when I hold her at my breast. I often notice her staring at me.

My baby could also hear very well at birth, too. She turns towards me when I speak. Loud voices or noises startle her and often make her cry. However, when I play the music I played her while I was pregnant, she seems to recognise it and quietens.

I've been told my baby can distinguish my breast milk from another mother's, and will also respond better to certain smells, being repelled by those she finds unpleasant. She's also able to distinguish certain flavours from birth, and I need to be careful what I eat as strong flavours, such as garlic, can make my milk less pleasant for her.

Like all babies, mine loves the feeling of being cuddled and held close; this usually calms and reassures her. I love the feel of her against my bare skin and she seems to like it, too.

TEMPERAMENT

My baby has her own individual personality. It seems to me that even at this age, she has likes and dislikes and reacts to things in a particular way. She is an enthusiastic feeder while other I know babies are more passive and suck more slowly. Right from the start, she snuggled close to me but I remember my sister's baby wriggling about a lot at first.

Psychologists studying babies' temperaments have found that 75 per cent of babies fall into one of three personality types, while the other 25 per cent share features from more than one type. A baby will either be:

- Easy-going and a pleasure to be with because she is very even-tempered and generally responds positively to anything that happens to her or around her. Such a baby is very adaptable to new experiences, welcoming them rather than avoiding them. Her mood and behaviour are regular and predictable.

- Hard-to-manage because she is fractious and easily irritated but very active for most of the time. It doesn't take much to unsettle her. Her moods are variable and her behaviour is not predictable. She doesn't like change and takes a long time to adapt to new situations or unfamiliar faces.

- Slow-to-warm-up and generally inactive with mild reactions to most things. She will lack enthusiasm for new experiences, but won't have intense negative responses. If, for instance, she doesn't like a new toy, she will simply turn her head away from it rather than actually physically reject it.

Does my baby need special care?

Babies who are born prematurely, or who have a low birth weight or a condition diagnosed while in utero, after birth or caused by the delivery, may need to be looked after in the special care baby unit (SCBU) until well enough to go home. Mothers of special-care babies must strike a balance between visiting their babies and getting sufficient rest to maintain health and energy. Initially, one visit daily of 2–3 hours' duration (if sitting down next to a baby's incubator) or less (if standing up) is plenty. Later on, a morning visit lasting between just before the first feeding time until just after the following feed, then a shorter visit in the evening is recommended. Some parents alternate trips to the SCBU, with dad arriving in the evening after work. Premature infants sleep even more than full-term babies (who sleep about 16–20 hours a day), so a baby is certain to be asleep for much of these visits.

PREMATURITY

An infant who is born at 36 weeks' or less gestation is considered premature. Twins are very often premature because the uterus is often incapable of carrying two infants to term. Not all premature babies of the same gestational age have the same competencies, so infants are usually not discharged from the SCBU until they can successfully be fed and are gaining weight steadily (no matter what their age).

CARE IN THE SCBU

A baby cared for in this unit will be kept in an incubator, where he will be shielded from the outside world in a heated environment but be open to observation. Feeding and bathing and procedures such as taking blood and starting intravenous therapy can be accomplished without removing his from his heated home. Via portholes, parents are able to comfort their infants by touch until the babies are big enough to be allowed out for hugging and holding.

Very small prem babies are fed initially using a narrow diameter feeding tube that goes in through the nose or mouth and ends in the stomach. Prem babies are usually incapable of strong sucking and the feeding tube bypasses the need for sucking. Expressed breast milk or premature formula is measured in a syringe and dripped or pumped into the baby's stomach via the tube. When a baby is older, bottle feedings can be given while he remains in his incubator.

Parents who spend time in the SCBU are shown by the nurses how to perform the little tasks involved in daily routines, so they become more competent and

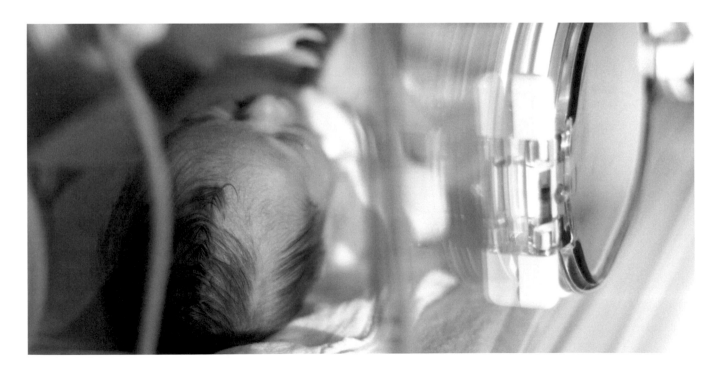

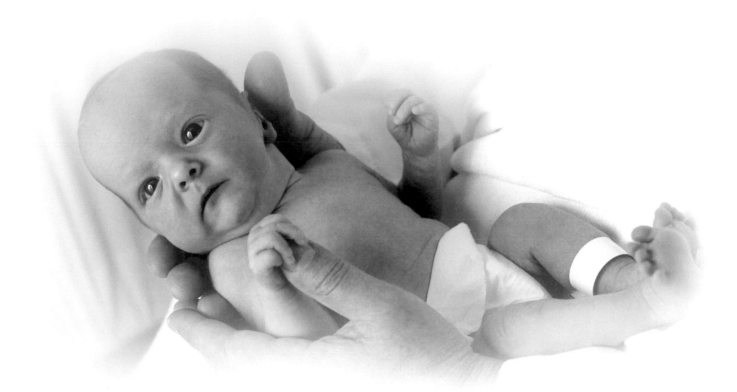

confident in their skills before bringing their baby home. Parents acquire proficiency in cleaning and changing, and measuring and giving vitamins. They also become comfortable picking their child up and holding him, as well as expert in feeding him.

Very premature infants are often quite ill initially due to the immaturity of their lungs, intestines, circulatory system, etc., and being pro-active and learning about a baby's medical conditions (and how to care for them) can be accomplished during the time she is in the SCBU.

JAUNDICE

Many newborn infants develop a yellow skin and yellowish whites of the eyes. This is due to a high level of bilirubin, a waste product of old red blood cells and is a result of a baby's liver being immature and unable to remove these unwanted cells. Jaundice occurs most often in newborns who were bruised during delivery, have a blood type different from their mother's or were born prematurely.

Generally, treatment is with phototherapy, in which a baby is placed under lights that impart energy to the bilirubin molecules in his skin and superficial blood vessels so causing a small structural change in the bilirubin molecules, which allow them to be easily excreted in urine. Phototherapy does not cure jaundice, but it does keep the bilirubin level in the safe range until the liver matures sufficiently.

If I do nothing else I will ... ✔

MAINTAIN CONTACT WITH MY PREMMIE

Even though she may be in an incubator, there are ways that I can care for her. I can:

✔ **Sing and talk** to her while she is in the incubator.

✔ **Fondle and cuddle her** through the portholes.

✔ **Provide skin-to-skin closeness** (kangaroo care) when she's allowed out of the incubator and the staff permit it. Research has shown that skin-to-skin contact can reduce stress levels even in the youngest baby.

✔ **Express breast milk** that can be fed to her.

✔ **Learn all I can** about her condition and physical care. If I keep a journal, this will help me record her progress (so I can tell her later on) and if I'm at her side while she's changed, bathed and massaged, I'll be able to perform these tasks as soon as possible.

Problems detectable at birth

Some conditions are transient and easily cured, such as having a high red blood cell count, low blood sugar or short-lived rapid breathing, but other problems may need significant treatment or prove unable to eradicate.

HAND, FOOT, LEG AND HIP PROBLEMS

Extra digits are common and range from extra skin without a nail or internal bones to a fully developed sixth finger or toe. Those on a thin stalk can be tied off with sutures, while more complete extra fingers or toes must be surgically removed.

A club foot may affect one or both feet. At birth, the affected foot flexes downwards at the ankle, turns in and tilts. Starting shortly after birth, the foot will be placed in plaster casts, which hold it in progressively closer to a normal position. Surgery can help infants whose feet are not adequately improved by casting or whose feet are more difficult to treat.

Hip dislocation may be apparent in some young babies if the socket that holds the ball-shaped head of the femur is too shallow and the head moves out of its correct position. A baby's hips will be examined at his newborn check and at 6–8 weeks. If a problem is suspected, he will be referred for ultrasound hip scanning and to an orthopaedic surgeon. In some cases, the condition will right itself over time as the socket develops. Other children will need to be fitted with a splinting device to keep the hips turned out so they develop normally over a period of time. Sometimes, traction followed by splinting or surgery is required.

TESTICLE PROBLEMS

Occasionally at birth one testis is undescended (not present in scrotal sac). Invariably it will arrive in its normal position within a few months. Sometimes, one testis will seem larger than the other because it is surrounded by fluid. Known as a hydrocele, most small- and medium-sized ones resolve in the first months of life. Those that do not disappear or are large may be treated with minor surgery.

HEART PROBLEMS

A heart murmur is a noise that can be heard when blood flow through an area within the heart or a major blood vessel is more turbulent than usual. Murmurs detected on the first day of life are often transient and are a normal variation. The most common cause of a significant murmur is when instead of the right and left ventricles being separated completely by a muscular wall (septum), there is a small area where the wall is incomplete and blood from the left ventricle can enter the right one. This murmur, known as a VSD or ventriculoseptal defect, typically is noted after 2–3 days of age. The majority of VSDs fully close as the heart grows

There exists a variety of less common heart malformations, some of which are serious.

Clues to a heart problem include blueness of the lips (not the hands and feet, which are normally purplish-blue in healthy newborns), rapid breathing, paleness and poor feeding. When a structural cardiac defect is suspected, your doctor will investigate further, possibly using tests – a chest X-ray, an ECG (electrocardiogram) or echocardiogram (sonogram of the heart) – or request a consultation from a paediatric cardiologist.

CLEFT PALATE

This is an opening in the roof of the mouth (palate) allowing communication between the oral and nasal cavities. In the newborn period, this defect can make feeding difficult for a baby, since the cleft prevents generation of the negative pressure needed for successful sucking. A temporary solution is to give bottle feeds using a very large teat (lamb's teat). A plastic device, like the plate often used with children being treated by orthodontists, can be made that artificially closes off the opening. Surgical repair of the cleft palate is usually recommended before one year of age and produces excellent results.

In severe cases, a cleft palate can be accompanied by a split upper lip (hare lip). More extensive surgery will be done to produce a pleasing result.

HYDROCEPHALUS

Caused by a number of situations, the result is the same – excessive amounts of spinal fluid press on the brain resulting in an abnormally large head circumference.

Hydrocephalus can occur in ill, premature infants when there is bleeding within the ventricles and blood clots block the path used by spinal fluid to exit the affected ventricle. Hydrocephalus may also be the result of an error in the formation of the ventricles or passageways during gestation, scarring following a brain infection occurring in utero, or a brain tumour compressing the ventricle or spinal fluid passageways. Hydrocephalus also can develop as the result of injury to the cells lining the brain following meningitis.

Treatment varies according to the severity. If hydrocephalus is not severe, spinal fluid can be removed by lumbar puncture (spinal tap) to lower the pressure. In other cases, a shunt will be inserted to divert spinal fluid or surgery done to enlarge the exit from which fluid from within the brain flows to the area surrounding it.

DOWN'S SYNDROME

Caused by an error in cell division early in the life of the tiny fetus, the typical facial and physical characteristics and associated medical problems all derive from an extra copy of chromosome 21 in each cell.

Children with Down's syndrome may have a host of medical problems. In the newborn period, congenital heart defects (which may require surgery) and intestinal blockage may occur. In childhood, there is an increased risk of ear infections and hypothyroidism (underactive thyroid). An affected child also needs to be examined for instability of the upper spine before playing vigorous sports activities.

Although intellectual disability and delay in reaching milestones are also prominent features, there is a wide variety of outcomes. Characteristically, children are sweet and happy.

SPINA BIFIDA

This condition covers a number of abnormalities in the formation of the posterior part of the spinal column (the bones or vertebrae which surround and protect the spinal cord) and overlying skin and soft tissues. The mildest cases, called spina bifida occulta, may be diagnosed only when an X-ray of the abdomen or pelvis is taken for unrelated reasons and the lower spine is seen to have no posterior closure of the vertebrae. The most severe cases, known as meningomyelocele, in addition to this vertebral abnormality, also lack a skin covering over the lower spine.

Spina bifida occulta requires no treatment. Sinus tracts and other soft tissue abnormalities near the lower end of the spinal cord will be corrected surgically as soon as they are detected. In the case of meningomyelocele, surgery in the newborn period will be done to close the spinal defect.

Spina bifida occulta typically has no complications, while in repaired defects of intermediate severity, some nerve damage may occur. Nerve damage is almost universally present in meningomyelocele. Injury to the nerves exiting the lower spinal cord can result in leg weakness, loss of sensation below the waist, and in males, impotency. Nerve injury may also affect the lower intestinal tract (stool incontinence, chronic constipation) and urinary system (incontinence and poor bladder emptying). Incomplete emptying of the bladder following urination can result in urinary tract infections and occasionally may lead to kidney damage.

SENSORY IMPAIRMENTS

A hearing impairment can be present at birth (congenital); premature infants have a higher incidence of hearing problems. Causes include in utero viral infections and inherited forms of hearing loss. Early detection and intervention – hearing aids, speech and language therapy, programmes designed for hearing-challenged children and, for some children, cochlear implants – have greatly improved the speech and language outcomes of infants with hearing disabilities.

Visual deficits apparent in newborns can result from inherited diseases of the eye, congenital cataracts, glaucoma and prematurity.

Glaucoma occurs when there is increased pressure in the fluid in the eyeball and is signalled by the combination of a larger iris and greater tearing in the affected eye, compared with the other one, and accompanying redness of the white of the eye. Treatment occasionally consists of medicated eye drops and often involves surgery to lower the pressure within the eye.

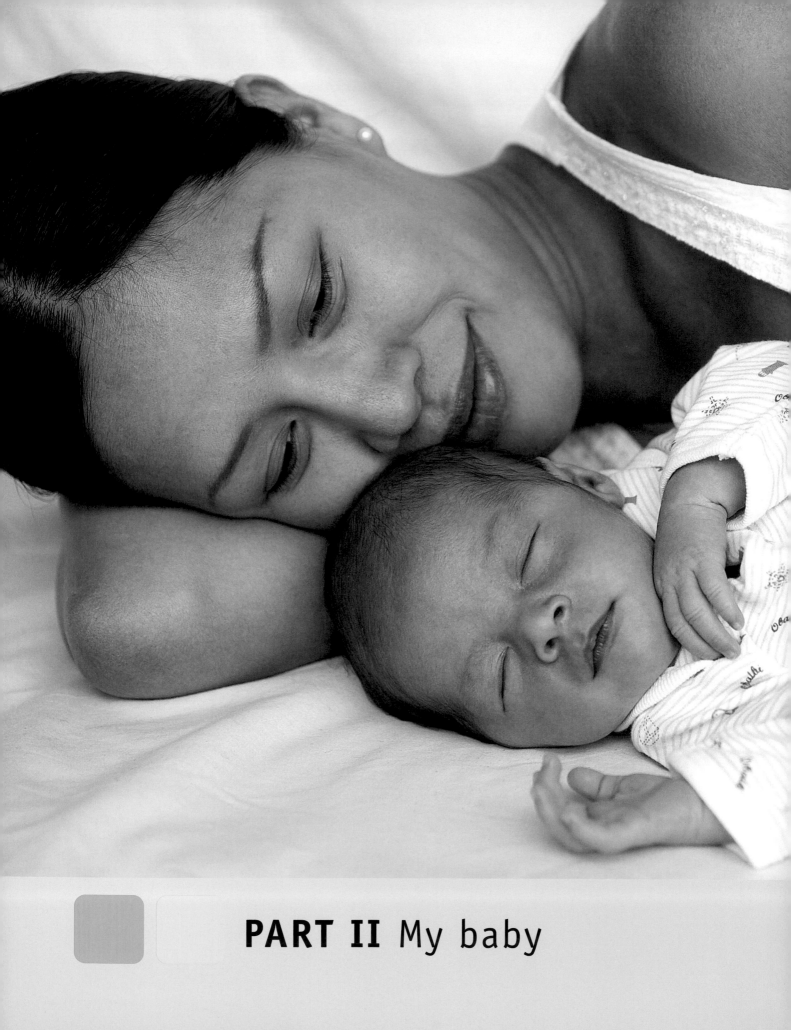

PART II My baby

Caring for my newborn

I've never been so busy in my life! I seem to be on a constant round of feeding, changing, dressing, cleaning, soothing and putting my baby to bed. I try to take things as easy as I can, which helps relieve some of the stress of not knowing whether I'm doing everything exactly right. Still, feeding seems to be going well and I enjoy the many moments of holding baby close and marvelling at the fact that she's here and I'm a mum.

Bonding

Like many parents, I fell in love with my baby the moment I held her in my arms. Other parents do not feel this immediate attachment but go on to develop strong feelings of affection and protection soon after birth. This is not surprising as maternal and paternal feelings are inborn and normally do not need any learning or teaching. In caring for my baby – holding, feeding, soothing and changing her – I find my attachment continues to grow so that now I believe that making her feel loved, secure and safe is the most important thing I can do.

Of course, I know that at birth my baby did not experience this same attachment to me. Although a baby is driven to obtain warmth, comfort and security from the earliest days of her life and is, in fact, 'pre-programmed' to solicit responses from her parents, it is up to the parents to satisfy these needs.

While my baby's total dependency evokes deep feelings in me, she is not sufficiently mature to become attached to me. This takes time and depends on our being able to communicate – both verbally and physically – how we feel about each other.

GETTING TO KNOW EACH OTHER

My baby, like all babies immediately after birth, began to communicate with my partner and me. She did this through crying, other noises, facial expressions, body movements and touches, and over time I am able to respond appropriately.

One thing that I try to do is to talk to her as I go about my daily activities. Even a small baby loves the sound of her mother's voice, so I make sure to give her a running commentary on what I'm doing and what is happening in the world around me. I make a special effort to talk naturally to baby so that she can pick up on the sounds and rhythm of words and normal conversation. When baby 'replies' with noises or gurgles, I respond to the sounds she makes with "Is that so?" or "I know" and try to respond effectively to any gestures that she makes. I always look into baby's face when talking with her and smile to make her feel secure and content.

Rocking baby and dancing together to music is something else we enjoy together.

Because my baby learns about me through all her senses – smell and touch being as important as hearing

EXPERTS ADVISE

Lack of attachment
Your interactions with your newborn should trigger warm feelings of attachment in you. If you feel that this is missing, speak to your GP or health visitor. You may be suffering postnatal depression (see page 130) or another ailment.

and vision – skin-to-skin contact and plenty of cuddles reassure her and make us both feel good.

I know that as my baby grows, she'll learn how to predict my behaviour and be able to work out what will make me smile and how to get me to pay attention to her. I can't wait until she is mature enough to smile back at me, stretch out her arms to be picked up and snuggle into my neck when I cuddle her.

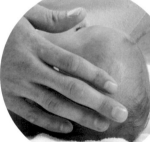

All babies and parents benefit from close contact, particularly skin to skin. Fathers don't often spend as much time with their babies as mums, so I'm encouraging my partner to put aside some time every day to hold and massage our baby, which will help him develop his handling skills and confidence.

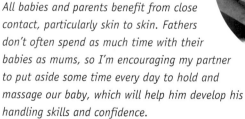

Feeding basics

Most of my time with baby is taken up initially with feeding and this is true of all new mums whether they breastfeed like me or bottlefeed with expressed or formula milk. It can take a couple of weeks to settle into a comfortable and reassuring pattern of feeding.

Breastfeeding gives baby the best start in life, supplying her with vital nutrients and protecting her from infection. It also helps protect me from various diseases and promotes a strong physical and emotional bond with my baby. A mother who chooses, however, to bottlefeed her baby – maybe because she has an existing medical condition, is taking medications or feels uncomfortable breastfeeding – must try not to feel guilty about this decision. Her baby will still receive adequate nutrition and there are techniques for ensuring closeness (see page 154).

HOW OFTEN TO FEED

While all babies need to feed frequently, especially initially, they can have different patterns. Mine likes feeding every couple of hours while others I've met feed in a random fashion. Like all mums, I soon got to know exactly when my baby is hungry. A newborn's tummy is tiny and can't hold much more than a couple of ounces at a time. In the first few weeks, on average, my breastfed baby wanted feeding every couple of hours, night and day (a bottlefed baby may want feeding every 3–4 hours). Breast milk is low in protein and high in milk sugar, and babies need to have little and often to grow well. Bottlefeeding also needs to be baby led so, if you are bottlefeeding, you should feed your baby whenever she seems hungry. Most normal weight babies can go only about 6 hours without a meal. When my baby has had a long sleep, I find it worth gently waking her and offering her a feed right away.

HOW MUCH TO GIVE

If, like me, you are breastfeeding, your baby will probably want to feed well from the first breast for as long as she can. I then offer a break for winding or a nappy change, and bring her back to my other breast for a second helping. My first breast refills while she is on the second side, so if she wants more, she can go back to the first side.

Just as each baby has a different personality and a different suck, each breast has a different capacity and works individually but frequent feeding will help to build the milk supply in the first few weeks.

If you are bottlefeeding, your baby will need 60–75 ml (2–2½ oz) of formula for each 0.5 kg (1 lb) of body weight. For a 3.5 kg (7.7 lb) baby, this would mean you need to give her 420–525 ml (15–18½ oz) of formula in a 24-hour period. Until your baby weighs about 5 kg (11 lb), she will need at least 6–8 bottlefeeds each day, as he only takes in about 60 ml (2 oz) per feed.

It isn't usually helpful to weigh a baby every week, as she may not grow at a steady rate, and it can make you more anxious; growth charts are available that show national averages.

If you are struggling with feeding, then it's worth getting help right at the start. If you're worried that your baby isn't 'getting enough', take a look at my checklist. If something seems amiss, discuss with your health visitor or other new mothers, family or friends.

SIGNS MY BABY IS THRIVING

- [ ] She is relaxed during feeding; she sucks and swallows slowly and pauses every now and then.

- [ ] Feeds actively only for about 30 minutes at a time, which indicates that she's latched on well. If a baby feeds for ages, something's not right and it may mean the attachment needs improving.

- [ ] Is contented or sleeps well between most feeds and is alert and usually happy when awake.

- [ ] Has poos that, in the first 5 days, change quickly from sticky black to golden yellow and are always soft (runny if breastfed, firmer if bottlefed).

- [ ] Has plenty of heavy, wet nappies.

- [ ] Is filling out and feels heavier.

Successful breastfeeding

Only a very small percentage of women are really unable to breastfeed fully; usually due to breast tissue damage or breast surgery, hormonal or endocrine problems, or restrictions by certain medications. But many women lack the confidence to breastfeed. Babies, however, do not have this problem. All babies are instinctively able to feed shortly after birth, if they are given the right opportunity and environment.

A comfortable position can be key to successful breastfeeding. Like most women, I generally feed sitting upright on a chair, often with my feet raised and a pillow supporting my arms, but sometimes I try other positions. Lying on my side is useful when I'm tired or find it uncomfortable to sit. I use plenty of pillows to support myself and hold baby close so that her mouth is in line with my breast. A woman who had a caesarean should bend her knees and support her back with a pillow.

Whichever position I use, I need to be able to bring baby easily to my breast and hold her there – close to me with her whole body facing my breast and her chest next to mine – firmly.

To make the atmosphere as calm and relaxing as possible, I take the house phone off the hook or close the door so I won't be disturbed. I keep a glass of water nearby in case I get thirsty.

I've been advised that when I want to stop breastfeeding altogether, it's best to do so gradually, interspersing breast milk with milk (or formula, depending on baby's age) in a bottle. Not only will baby need time to get used to feeding from a bottle, but my body will need time to readjust. If I stop suddenly, there's a chance that my breasts may become engorged and painful (see page 158).

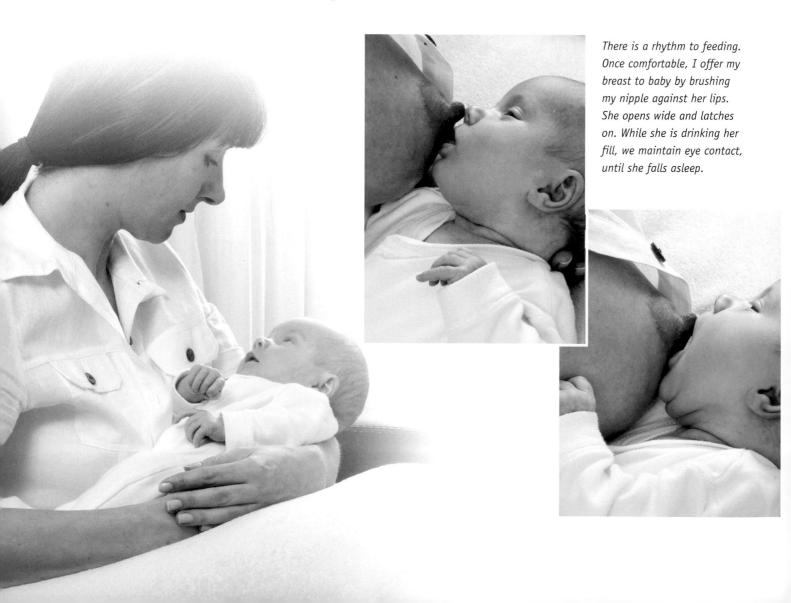

There is a rhythm to feeding. Once comfortable, I offer my breast to baby by brushing my nipple against her lips. She opens wide and latches on. While she is drinking her fill, we maintain eye contact, until she falls asleep.

OFFERING THE BREAST

I find it helpful to cup my breast with my hand or to support it by placing my fingers against my ribs just underneath it. I need to ensure that my fingers are not in a 'scissor grip' around my nipple, as this can prevent baby feeding properly. My baby's nostrils are flared, to allow her to breathe and feed at the same time, so I don't have to press my breast away from her nose. If she doesn't start to suck as soon as she feels my breast against her cheek, I brush my nipple against her lips to trigger the rooting reflex. Once she opens her mouth, I draw her to my breast.

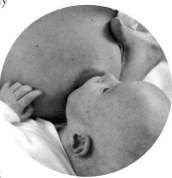

Latching on

When she is fully on my breast, much of the underside of my areola as well as my nipple will be in her mouth – near the soft part at the back – and her jaw muscles will work rhythmically. Every part of my breast releases the milk similarly and when it flows, baby drinks it slowly and steadily, and I can hear her swallowing.

If her mouth isn't sufficiently open to take in part of my breast as well as my nipple, or her tongue doesn't come well forward so she can hold on to my breast comfortably while feeding and press the milk from behind my nipple, or if her cheeks cave in when sucking, she needs repositioning. I insert my little finger in the corner of her mouth to break the suction.

If I do nothing else I will ...

ENSURE A GOOD MILK SUPPLY

To guarantee there is plenty of milk, I need to:

✓ **Encourage my baby to feed** within the first few hours of birth or start expressing milk if she can't take it directly.

✓ **Make sure baby is fully attached** to my breast at each feed; I'll get help quickly if this is difficult.

✓ **Encourage frequent feeding,** day and night, for the first few weeks; I will use a sling to carry baby around, and have her sleep close by.

✓ **Take in sufficient food and drink** and get plenty of rest; the let-down reflex works best when I feel relaxed.

Drinking her fill

My baby's sucking pattern alters while she feeds – from short sucks to longer bursts, with pauses in between. She lets me know when my breast is empty by letting the nipple slide out of her mouth, playing with the breast or falling asleep. It's important that she empties the breast to prevent blockages and ensure she gets sufficient fat content. When my breast is full, the milk is lower in fat, but as milk is released, the fat level rises. When she stops sucking, I usually offer the other breast. She doesn't always want it so I start with the second breast at the next feed. To remove her from the breast, I break the suction with my little finger.

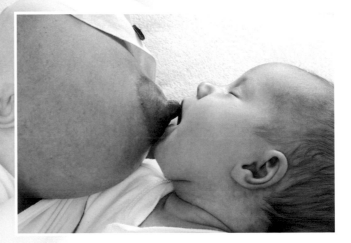

Breastfeeding twins

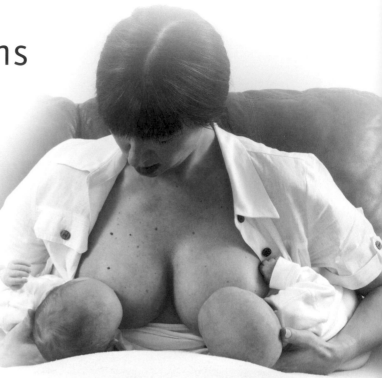

If both twins are well, feed them as soon as you are able. If one or both of the twins needs some extra care, you may need to express milk for them as soon as you can. Even if both twins latch on successfully straight away, you will need some help at first, particularly if you have had a caesarean, because finding a comfortable position and holding one or both new babies is very difficult to do without someone actively assisting you. Your partner, birth companion, nurse or midwife can cuddle one twin while you feed the other.

Most twin mothers build up a very good milk supply, as long as the babies are fed frequently, which 'orders' the milk to be made in sufficient quantities for two. Feeding twins provides double the stimulus to the breasts as a singleton, and therefore if one twin is a poor feeder or becomes ill, the breasts continue to be stimulated by the other.

MANAGING FEEDING

Most twin mothers have no fixed pattern for feeding both babies together or separately; at times, one way may just seem easier than the other. Some mothers breastfeed both babies and others breastfeed one and give expressed milk to the other – either rotating between the babies or always giving one expressed milk. Either way will ensure you have sufficient milk but you may need to keep a record of which twin you've been feeding in which way.

Feeding both twins at once can make things easier. Because new babies need feeding frequently at first, feeding separately can mean almost continuous feeding/changing/settling without a break. One drawback to breastfeeding both twins at once, however, is that if you have no spare hand when your babies are still learning to latch on and stay on, which may mean you feel uncomfortably trapped; you'll have no free hand to scratch your nose, move your hair or sip a drink. If one baby loses her latch, it can be hard to get her back on again. Some mothers find a V-shaped pillow helps

Many twin babies eventually develop a preference for one breast over the other, so if you don't want this to occur, it is better to alternate your babies at each feeding during the early weeks. Bear in mind, however, that many twins have unequal skills at breastfeeding, at least at first, so making sure each breast gets the stimulation of the better feeder is also a good idea. Creating a routine is easier when both babies are of a similar size and have similar feeding patterns. It can take up to 6 weeks to establish a routine, but once you have one it will be much easier on you.

Keeping a written record at first may be helpful and some women use different-coloured ribbons pinned to their bras as reminders.

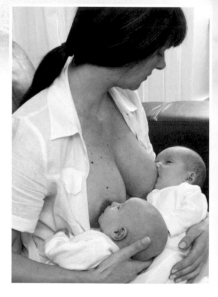

DIFFERENT POSITIONS

Feeding two at a time can be done in a number of ways – though the time to experiment is not when either of your babies is eager to be fed or when they're sleepy. You may find that a position that didn't work when your twins were new becomes easier when they're older.

The most popular positions include the football (top) and parallel (bottom) holds. Another common position with young infants is to hold them in a V shape with their feet either touching or crossed over each other. Or, you can hold one baby in the football hold and the other across your lap. Whatever position you choose, it's likely that you'll need some support for your back or to raise your babies to your breasts.

Expressing milk

There are a good number of reasons to express breast milk; I find it helpful to relieve some of the pressure of overfull breasts and to enable my partner to bottlefeed our baby occasionally at night or when I am out. It's essential if I want to maintain breastfeeding when returning to work. Expressed milk can be fed to premature babies, which not only gives them vital protective nourishment but enables their mothers to maintain their breastfeeding capabilities.

I was advised, however, not to try and intersperse bottlefeeds with breastfeeds in the early days; my baby needed time to get used to feeding from the breast and she would have had to learn a new sucking action if I fed her from a bottle. But once I was able to establish a successful routine, I tried feeding her expressed milk. Like most babies, she was reluctant to feed from the bottle at first, so it was easier to let my partner give her the bottle when I was out of the room. Some women feed expressed milk from a dropper or spoon.

Breast milk should be expressed straight into a sterile bottle for feeding or a glass or plastic container or breast milk freezer bag and stored in the fridge up to 8 days, or frozen and used within 3 months. To thaw frozen breast milk, hold the container under warm running water. Or, for a larger container, place it in a bowl of warm water. After the water cools, replace it with more warm water until the milk is thawed and warmed to body temperature.

EXPERTS ADVISE

Proper storage

Freezing destroys some of the immune properties in human milk, so it's best to give your baby fresh milk (which can be left at room temperature [up to 25°C/77°F] for 4–6 hours) or expressed milk that has been refrigerated (0–4°C/32.7°F). Label each container with the date you express it, so you can use the oldest milk first and avoid wasting any. Hard-sided containers provide the best protection for nutrients and immunities; they do not need to be sterile. Once milk has thawed, do not refreeze it.

HOW TO EXPRESS MILK

Like many women, I find it quicker, more effective and easier using a pump than expressing by hand. There are a number of pumps on the market – manual, electric and battery operated. I had to try several before I found the one that suited me. It is possible to hire a pump or like me, you could ask another breastfeeding mum whether you could try out her pump.

To use a syringe-style hand pump, simply place the funnel over your nipple, forming an airtight seal, and then draw the cylinder in and out a few times to draw out the milk. With an electric or battery-operated pump, you just need to position your breast then turn the machine on. It will draw out the milk.

To express milk by hand, stimulate your milk flow by gently stroking downwards from the top of your breast toward the areola. Then place both your thumbs above the areola and your fingers below and begin rhythmically squeezing the lower part of your breast while pressing towards your breastbone.

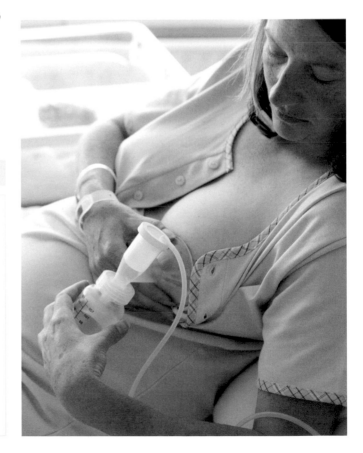

Bottlefeeding

When feeding expressed breast milk or if you feed formula milk from a bottle, good hygiene is essential (see Making up formula, below). Bottlefed babies are more prone to infections than breastfed babies.

FORMULA

Until a baby is at least a year old, she requires formula milk, which is carefully produced under government guidelines to ensure that it replicates human milk as closely as possible and contains the needed amounts of fat, protein and vitamins. Ordinary cow's milk contains high levels of protein and minerals, which can put a strain on a young baby's immature kidneys and cause dehydration, and it also lacks sufficient iron. Goat's milk and condensed milk are also unsuitable.

If you're unsure as to which formula is best for your baby, your health visitor will be able to give you guidance. Formula is available in powder, liquid concentrate and ready-to-feed forms at most supermarkets and chemists. Powdered formulas are usually the cheapest of these, but ready-to-feed forms, while the most expensive, can be useful in the first few weeks, while you're getting used to feeding. Ready-made bottles come in handy for night-time feeds, or when you're short of time or travelling. With all forms, the manufacturer's instructions must be followed carefully for your baby to receive the proper nutrients.

Don't buy or use outdated infant formula. Make sure, too, that the container is free of bulges, dents, leaks or rust spots; formula in a damaged container may be unsafe.

Full-term, bottlefed babies who are diagnosed as intolerant to lactose or protein in cow's milk, or who have other feeding or medical problems, will be prescribed one of a range of specialised formulas. These include hypoallergenic formulas and soya milks, which have been formulated to provide these babies with all the nutrients they need.

MAKING UP FORMULA

It is vital to feed a baby freshly made up formula milk, as stored milk can increase the chances of making her ill. Anti-reflux formulas are made up differently from other types. Ask your health visitor for information.

Before you begin, make sure your work surface is clean and disinfected and your hands are thoroughly washed. Bottles, teats, rings and caps must all be sterilised (see page 155). The top and lids of formula containers should be washed with soap and hot water.

Boil the water

Fill a kettle with fresh or filtered water and boil. Do not use mineral water or softened water, because the level of mineral salts can be unsuitable for babies. Pour the correct amount of cooled (but still hot), boiled water into a bottle.

If using liquid concentrate, pour the the equivalent of 1 can into a clean lidded container.

Measure the formula

Use the scoop provided to measure out the required amount of powdered formula, then level off any excess with leveller or a knife – scraping across the scoop, not patting down.

For liquid concentrate, pour 1 can into the container of cooled-down water.

Mix

Double-check the number of scoops you need and add them to the bottle. Hold the edge of a sterilised teat and place it on the bottle then screw on the retaining ring. Cover with a cap. Now shake the bottle hard so that the water and powder are thoroughly mixed.

With liquid concentrate mix, stir well with a clean spoon then store in covered container for up to 48 hours in the fridge or pour into bottles.

FEEDING MY BABY

In these early weeks, I find it useful to have commercially prepared ready-to-feed bottles on hand so baby can be feed as soon as she is hungry. This helps prevent her getting upset while waiting and then refusing to feed.

Feeding baby can be a messy business even at this stage, so I usually lay a towel over my lap to protect my clothes and put a bib on baby to avoid having to change her outfit afterwards.

It's important to be comfortable before starting and to pay attention to baby throughout. I need to hold her securely in my lap with her head in the crook of my elbow and her back supported along my forearm. I cuddle her close and talk or sing to her and also watch her all the time and respond to her demands. Occasionally she likes to pause for air or to bring up some wind; other babies may prefer to keep on feeding until all their formula has gone. I like to treat feeding times as relaxing and enjoyable occasions. I know that by the time she is 3 months old, I'll see her start to get excited when she knows her bottle is on its way.

Before feeding I always check the temperature of the milk. I shake a few drops onto the inside of my wrist; it should feel warm but not hot. If it's too cold, I either heat it gently in a pan of simmering water or hold it with the cap covering the teat under running warm water; I never warm a bottle in the microwave as it will continue to heat when it's removed and can scald baby or will heat up unevenly. If I want to cool it, I hold the bottle under running cold water.

Offering the bottle

I let baby see the bottle then stroke her cheek to prompt the rooting reflex; she automatically turns to me with her mouth open ready to suck.

I hold the bottle at an angle of about 45 degrees so that its neck is full of milk and there are no air bubbles. Then I offer the teat to baby and allow her to take it

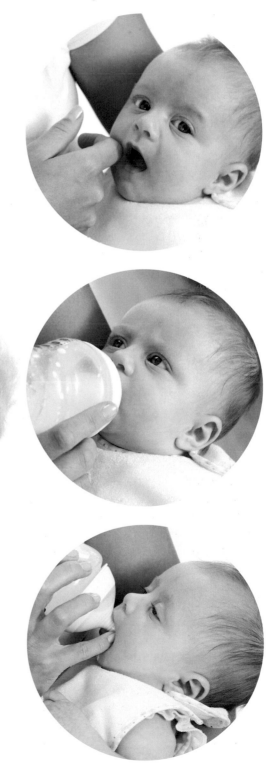

If I do nothing else I will ...

MAKE BOTTLEFEEDING MORE INTIMATE
In order to make the experience more similar to breastfeeding, I will:

✓ **Hold my baby skin to skin,** opening my clothing so the bottlefeed becomes more like a breastfeed.

✓ **Cradle my baby in my arms** rather than having her lie flat, or hold baby so she's lying back on my thighs facing me in order to maintain eye contact and physical closeness.

✓ **Try holding the bottle in my armpit,** which allows baby to be snuggled in very close, into a position similar to breastfeeding.

✓ **Talk to my baby reassuringly** while she feeds. When she seems to stop feeding, or shows she wants to slow down, I'll take the teat part way out of her mouth and watch for mouth movements that mean she's ready to re-start.

✗ **Not make my baby take her milk at too fast a pace** or more milk than she seems to want.

✗ **Not 'poke' or 'screw' the teat** inside baby's mouth if its closed. This can cause her to choke and splutter, and takes some of the control of the feed away from her.

✗ **Not let too many different people feed her;** my baby needs to get used to my partner and me first.

deep into her mouth and to begin sucking. I keep the bottle steady so that she can latch on properly.

Drinking her fill
I like to feel her sucking on the bottle. So that the top of the bottle is always full of milk, I adjust the angle, when necessary.

When baby has finished feeding or I need to wind her, I remove the bottle by gently slipping my little finger into the corner of her mouth to break the suction. Once she has finished, I throw away any unused milk. I always start the next feed with a freshly made-up bottle.

WINDING
My baby will usually swallow some air while feeding, especially when taking milk from a bottle because it is not always easy for her to make a tight seal around the teat with her mouth. Air can form bubbles in baby's stomach, causing discomfort and a feeling of fullness, so I need to help her expel the air.

Some babies need winding more than others, and sometimes a differently shaped teat can ease the problem. But if a baby simply falls asleep after a feed, there's no need to disturb her. In fact, a baby will often drift off to sleep after feeding; her eyes will start rolling and she'll give the appearance of being intoxicated but it's a perfectly normal reaction.

As well as expelling air, baby may also bring up milk that she has swallowed (known as possetting). Unlike vomiting, this spitting up is usually a dribble of milk from the mouth, which the baby hardly seems to notice. Sometimes it happens because of overfeeding, but generally it's a result of the valve at the top of the stomach not yet being strong enough to prevent fluids from rising back up. By holding baby's body straight at a 30° angle during and after feeding, I help ease the problem by making it less likely that fluids will 'run out' from the top of her stomach.

On my shoulder
I lift baby up so that her head is over my shoulder and faces away from my neck. I use one hand to support her bottom and the other to gently rub or pat her back – generally starting at the base

of her spine and moving upwards, to literally 'bring up' the trapped air.

Sitting up
Alternatively, I can raise baby into a sitting position on my lap. Supporting her neck with one hand, I use the other to gently rub or pat around her shoulder blades.

Across my knees
Sometimes, I lay baby down so that her chest and stomach rest on my knees (or her chest on the crook of my arm) with her head facing away from me and her mouth unobstructed. Then I gently rub or pat her back.

STERILISING THE EQUIPMENT
Until baby is at least 6 months old, her feeding equipment needs to be sterilised whether she is being fed expressed breast milk or infant formula. Different sterilising units are available and it's important to follow the manufacturer's directions. Before sterilising, the equipment must be thoroughly washed.

Washing bottles and teats
I always use hot soapy water and a clean bottle brush and pay particular attention to the areas where hardened milk can easily become lodged – the screw thread at the top of the bottle and the inside of the neck. When I've finished washing the outside of the teat, I turn it inside out to finish the job before rinsing everything thoroughly with cold water.

TWIN FEEDING
Although it will save time and effort to feed both babies at the same time, this can be difficult to do without an extra pair of hands to help. When the babies are young, it may be possible to feed them together – lying parallel supported in the crook of one arm (so you have two hands free to feed them) – or with their heads on your lap under your arms and their bodies facing away and supported by pillows. Later on, you may want to feed them both at the same time but with one or both sitting in an infant chair or bouncer or propped up against cushions facing outwards so you can maintain eye contact.

FEEDING WHILE OUT AND ABOUT
When I need to transport a feed, I use ready-made formula in cartons or I take some boiled water in a sealed flask and pre-measured formula in a sterile container along with a sterilised bottle.

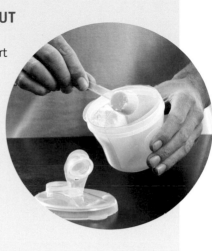

Steam sterilisers
These can be either electrical or microwave versions. Add water to the unit as per the manufacturer's instructions. Place the washed bottles upside down onto the locators on the base, the retaining rings onto the teat tray. Place the teat tray onto the central stem and position the caps over locators on the cap tray and place over the teat tray. Cover the unit, plug it into the mains socket and then switch on the mains power. Press the power button on the machine to start. The unit will heat up for sterilising then cool down. After cooling is complete, bottles are sterile and ready to use. Re-sterilise any equipment not used right away.

Cold water steriliser
Make up the sterilising solution as per the manufacturer's instructions. Loosely place the retaining rings over the neck of the bottles (do not screw on) and add to the solution along with the teats and caps. It's important that all the equipment be submerged in the water without air bubbles trapped inside. Place the sinker on top of the items – to ensure that they remain submerged in the solution – then place the lid on top. After 30 minutes the items will be sterilised and ready to use. Before use, the items must be rinsed in freshly boiled, cooled water. Do not leave anything in the sterilising solution for more than 24 hours. After 24 hours, the solution must be changed.

Overcoming difficulties with feeding

Babies are born to breastfeed; nature intends a baby to get all her food at the breast for around 6 months, then to carry on breastfeeding as she gets used to solid food. This will keep both mum and baby as healthy as possible. It may also give mum a break from menstrual periods for several months, and can reduce the chance of an unwelcome pregnancy while baby still needs a lot of attention.

Generally, if the birth was normal and a mum holds her baby straightaway, breastfeeding is likely to get going well. But for some mums, feeding can take some time to get going well. While most start breastfeeding, many women encounter problems and stop long before they had planned. The most common reasons given for stopping are:
• Baby rejects the breast.
• Breastfeeding is painful.
• Milk supply seems low.

ENGORGEMENT
Starting shortly after birth, hormonal changes prime the breasts for breastfeeding. The pituitary gland begins the process of lactation (milk production) by producing and releasing the hormone prolactin. Once this process has begun, a baby encourages milk production by her frequent sucking. Whether you're breastfeeding or not, 2–4 days after the birth, breasts become larger and firmer and may be painful as they prepare to provide milk. This is referred to as engorgement.

To ease the discomfort of engorgement, I found wearing a well-fitted, supportive bra made me feel much more comfortable; some experts recommend wearing a bra 24 hours a day during the engorgement period. Before breastfeeding, it helped me to stand under a very warm shower or put warm compresses on my breasts. (The moist heat dilated the milk ducts and, when baby sucked, the milk flowed more freely and my breasts were relieved of pressure.)

If you're not going to breastfeed, try putting a cool compress on your breasts and taking an analgaesic such as paracetamol or ibuprofen. Don't stimulate your breasts or try to express milk to relieve pressure, as this will only cause your body to produce more milk.

Engorgement lasts around 2–5 days – lack of stimulation by a sucking baby will gradually slow and then stop the production of milk. There's no need for

If I do nothing else I will ...

PREVENT PAINFUL BREASTS
By taking a few self-help measures, I can ensure that feeding remains comfortable. I need to:

✓ **Ensure my breasts aren't too firm** for baby to grasp. Before offering to baby, I should press my fingers against my breast, about 5 cm behind the nipple, and push into my chest wall working all around the darker areola until it gets softer. Pressing a little milk out first with my fingers may also help.

✓ **Lean back comfortably** and let baby lie face down on me, which may improve her feeding reflexes so she can open her mouth wider. While holding her this close, I need to support her shoulders and bottom but not her head; her chin should press into my breast so her nose is free.

✓ **Carry baby around** in a sling and offer the breast as soon as she looks interested, rather than waiting for her to cry – she won't attach so well when upset. I may have to give expressed milk to keep up my supply.

✓ **Slide baby off carefully** if my nipple starts to hurt a lot during a feed, and try again or offer the other side. I can dab my nipples with a little expressed milk or a tiny smear of pure lanolin to soothe and heal them.

✓ **Keep my breasts well drained** by offering alternate breasts at each feed. If I find any lumps after a feed I will gently massage my breasts to prevent blockages.

✓ **Express milk correctly.** My nipple has to fit the pump funnel well – some mothers need a larger funnel – and I may have to soften my breast first.

special care for healthy breasts; just wash your breasts with mild soap and rinse well.

BABY SEEMS DISINTERESTED IN FEEDING

Newborns feel safest when they are close to their mothers. Right after birth, when I held my baby close to me, skin-to-skin against my chest, this helped relax baby and made her ready to feed within an hour or so. If you were unable to do this for any reason, early feeds may be less easy, but you can correct the situation now.

If your baby appears to reject your breast, there'll be a good reason. You may feel that your baby is rejecting you, and that it might be better to switch to a bottle but your baby isn't saying 'I don't want to breastfeed' but only 'I can't manage to feed yet'.

To help your baby to become more interested in breastfeeding, hold her close as often as you can using a soft sling, if necessary, or you could put your baby inside a low-cut stretchy top to hold her against your chest. Your partner can carry her, too.

Express your milk and give it to her in a little cup. (Ask your GP or health visitor to show you how to do this safely.) When you wash the top half of your body, use plain water, so that your natural odour (which your

If I do nothing else I will ...

INTEREST MY BABY IN FEEDING

It's important that baby gets off to a good start. I can help this if I:

✓ **Keep her close,** in skin-to-skin contact, or wearing light clothing so she will be soothed by my familiar scent, voice and heartbeat.

✓ **Maintain peace and quiet** by keeping the room dimly lit, playing music that I played during pregnancy and handling my baby gently.

✓ **Give small feeds of expressed milk** by syringe or cup every couple of hours but avoiding dummies, as they might make breastfeeding harder.

✓ **Co-bathe** in a deep, warm bath with my baby face down on my chest and her tummy on my tummy.

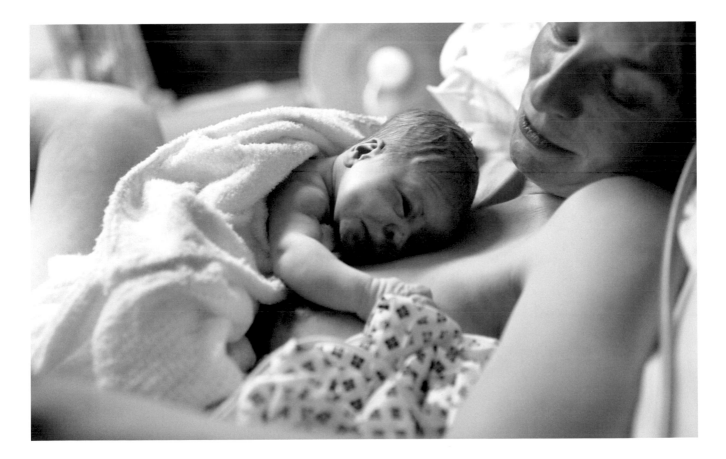

baby recognises) won't be changed. Your breasts produce a scent to attract your baby, and she will start looking for the source of your delicious milk.

If your baby is finding feeding difficult and seems fretful, it's best to keep her with you and your partner as much as possible until she settles down. Your family and friends will understand that it may be better for them to wait a bit before they give her a cuddle.

If your baby wants to feed but can't attach well – perhaps because your breast is swollen – she may become very frustrated and not want to try next time. You'll need to be very patient and gentle, and avoid pushing her head. Keep calm and offer expressed milk frequently, to help get your supply going until she's able to attach himself.

If you give expressed milk in a bottle, it will help your baby if you hold her close to your breast (with some skin contact, if possible) while you feed her.

REJECTING THE BOTTLE

Sometimes, babies used to breastfeeding reject the bottle. This can be a challenge if you are returning to work or if you have to leave your baby, and know the bottle is essential – if only she'd take it. Some parents find the solution is to offer the bottle in a way that's very different from a breastfeed.

Try positioning your baby so that she's facing you – maybe in her infant or car seat – and gently place the teat in her mouth, letting her explore it with her tongue. Stay calm and playful, and don't insist on the feed if your baby starts to show distress. Try again later.

PAINFUL BREASTFEEDING

Breastfeeding should give mothers and babies pleasure for many months. It should never hurt; any pain is a warning sign that something's not quite right. If it isn't comfy, it won't be right for your baby, so it's worth getting help quickly. With good support, the pain will go, and you will soon be able to enjoy breastfeeding.

If your nipples are sore during feeding, your baby probably isn't fully attached to your breast (see box). For baby to attach well and to get the milk to flow easily, you need to be comfortable and your breasts sufficiently soft. If your baby is lying close to you when she is ready to feed, she can move herself around to find your breast. If she can't self-attach, you may need to help her a little, but don't use any force.

It's vital that all breast parts get well drained; over-fullness can lead to painful feeding and other problems including infection of the mammary glands (mastitis).

REASONS FOR ATTACHMENT PROBLEMS

Swollen breasts. Temporary fluid retention that develops at the end of pregnancy or in labour, or from engorgement (enlarged and firmer breasts) as the milk increases a few days after birth, can make attachment difficult.

Enlarged or inverted nipples. Nipple shape may be genetic or just caused by temporary swelling; you may need specialist help for a while until your baby can manage to attach.

Baby not opening wide: If baby doesn't open her mouth well, she can't fully attach; this is common after a difficult birth.

Tongue-tie: If there's a restriction under her tongue, baby may not be able to put it out far enough to attach well. A minor procedure to snip the tie may be needed; get a breastfeeding specialist's opinion.

Check your nipples after your baby has finished feeding; they should look the same shape as before. If they're squashed, pulled out, grazed or blistered, your baby needs to get further on next time, or your nipples may then crack and bleed. One reason may be that your baby may not be close enough to your breast. Her feeding reflexes may be reduced and she may then squeeze or pull on your nipple. Your nipple then will get rubbed by the hard part of your baby's mouth.

LET-DOWN FAILURE

Being unable to produce adequate milk or milk that does not flow freely is due to failure of the let-down reflex, usually a result of unrelieved breast engorgement in the first week after birth. Sometimes let-down failure occurs if a baby has problems immediately after birth and stays in the nursery, or is very small or premature and cannot or will not suck vigorously. Depression and emotional upset also can reduce milk production. You can begin to suspect let-down failure if:
• Your breasts don't leak between feeds.
• There is no let-down sensation (mild uterine contractions immediately after birth, then pins and needles in breast after two weeks).

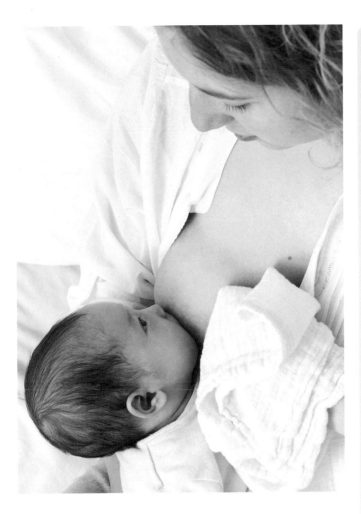

• Baby seems unhappy and appears hungry.
• Baby does not gain adequate weight.
• Baby urinates infrequently.
Feeding frequently in a quiet and relaxed place while sitting in a comfortable position with baby correctly latched on can help address the problem. Use a breast pump if your baby isn't providing adequate stimulation in terms of pressure or time at the breast. Discuss depression or emotional problems with your GP.

EXPERTS ADVISE

Pain or vomiting

If your baby seems to be in pain or vomits after every feed, then she may have a treatable condition such as reflux or gastroenteritis. Both these conditions need medical help, so contact your GP or health visitor for advice.

SUPPORT WITH FEEDING

Information on infant feeding is widely available from books, websites, professionals and friends and relatives, but not all is equally valid. It's important to ask yourself on what is the individual basing his or her advice. Grandmothers, for example, are experienced in baby care, but may be advocating routines which are out of date and no longer recommended. Midwives and baby nurses have a basic grounding in infant feeding, but may recycle outdated knowledge. Doctors get little if any teaching on this subject, even as paediatricians, and may have only been given training by a formula salesperson.

A number of organisations aim at supporting parents by enabling informed choices. Often, they provide online information, books and other resources, and run support networks. Their publications on child care and feeding issues are based on the latest evidence.

International Board Certified Lactation Consultants (IBCLC) are breastfeeding specialists with a professional qualification, which is regularly updated. Many have midwifery, nursing or other health qualifications, and some specialise as infant feeding advisers in maternity units or primary care trusts (PCTs). Others are breastfeeding counsellors with voluntary organisations and a growing number are in private practice. The UK's professional organisation for IBCLCs is Lactation Consultants of Great Britain or LCGB. Its website lists practitioners around the UK who are available to support parents in various ways.

Accredited voluntary breastfeeding counsellors (BFCs) have personal experience of breastfeeding, and take a course of training in listening skills and in helping to get breastfeeding going well and overcome any difficulties.

Peer supporters are mothers who have breastfed and have been through a short training programme. They work voluntarily in their own communities to encourage mothers by being alongside them. They refer mothers who have complex or unresolved conditions to health professionals or other breastfeeding specialists. They provide hospital and home visits, telephone counselling and support groups.

Handling my baby

Lifting, holding and carrying my baby was quite daunting at first; newborns can seem so fragile and I was concerned about providing adequate support – particularly when putting her in and taking her out of her bath. However, the more I cared for her the easier these tasks became.

HOLDING AND CARRYING

Like all new babies, mine loved – and pretty much demanded – being held a lot. I found a sling was vital in the early weeks; it enabled me to keep my hands free while baby could snuggle close and be well supported. She could also breastfeed while being in it.

Some safety issues have been raised over slings and certain models are no longer recommended (see page

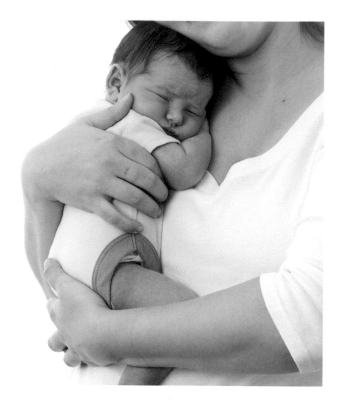

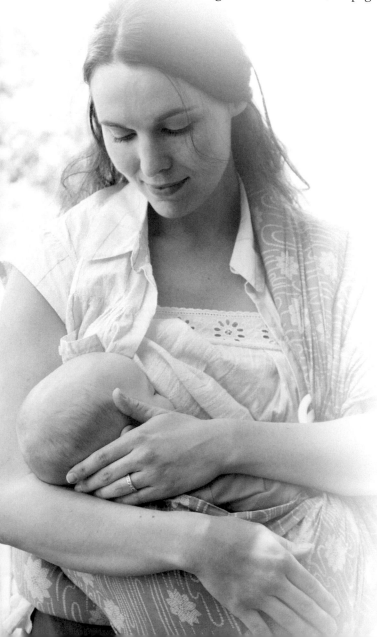

170). As I did, it's important to become acquainted with this essential advice.

When I was not using a sling, I most often held my baby resting against my shoulder; not only was this comfortable, but she was able to nestle closely against my body, where she could hear my heartbeat, which was comforting. This position also protected her from accidental knocks and bumps and bruises as I moved around my home.

At other times I would cradle baby in my arms – either face up, head nestled in the crook of my elbow or face down with his body supported on my forearm and my other hand supporting her underneath her tummy. (This latter position can be helpful if baby suffers from colic [see page 176].)

Of course, I was very careful to protect baby's head with my hand or to ensure it was tucked into my body while walking around with her to prevent it being knocked by obstacles at that level.

LIFTING BABY

Assuming the right position for lifting (and laying down) baby when she is tiny prevents backache later on when she becomes much heavier. It is important to stand with my legs slightly apart, knees bent and back straight and to lift baby close to me. Just as important is to ensure that baby's neck and bottom are supported throughout the procedure.

When lifting, I slide one hand under her neck to support her head and the other underneath her bottom. Then, taking her weight in my hands, I slowly raise her from the surface, keeping her head slightly above the level of the rest of her body. As I bring her in close to my chest, I move my bottom hand up her back to support her head as I bend the other arm to support her head in the crook of my arm. My wrists cross over each other near the middle of her back, and her bottom rests on my forearm.

LAYING DOWN
When laying baby down from a cradled position, I gently slide my arms apart so that one hand supports her head and neck, while the other supports her bottom. I then slowly move her away from my body keeping her body in line with my own. Then I bend close to the changing mat or mattress and slowly lower her, bottom first, onto the surface.

Once baby has made contact with the surface, I gently ease my supporting hand from underneath her bottom, then lower her upper body and head – making sure her head is well supported until it is resting comfortably on the surface. Finally, I gently slide my hand away.

If I do nothing else I will ...

LIFT AND HOLD MY BABY CORRECTLY
A newborn can't support her head, and getting into the wrong habits can lead to backache later on. Therefore, I must always:

✓ **Support** baby's spine, head and neck.

✓ **Protect** baby's head when walking with her.

✓ **Keep baby's head in line** with the rest of her body.

✓ **Keep baby close,** talking to her and stroking her as often as possible.

✓ **Gently wake baby** if she's sleeping so as not to startle her when I lift her.

✓ **Look into her eyes** as I lift and lay her down.

✓ **Bend my knees** when lifting.

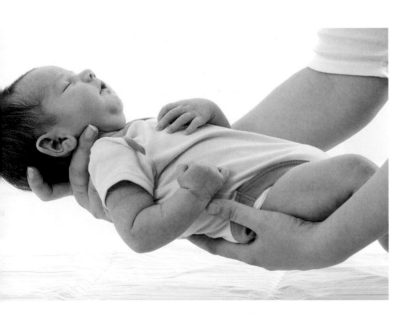

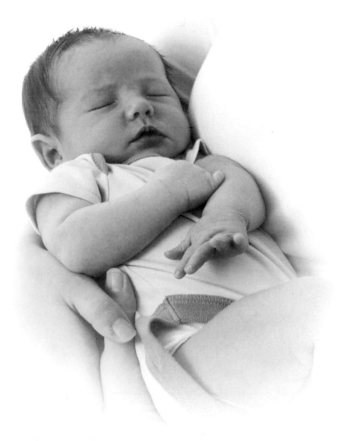

Nappy choice and changing

It's been estimated that the average baby needs around 6,000 nappy changes between birth and being toilet trained, so it's important to choose the type that best fits one's lifestyle.

TYPES

Disposables have greater absorptive capacity, will keep baby drier and are more convenient, but they also are more expensive than fabric nappies in the long term. Disposables need to be disposed of carefully but fabric nappies, while reusable, need to be rinsed, sterilised, washed and dried. In addition to fine muslin squares for a newborn and standard square cotton or terry-towelling ones for an older baby, plastic pants, nappy pins and optional liners may be needed – though some fabric nappies have a plasticised outer layer – as well as cleaning equipment (see page 164). Fabric nappies should be pre-washed before use but avoid fabric softeners as these can make the nappies less absorbent.

Pre-shaped nappies come already tailored to fit a baby's bottom, so you don't have to fold them or fiddle about with nappy pins. Most have elasticated legs and waist, as well as self-stick tabs or snap fastenings and a separate waterproof cover. You may also want to use a nappy liner. They wash and wear like ordinary fabric nappies, although you should check the care label before soaking them in sterilising solution, as the elastic around the legs and waist of some brands may be affected.

BOTTOM CREAMS, OINTMENTS AND POWDERS

Whether or not you use a cream or ointment should be on the recommendation of your health visitor or GP. Some parents regularly apply an ointment or cream in the hope of preventing rashes (see page 164), and switch to a different ointment or cream if a rash should appear (returning to the original formulation when the rash has healed). Other parents, including myself, don't use any bottom cream or ointment unless a rash appears. Baby powders, however, should never be used as they neither provide a barrier against moisture nor are effective in removing it from the nappy area. Inhaling powder aerosolised during application is potentially harmful.

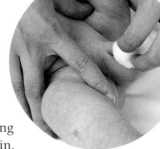

CLEANING THE NAPPY AREA

This is the first step in changing. I use cotton wool or a soft facecloth moistened in cooled, previously boiled, water or commercially available unscented baby wipes to remove any remaining stool or dried urine from baby's skin.

When cleaning my girl, I lift her bottom slightly by raising both her ankles gently with one hand. Wiping downwards, I clean the outer lips of her vulva – but not inside. Then, keeping her bottom raised and with a piece of fresh cotton wool, I clean her buttocks, the backs of her thighs and up her back, if necessary. Then I pat dry the whole area thoroughly.

When cleaning a boy, I wipe his penis using a downward motion, but I don't pull the foreskin back, and clean around his testicles. Holding baby's ankles, I lift his bottom gently and clean his anal area and the backs of his thighs. Then I pat dry the whole area thoroughly.

MY NAPPY CHANGING ROUTINE

Before I bring baby over to the changing table or mat, I make sure I have everything I need, open and ready to use. I keep a few small toys close by to help distract her for the final few seconds of the job. All the time I am changing her nappy, I talk and sing to baby, rubbing and tickling her arms, legs and feet in a gentle massage and maintaining as much eye contact as possible.

This method works for both disposables and for shaped, Velcro® or popper-closing cloth nappies.

1 I lay baby face up on the mat, making sure that I'm supporting her head and the base of her spine as I lower her down. If she's dressed, I take off all her clothes down to her vest or just her nappy.

2 I then unfasten the tabs and slide the nappy away, using an unsoiled area to give a first wipe. (Baby boys are likely to urinate shortly after a nappy is removed, in reaction to the cooler air, so I drop a tissue or wipe onto the penis to deflect the flow or, if the nappy is only wet, hold it over the genital area until the danger time has passed.)

3 Using one hand (I keep the other on baby), I roll up the nappy and place it where baby can't kick it. Now I carefully clean (see opposite) within all the skin folds, using separate pieces of cotton wool or different wipes for the genital areas and bottom to avoid spreading infection. With another piece of dry

cotton wool, I pat dry, particularly in the folds where soreness can develop.

4 Then I spread out a fresh nappy and, while gently lifting baby's legs, carefully slide it underneath her. If I was using a bottom cream or ointment (see page 162), I would apply it now to those surfaces coming into direct contact with the nappy, for these are the areas most likely to be affected with nappy rash.

5 I bring the nappy up between her legs. (If I'm changing a boy, I'll make sure that his penis points downwards so he doesn't urinate into the waistband.) Then I'll secure the nappy at the sides and tuck in the top edge neatly.

6 Once baby is removed to a safe place, I place the disposable into a bag and throw it away or place the cloth nappy into the appropriate holding bucket.

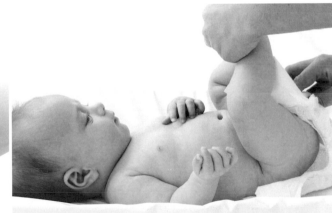

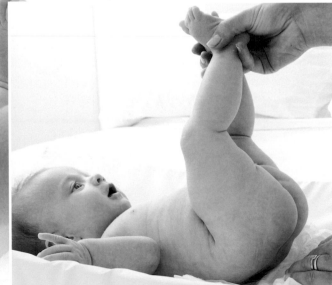

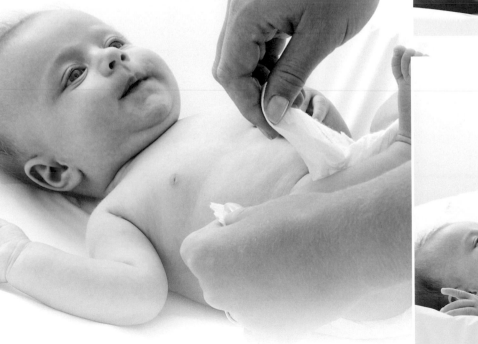

DEALING WITH SOILED NAPPIES

Both for the sake of the environment and baby's wellbeing, it is vital to dispose of or clean her soiled nappies properly.

Disposables

Soiled disposable nappies should be wrapped up so the contents don't leak and be transported as quickly as possible to an outside bin so that their odour doesn't remain in the house. Special scented sacs are available that contain the odour until the nappies can be taken outdoors; these are very useful when you can't get to an outside bin quickly.

Fabric nappies

Sterilising, washing and drying nappies are laborious processes and if incomplete, can leave waste ammonia or bacteria on the nappy that can lead to nappy rash and infection. Using too much detergent with nappies, however, will irritate baby's sensitive skin. Therefore, measure the amount of soap carefully and rinse everything twice. A nappy service will do all the hard work – but at a cost.

Vital equipment: 2 plastic storage buckets are needed – one for urine-soaked nappies the other for dirty ones – tongs, a plastic bowl and sterilising solution. A washing machine is essential and a tumble dryer is a good idea unless a nappy service is being used.

To thoroughly sterilise, nappies must be left to soak for at least 6 hours in a bucketful of sterilising solution. Using different-coloured buckets for urine-soaked and dirty nappies will make things easier and prevent mistakes. The buckets should be big enough to hold at least six nappies, but not too heavy to be picked up when filled with water. They should have sturdy handles and tight-fitting lids.

With soiled nappies, as much excrement as possible should be scraped into the toilet bowl, then the nappies should be rinsed. Biodegradable nappy liners can be removed with the stool and flushed down the toilet. Then, unless washing right away, the soiled nappy must be left to soak in the bucket with the lid tightly sealed.

Urine-soaked nappies should be rinsed under a tap then wrung out before washing or soaking.

Plastic pants should be washed in tepid water and some washing-up liquid; they will harden if the water is too hot or cold. If they do stiffen, they can be softened by tumble drying them on a low setting for 10 minutes.

NAPPY RASHES

Nappy rashes are quite common and are caused primarily by irritation from urine and faeces. Wetness from urine interferes with the skin's barrier capacities

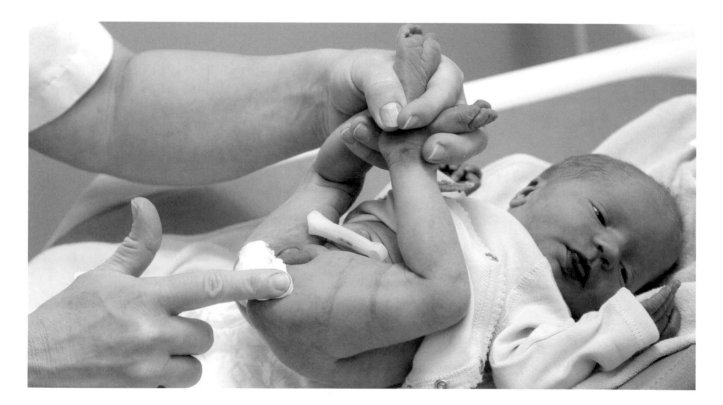

If I do nothing else I will ...

TREAT NAPPY RASHES
Self-help measures can prevent or help heal rashes. I need to:

✓ **Change nappies often.**

✓ **Clean baby's skin gently** with water and a soft facecloth or with an alcohol-free wipe.

✓ **Expose her skin to air** as often as possible. I either let her lie on a mat with no nappy on or hold her on my lap so she sits on an open nappy.

✓ **Use a barrier ointment or cream** (zinc oxide or petroleum jelly).

against other irritants. One plus for disposable nappies is that highly absorbent ones are much better at keeping the wetness off the skin's surface than fabric nappies.

Friction between the skin and the nappy exacerbates irritation so that rashes occur most frequently in the skin areas that are in closest contact with the nappy and rarely occur in the thigh creases. Waste products from both urine and faeces can damage the skin as well. Preventing and treating nappy rashes involves minimising the factors that go into making a nappy rash.

In order to lessen baby's chances of contracting a rash, I use highly absorbent disposables and change them often. I make sure the nappies aren't put on too tightly as this increases the friction between the material and her skin.

PERSISTANT NAPPY RASHES
Even if appropriate steps are taken, a nappy rash may persist. It is hard to prevent irritation if a baby has diarrhoea or is sleeping through the night and is exposed to urine for long periods.

Another cause is a Candida infection of the skin. This yeast, which lives in the intestinal tract, reaches the nappy area in faeces. It also is present in higher numbers when a baby takes an oral antibiotic. The higher number of organisms, combined with diarrhoea that is likely to result from the antibiotic's effect on beneficial intestinal bacteria, make a rash more likely. Usually, a yeast infection occurs in skin already

irritated, so a baby may have a secondary infection. If you believe your baby has a Candida rash, call your GP. Although treatment varies, an ointment effective against yeasts, such as clotrimazole or terbinafine, is typically prescribed. Some GPs also recommend adding hydrocortisone cream to the regimen to treat the underlying irritant rash as well.

CIRCUMCISION CARE
Once the original dressing has been taken off, you can clean the circumcised area at nappy changes. While the rest of the nappy area can be cleaned with a facecloth or wipe, do not use these on the penis until the circumcision has healed. The bright red colour of the head of the penis gradually becomes less red and, when healing is finished, ends up being a light purplish-blue. You will have been prescribed ointment-soaked gauze or ointment.

Using clean cotton wool soaked in cooled-down boiled water, gently dab the head of the penis. Remove any attached crusty material if it comes off easily. Let the penis dry in the air. Then apply either the ointment-soaked gauze or the ointment with your finger. When reapplying the nappy, put it on so that it fits snugly against the penis. You may think that this will be uncomfortable for your son, but a snug nappy prevents the penis from moving around in the nappy (which is much more irritating).

It is good practice to clean the groove where the head of the penis meets the shaft. It is there that thick white mucus secretions produced by skin glands can, if not regularly removed when changing nappies or at bath time, cause adhesions (when the skin at the end of the shaft sticks to and grows together with the skin of the glands).

Infection following circumcision is rare, but if your newborn develops a fever and is especially fussy, this could indicate infection. The shaft of the penis, which is not involved in the circumcision, should retain its normal colour; redness of the skin of the shaft closest to the head of the penis also may signify infection. Call your GP immediately if you are concerned that an infection is possible, as this has the potential to become quite serious.

Keeping my baby clean

My baby doesn't really get dirty – save for the nappy area (see page 162) – so most of the time I just give her a quick once-over to clean the more exposed parts of her body, making sure I pay special attention to her numerous skin folds, where dirt and perspiration are easily trapped.

Her naval needs cleaning daily until the umbilical cord remnant falls off and the area surrounding it is completely healed.

I don't give baby a bath every day, but when I do I do it quickly as she doesn't much like being naked. Neither do I shampoo her hair frequently; I just wipe it with a damp cloth and sponge.

MY TOPPING AND TAILING ROUTINE

Before I begin I lay out everything I need within easy reach – a bowl of cooled boiled water, cotton wool, a soft towel or cloth and a bowl or bin to hold the used cotton wool.

Eyes and ears: I wipe each eye, above and below, from the inner to the outer corner, with some cotton wool dampened with cooled boiled water. I use a different piece of cotton wool for each wipe and each eye, to reduce the chances of spreading infection. I then wipe around and behind the ears – not inside – with more cotton wool.

Neck: I wipe this clean with wet cotton wool and pat dry with a soft cloth.

Hands and feet: I unclench baby's hands to check for dirt between her fingers and underneath her nails. I wipe everything clean and pat dry as before. Then I clean the top and bottom of baby's feet, and between her toes, gently easing them apart, where necessary. before patting them dry.

Stomach and legs: If these are dirty, I wipe her tummy with more wet cotton wool then use new cotton wool to start on the folds where her legs meet her torso. I wipe down along the creases and away from her body to avoid transmitting infections to the genitals. Finally, I pat dry with the towel, checking that no moisture is trapped in the folds.

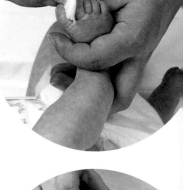

Umbilical cord area: I use clean cotton wool, moistened with rubbing alcohol, to gently wipe the stump, the area around it, and the crevices of the navel. I then pat dry the area gently.

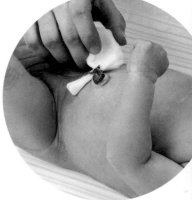

Umbilical cord

The stump will dry and heal much faster if you expose it to air as much as possible. In particular, don't cover it with plastic pants or nappies and, if it does get wet, make sure it is thoroughly dried.

MY BATHING ROUTINE

I use a plastic baby bath, placed on the floor or other well-supported surface, with a plastic sheet underneath. Before giving baby a bath, I make sure the room is sufficiently warm and that baby's face cloth, fresh clothes and clean nappy are within easy reach, but not so close that they can be splashed. I place a soft towel on top of her changing mat close to the bath. I also have a gentle baby wash to hand, though it's possible to just use water. Shampoo is not needed until she's older.

I add about 5–8 cm water to the bath. The water temperature is essential – 30°C (86°F) on a bath thermometer – you don't want to scald or freeze her.

Until she gets to love her bath, I talk and sing to her all the time to help keep her calm. When I want to clean baby's hair, I do so just before I put her in the bath. After her bath, I lift her straight out onto her towel, which is a soft, safe surface for drying.

Into the water: Kneeling close to the bath, I cradle baby in my arms, supporting her bottom with one hand and her head and shoulders with the other. I lower her gently into the water, bottom first.

Chest and stomach: Keeping baby's head and shoulders supported – I grip her gently under the arm to prevent her from slipping down into the water or rolling over – I gently wash water over her chest and stomach.

Neck and back: I sit her up, supporting her chest at the front, and gently pour water down the back of her neck and upper back.

Lower back: I then tip her further forwards, taking care to keep her face out of the water, and wash water over her lower back and bottom.

Drying: I lean her back so her head, neck and shoulders are now resting on my hand and forearm and, using the

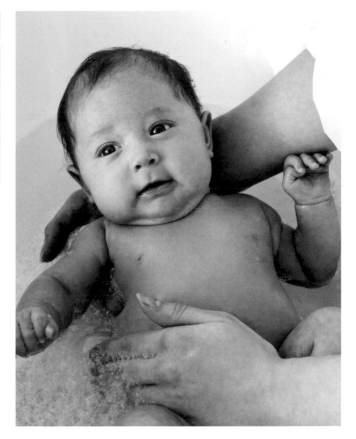

same grip as I used to lower her in, I lift her out, supporting her bottom as well. Then I place her on her towel and wrap her up to keep her warm. I make sure I don't cover her face. Then I dry her all over, paying special attention to her body creases. Sometimes, I lean her against my shoulder to pat her dry.

MY HAIRWASHING ROUTINE

The simplest way of doing this is to first wrap her in her towel and then lay her face up along one arm. Her head should be over a bath filled with warm water. I use my free hand to scoop up some water to rinse her hair, making sure that no water runs onto her face and eyes. Then I pat her head dry with a towel. I finish by brushing her hair with a soft baby brush.

Fontanelle

On the top of baby's head near the front is a diamond-shaped patch. Known as the fontanelle, this area of skin covers a tough membranous layer, underneath which lay skull bones that have not yet fused together. (This eased her journey through the birth canal.) Although it may move as baby breathes, I don't have to worry about touching it. In about a year, the skull bones will close.

Dressing my baby

Most of the time, my baby wears a one-piece babygro with a short-sleeved vest underneath. My favourite garments are those made of soft, natural fibres, which are hardwearing but comfortable, and have room for growth. Before I buy or put anything new on baby, I check for raised seams and scratchy labels. I can cut the labels out but raised seams will annoy her.

Like other babies, mine doesn't like having her clothes changed; she fusses when she feels air on her skin and garments being placed over her head. When I dress her, I always have everything within reach so I never have to leave baby alone on her changing mat, even though she can't turn over yet.

HOW MANY CLOTHES DOES SHE NEED?
It's important that my baby not be too hot or too cold but 'just right', so the correct number of garments is important. As a guide, my baby needs about the same number of layers that I'm wearing, and to ensure that I can more easily control her temperature by reducing or increasing the layers as necessary, thin garments are better than one thick item. Had she been born premature or is small for her dates, I would put one more layer on her. When I'm wearing a sling or using a carrier, I have to count it as a layer of clothing.

In hot weather, I may dress her only in a vest and a nappy, or perhaps just a nappy; in cold weather, I usually put a jumper over her babygro (unless she is in a sling) and add a hat. In order to check if my baby is warm enough, I place my (warm) hand under her vest and touch her chest or back – she should feel just warmer than my hand.

Baby mittens
My newborn's nails are very sharp so to prevent her scratching herself, I cover them with a pair of soft, cotton mittens, often called 'stratch mitts'.

USING A VEST
I like vests that join at the crotch with poppers – because these don't ride up letting my baby's back become cold – and that have an envelope neckline – because these are easy to slip over baby's head and can be pulled down over her shoulders and off her legs, which is ideal when the bottom of her vest is soiled and I don't want to pull it over her head.

I try and talk to her throughout and always gently ease the garments over her head and limbs.

Over her head: Keeping the vest at the back of her head, I gather up the material at the bottom then stretch the neck opening wide. I gently raise her head, manoeuvring the opening over the crown of her head, and gently pull the vest down over her head and neck.

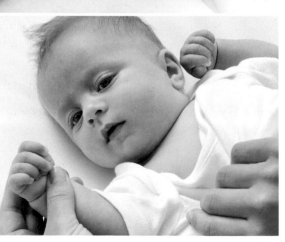

Putting her arms in the sleeves: I straighten the fabric around her neck then take one sleeve and gather up the material in one hand leaving my thumb and forefinger just inside. I gently take hold of baby's wrist with my other hand and place it inside the sleeve (using my thumb and forefinger to ease her hand through). Then I

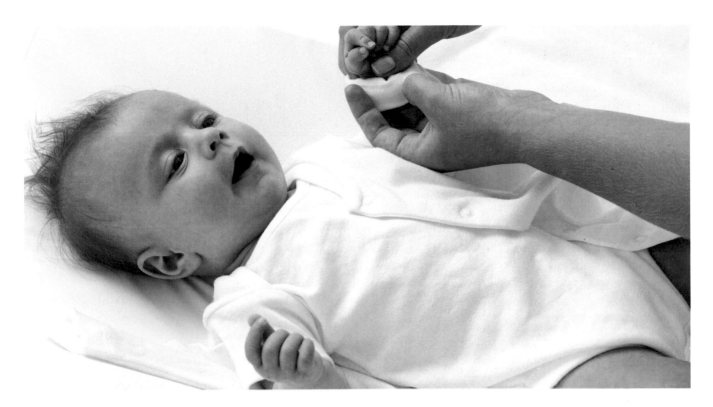

gently pull the sleeve down her arm. I repeat this with the other sleeve.

Doing up the poppers: Once both arms are free, I gently smooth the fabric over her front, lifting her bottom slightly in order to slide the tail of the vest underneath and up through her legs. I then join the front and back poppers.

Removing a clean vest: After undoing the poppers, I slide the vest up her body. Gathering up a sleeve in one hand, I use my other hand to gently guide baby's arm out of each sleeve. Then I gather up the vest at her neck and stretch the opening as wide as possible to avoid dragging the material over her face. I pull the vest up over her face to the crown of her head in one smooth motion then gently lift her head to remove the vest.

Removing a dirty vest: Having removed the soiled nappy and given baby's bottom a quick clean, I gently lift up her head. Then I stretch one corner of the neckline over her shoulder and repeat this on the other side. Laying her back down, I slide the neck opening down each arm. Then I stretch open the neckline again and gently lift her arms from each sleeve. Finally, I gather up the material and slide it down her legs.

USING A BABYGRO
While my baby is young, she wears an all in one suit 24 hours a day. Before putting one on, I open all of the poppers and spread the babygro out. Then I lay her on top of the suit.

Putting in her arms: I gather up the sleeve material and gently slide it over baby's wrists, making sure that I don't catch her fingers or nails. With some suits, I have to stretch the wrists if they are too tight to fit her hands through them.

Putting in her legs: Taking each leg in turn, I gather up the material and slide in her foot until her toes reach the end. Then run the material fully up her legs.

Fastening: I line up the two sides of the bodysuit on baby's front and fasten the poppers from the top down to the crotch. I then fasten the leg poppers on one leg from the ankle up to the crotch, and then do the other leg, again starting from the ankle.

Removing: I undo all the poppers and support one knee at a time as I ease the material off the legs. Then I lift up baby's bottom and slide the lower half of the suit up her back. Supporting baby's elbow, I gently remove each arm from its sleeve without tugging. If the bottom half is soiled, I start at the arms and work downwards.

Going out...or staying in

I know it is important to allow myself to rest and recover from labour and delivery so, during these first few weeks, I only take baby out for brief walks rather than any long outings. Being outdoors is therapeutic as well as enjoyable. I make sure that baby is dressed properly but am aware that if I feel uncomfortably cold or hot, then baby feels the same, so I either go back inside or to a place where the temperature is more suitable, perhaps adjusting my layers of clothing.

Because the vast majority of infections are spread by face-to-face interactions, I avoid cramped, closed-in spaces (such as busy shops or crowded restaurants) but take walks in the park, around my neighbourhood or a nearby shopping centre.

Some of the time I take baby out in her pram, but for short walks or excursions I 'wear' her in a sling or carrier, which, while keeping her close, enables me to keep my hands free. It's important to remember that a carrier or sling counts as a layer of clothes, so baby should be dressed in one layer less than I am wearing when I take her out in a sling or carrier.

USING A SLING

Like lots of mums, I find slings are great for keeping baby close. As well as using them for taking baby out, I often put her in one when I'm home doing chores or when she's crying. Wearing a sling also means I can breastfeed my baby discreetly when I'm in a public place or restaurant.

Slings are essentially lengths of fabric or shawls, without the padding that carriers have. They are most suitable for babies up to 3 months but seek advice before using if your baby was premature or suffers from breathing problems or has a cold.

It's very important to use one in the correct way. If the fabric blocks a baby's nose and mouth, he could suffocate. So, of course, a baby must never be put face down in a sling or held so that his chin curves down to his chest, which can also restrict breathing. When I use a sling, I am always extremely careful to be aware of baby's position and to protect her head with my hands when bending forward or to the side. I also try and avoid any bumping or jarring movements.

To ensure my baby's safety, it's important that:
- The sling should fit snugly against my body so that baby is kept high and tight against my chest, not around my waist or hips.
- Baby's face and the front of her chest should always face upwards and her body and chin must be held high off her chest.
- Her face must be completely clear and uncovered.
- I am always able to see my baby's face without opening any of the fabric, and I need to check on her regularly. Her face should be close enough to mine so that I can bend down and kiss her frequently.
- If wearing her in the sling, I must take care not to fall asleep with her in it.

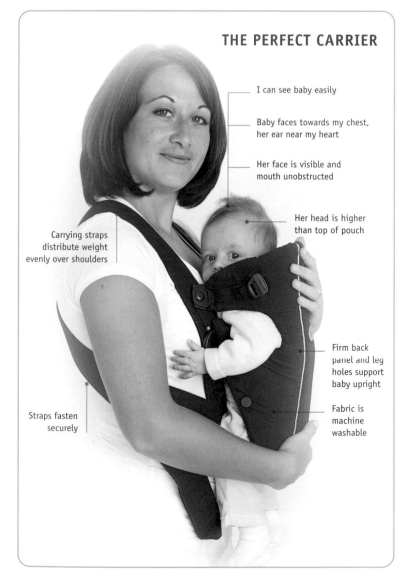

THE PERFECT CARRIER

I can see baby easily

Baby faces towards my chest, her ear near my heart

Her face is visible and mouth unobstructed

Her head is higher than top of pouch

Carrying straps distribute weight evenly over shoulders

Firm back panel and leg holes support baby upright

Fabric is machine washable

Straps fasten securely

USING A CARRIER

Some styles leave a baby's legs and arms free, others form more of a cradle. Before buying a carrier, make sure that the sling offers good head and back support, has wide shoulder straps, is comfortable and can be put on easily without help. All buckles, zips and fasteners should work smoothly and the fabric should be washable and shrink-proof. It should also have a 'meets safety standards' tag.

A model should be chosen according to baby's weight – many carriers aren't suitable for newborns or prem babies (though there are some models for very small babies) – and the manufacturer's instructions need to be followed carefully when putting it on.

HATS

In the cooler months, I always put a hat on baby – a light one most of the time and a heavier one when my head feels a little cold. In the summer, a sun hat is essential in the sunshine to shade her from the rays.

VISITORS

Shortly after delivery, my relatives and friends began arriving, hoping to see and perhaps hold my newborn. Although I was happy to see my close friends and relatives, I tried to keep the visits short. After all, I need time to recover, rest and relax and want some privacy when breastfeeding – at least until it is well established. I rely on my partner to keep a close eye on me and advise guests and would-be-visitors that I have to rest.

I am also worried that visitors will bring germs that could spread to my newborn. Young babies are more susceptible to severe bacterial infections than older children and adults, and if such an illness occurs, it can progress rapidly. However, it is more likely that visitors will more readily introduce colds and flu germs, which I also want to avoid. As most infections are spread by close contact and touching, I do the following:

- Tell people with coughs and colds to put off visiting until they are well.
- Only let a few close family members and friends hold baby – and only after they have washed their hands. Other visitors are allowed to look at, but not touch or kiss, baby.
- Refuse to let anyone smoke near my baby or in my home.

I know there are some people who think I'm being neurotic, but I am determined to keep baby safe. It is easy to do as I want if I say that I am taking my health visitor's or GP's advice.

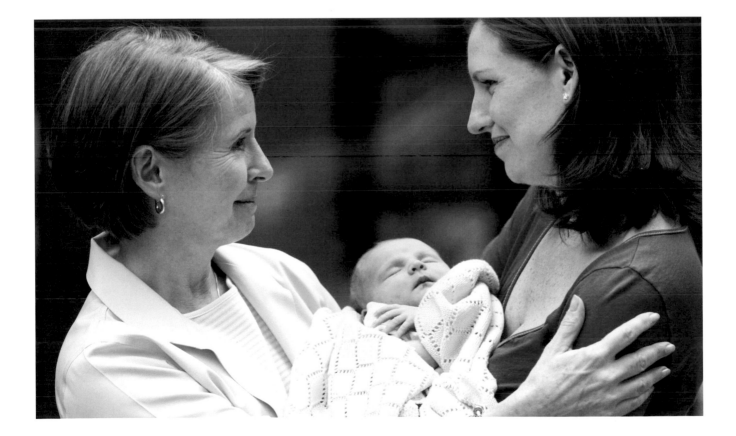

Putting my newborn safely to bed

WHERE AND IN WHAT?

For at least the first 6 months, my baby will sleep in my bedroom next to my bed. This makes it easier to feed her and I'm better able to respond if she has trouble breathing or stops moving (see SIDS page 174).

While she is small, I am putting her to bed in a Moses basket, which I can move to different parts of my home so she can keep me company or come with me when I go out. Some parents have their babies sleep in a cot from the start since they'll quickly outgrow the basket. If my baby was born pre-term (before 37 weeks) and/or had a low birth weight (less than 2.5 kg) my doctor would probably have recommended that she sleep in a cot. My baby will probably use her cot (which I will select using the checklist on page 185) until she is at least 2, after which she'll need a bed. I may try to find a cot that can be converted into a junior bed, which she may be able to use up to age 6 or so.

Safety considerations

When I leave my baby in her cot, I always secure the cot side in the 'up' position, ensure that there are no toys in her cot that could present a risk of choking or suffocating, or leave my baby alone in her cot with a bottle as this presents a choking risk, too.

Once she can stand or kneel, I must move toys hanging over the cot, such as mobiles, out of her reach. And once she can kneel and later stand, I need to start checking the height of the cot side to ensure it reaches her chest and there is no risk of her falling out. Once the cot side is below her chest, the mattress base needs to be lowered. When the cot side comes to below the level of her chest and the base is at its lowest level, my baby will need to be moved to a bed.

SAFE SLEEPING

My baby's position, sleepwear and bedding and the temperature of her room are all vital in ensuring she is at low risk for SIDS (sudden infant death syndrome (see page 174). My baby must always be put on her back to sleep and neither her nightclothes nor her bedding be overly warming (see below for gauging body temperature). It's important, too, that her room is kept at a temperature of about 18°C (65°F). I always ensure that:

- Covers are no higher than baby's shoulders.
- Baby's feet touch the foot of her cot.
- Cot is free of bumpers, sheepskins, duvets and pillows.
- Fitted cotton sheets are used; they won't crease when my baby moves around.
- Cotton cellular blankets are used; I can add or take away a blanket, as necessary.
- Baby's head is left uncovered; this enables heat to be lost as necessary and avoids overheating.

To check whether my baby is sufficiently warm, I feel her tummy, not her hands and feet, as the hands and feet tend to feel cool most of the time.

CHOOSING A COT

- [ ] The cot is new or, if second-hand, I know its history and that it meets current safety standards.

- [ ] The bars should be spaced appropriately and there should be no sharp edges.

- [ ] The side can be lowered so I will be able to put my baby into bed and lift her out easily without straining my back.

- [ ] The mattress is new and carries a Kitemark® tag. It has a waterproof cover, which can be easily wiped after leakages.

- [ ] It will either be made of foam, natural fibre or with coiled springs, depending on how much I want to spend (foam is cheaper than natural fibres) and whether I want it to be hypoallergenic.

- [ ] There will be no more than a 2.5 cm gap between the mattress, the cot sides and the ends – to prevent my baby becoming trapped.

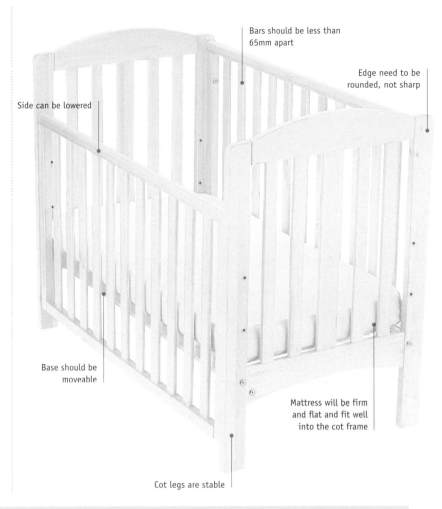

Bars should be less than 65mm apart

Edge need to be rounded, not sharp

Side can be lowered

Base should be moveable

Mattress will be firm and flat and fit well into the cot frame

Cot legs are stable

Monitoring my baby

Like all new parents, I feel it is completely natural and normal to want to keep an eye on my sleeping baby and will want to check on her frequently. By using a baby monitor, I will keep in constant contact with her, which will be reassuring. I will be able to listen to her when she is in another room.

There are many monitors on the market; the most basic will allow me to simply listen to my baby, others have lights to represent my baby's sounds or show the temperature in her room. I need to check out the various options to find the one that meets all my concerns and needs.

I may also use a breathing monitor that sounds an alarm if my baby stops breathing.

Nightclothes

While my baby is small, I put her to bed in a vest, nappy and babygro or sleepsuit, but when she's a bit bigger and more active, I'll put her in a sleeping bag, which cannot be kicked off as sheets and blankets can. The best one to choose will be based on my baby's weight – not age. If I choose too big a bag, there is a risk of her slipping down inside. Sleeping bags usually have a tog measurement or warmth rating; the higher the tog, the warmer the bag. A 2.5-tog bag is recommended for standard conditions (a room temperature of 16–20°C [61–68°F).

As my baby becomes more active, she may want to move around more than a bag allows, in which case it will be time to change the bag for sheets and blankets.

SLEEP STRATEGIES

Like most babies, mine sleeps for about 4–5 hours at a time, and because I'm breastfeeding I expect this to continue for some months. If I were bottlefeeding, my baby might start sleeping for longer periods sooner (as formula milk is more filling. In all, my baby sleeps for around 16 hours per day, but wakes frequently in the night. Because she wakes so frequently, I'm finding it hard to get sufficient rest myself and therefore have resolved upon two courses of action: establish different routines for nap times and bedtime and make sure I try and get some sleep then.

Nap times

Although my baby sleeps a lot during the day – since she doesn't recognise day from night – this will gradually decrease over the coming months, so that by 6 months of age she may sleep for an hour or two twice a day and by the age of 1, she may have only a single nap. To help her recognise day from night, I make sure that when she is awake, I spend time playing, singing and massaging her and when she falls asleep, I treat these nap times differently. For example, I:

• Let her sleep wherever she happens to be – in her Moses basket, chair or playmat – as long as its safe.

☥ EXPERTS ADVISE

SIDS (Sudden Death Infant Syndrome)

Every parent's nightmare, this is said to occur when a baby dies suddenly and unexpectedly before the age of one and no detectable cause can be discerned. The baby usally dies painlessly in her sleep in her cot (hence its old name, cot death), but may also die in her pram or even while being held. Premature and low birth-weight babies and boys are at greatest risk but it can affect any baby. Death normally occurs during the night, between midnight and 9 am.

Although the exact cause is unknown, recent research has led to a better understanding of the risks and preventative measures (see page 172). One vital preventable risk factor is smoking – both during and after pregnancy. Exposure to one parent's smoke doubles the risk of a baby dying of SIDS. Don't let anyone smoke in the same room as your baby and don't burn incense in your baby's room.

SWADDLING

Wrapping my baby so that her limbs are unable to move freely and disturb her can ensure she will drift off to sleep. The trick is to make her feel secure without wrapping too tightly or completely restricting her movements. I check to see that the blanket is not too tight around her neck and I wrap her so that she has access to her hand and fingers, which can be comforting.

- Not try to dim the lights or cushion her from normal household noises.
- Stop her sleeping more than 4 hours to begin with and fewer hours later on.

Bedtime routine

Although she won't settle into a recognisable pattern for at least 3 months, I am going to try and establish a regular pattern of events that may help my baby to know when it's time to sleep. Among the things I will do leading up to bedtime are to:
- Feed her in a dimly lit and quiet room.
- Engage in some relaxing activities, such as giving her a bath, trying some gentle baby massage or rocking her with some soothing music – especially the song I played her when I was pregnant.
- Dress her in nightclothes different from those she wears in the daytime.
- Put her down in her night-time bed in a dimly lit room.
- Give her a cuddle and kiss, gently say "good night".
- If she finds it difficult to sleep or wakes up and cries, I'll return to gently stroke her and talk quietly to her, but not pick her up.

If I do nothing else I will ...

SAFEGUARD MY SLEEP
To take care of my baby I need to be reasonably alert, relaxed and rested! Therefore, I have resolved to do the following:

✓ **Grab some sleep when baby does,** even though there's lots that needs to be done.

✓ **Take up any offers of help.** Someone else may volunteer to do some chores while I get some rest.

✓ **Go to bed early.**

✓ **Feed baby just before I go to bed.**

✓ **Get partner to help.** He can give baby at least one night-time bottle (if using expressed milk or bottle-feeding).

✓ **Keep her changing supplies close to my bed** to minimise night-time disturbances.

1 On a flat a surface, I lay a soft blanket so that it forms a diamond. I fold down the top corner to meet the bottom, forming a triangle, and place baby in the centre with her head above the fold.

2 Holding baby's right arm by her side, I gently pull the right side of the blanket across her body and tuck the corner under baby's left side.

3 I then bring up the bottom of the blanket to her chest making sure her toes have some wiggle room before gently pulling the right-hand corner of the blanket over baby and tucking it in under her left side.

4 If it's not already out, I reach in and gently pull baby's right hand free of the blanket.

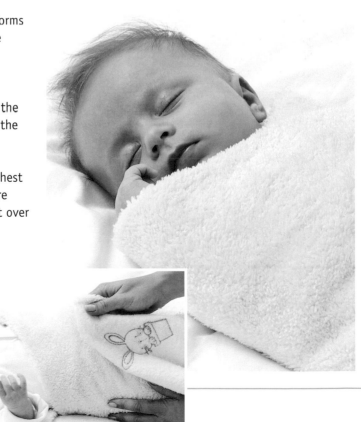

Responding to my baby's cries

I know that in crying, my baby is trying to tell me something – even if it's only that she's bored. I'm slowly beginning to understand her different cries – that she needs food, a drink, relief from discomfort (wind, heat, coldness, wetness, noise, bright lights) or someone to comfort her. Of course, over time, I'm hoping to be able to respond more effectively by learning to predict her needs, getting to know how she will react to certain situations and stimulants, observing her daily patterns of behaviour or by recognising her body language as she builds up to another bout of tears.

COLIC

Some babies cry for long periods for no discernible reason. Known as colic, as many as 20 per cent of infants suffer from screaming fits associated with

Movement often soothes baby's cries. I try putting her in a bouncy chair, holding her against my shoulder or in my lap while I move, dancing with her in my arms or swinging her in a hammock.

CAUSES OF PERSISTENT CRYING
Although colic is not considered to need medical treatment – you just have to wait it out – there are some other conditions that may need a doctor's attention:
- Immature digestive system or nervous system.
- Intolerance to cow's milk (delivered through breast milk or in formula).
- Lactose overload.
- Infection or illness.
- Birth injuries.
- Stressed mother.
- Difficult birth.

Other things to consider are that your baby's nervous system is still developing and she cannot yet cope with loud noises, bright lights or even the general stresses and sounds of home life going on around her.

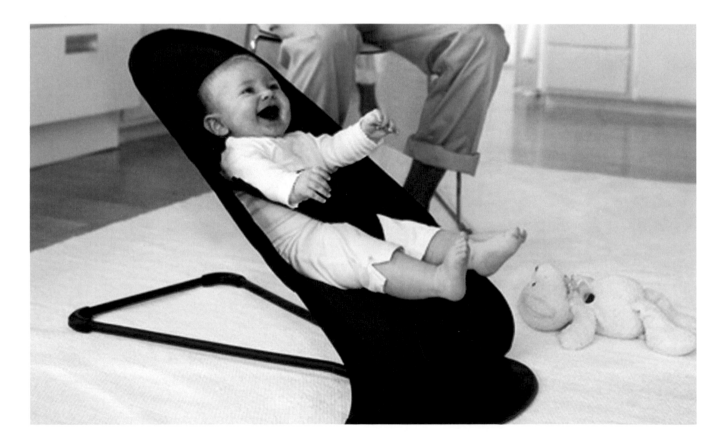

clenched fists and knees held up to the abdomen. Typically these crying spells start at 2–4 weeks of age, gradually increase in duration and intensity, and peak at about 6–8 weeks of age. Once the peak is reached, episodes gradually become milder until they go, usually at about 3 months of age, but occasionally lasting up until 6 months. Colic most often occurs in the evening, ending somewhere between 11 pm and midnight. There seem to be few distinguishing factors, as it occurs equally in girls and boys, in breastfed and bottlefed infants, in rich and poor, in firstborn and subsequent family members, and in those born vaginally and by caesarean section.

SOOTHING MY CRYING BABY

I try never to leave my baby to cry for more than a few minutes, as she becomes even more distressed and then

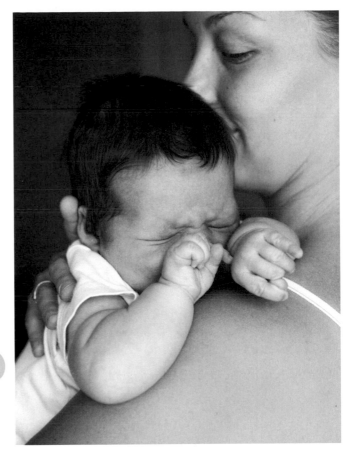

If I do nothing else I will ...

LEARN TO LIVE WITH CRYING

As not all crying can be 'cured', it's important I try and deal with my reactions. I will:

✓ **Find some way to direct any anger away** from baby. Deep breathing or listening to music with earphones often proves calming.

✓ **Learn to cheer myself up** by thinking about a joke or watching a funny movie.

✓ **Ask my partner to allow me some free time** away from baby or give me a relaxing massage.

✓ **Ask for help from my GP** or health visitor; there may be a problem.

✓ **Remember to 'pat myself on the back'** when I do something right and leave notes around the house that offer a positive message.

✓ **Leave baby to cry in a safe place** if it all gets too much.

✓ **Call my doctor** if I feel very sad or hopeless or am lacking in energy or tearful.

I find it difficult to know why she began crying in the first place. Young babies can't be 'spoiled' but they can become non-responsive if their cries are ignored. In responding to my baby's cries, therefore, I am letting her know that her needs are important to me and that they will be met.

So, generally, when my baby cries, I think whether she might need feeding, picking up, cuddling, talking to, having her nappy changed or being in a dark, dimly lit room. Naturally, once I've decided on the reason, I do what I think will stop it. If baby cries when I put her to bed, I usually wait a little while to see whether she will stop crying by herself. If not, I will go in to her.

Sometimes, however, none of the usual responses seems to work, so I have a repertoire that includes:
• Rocking and swinging.
• Firm, rhythmic bottom patting.
• Massage.
• Distraction (bathing and toys).
• Swaddling (see page 174).
• Gentle crooning.
• Going out with her in a buggy or car.

Looking after a prem baby or twins

Parents of premature or twin babies face additional challenges in mastering all the essential chores of baby care. Parents of premature infants often feel overwhelmed initially by the responsibilities that go along with caring for their infants at home while parents of twins commonly complain of the physical strain of managing two sleeping and feeding schedules simultaneously. Breastfeeding, while especially important to premature and twin babies (who are often premature) can be more difficult to establish – a prem baby may be unable to feed at the breast at birth and for weeks after, and managing two babies at the breast takes some effort (see page 150).

PREM BABY CONSIDERATIONS

You will not only need to stock up on smaller nappies, vests and outfits (easily found on the internet if not in baby shops), and a specially designed car seat but you may need to adjust your 'nursing skills', when dispensing medications and vitamins (see page 252), and be able to follow very specific instructions about feeding schedules or caring for ongoing medical conditions. While discharge instructions will be relatively short for a late preterm infant whose only problem is slow feeding, there may be a great deal more for you to do at home if your baby was much more premature or experienced complications.

Very premature infants often have continuing medical issues, so you will have to learn from the SCBU staff the special care your baby requires at home. In addition to giving vitamins and perhaps other medications, your baby may require oxygen or other special equipment or monitors with which you must become familiar. If your baby had major respiratory problems or apnoea (occasional long pauses in between breaths), you may be taught special CPR (resuscitation) techniques (see page 265) in the unlikely case that you will need to use them.

Maintaining body temperature

Although when he comes home your baby will have reached the point where he can keep himself warm if dressed properly, you will have to minimise the times he is undressed or cold. The rule of thumb for dressing

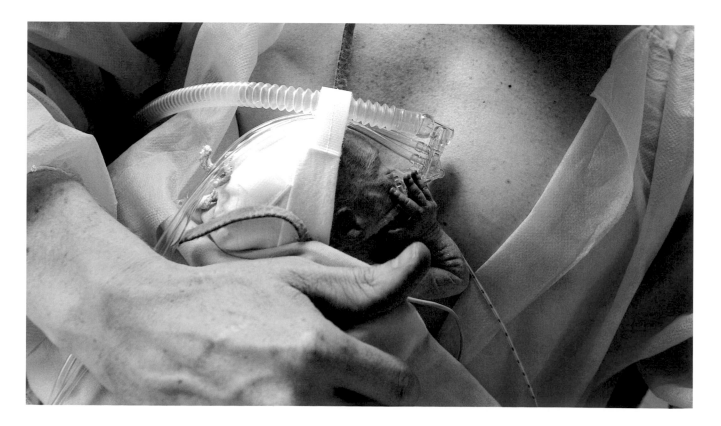

a prem baby is to add one more layer of clothing than you need for yourself. At home, hats are needed only when the thermostat is set below typical living temperatures (21°C [68°F]).

Germ control

If your baby was born before 34 weeks of gestation, he will be deficient in maternal antibodies that protect him from germs, so it is vital to limit touching, holding and close contact with your baby to only a few close relatives or friends – and only after they have washed their hands thoroughly and are free from infection. Do not allow anyone with a contagious illness to visit and be sure to avoid public places where people are in close proximity. It is also important that your baby receive his immunisations and that you surround him with family members who are immune to certain viruses and bacteria. For example, it is recommended that parents and all other adults in your household, including babysitters and frequent visitors as well as other children, are immunised against pertussis (whooping cough) and influenza ('flu').

Handling

While prematurely born infants are smaller than full-term babies, they can be picked up and held the same way (see page 160). A prem baby should be carried in a special prem baby carrier, so he can hear your heartbeat and feel your breathing and moving; this can help him to thrive as well as develop a stronger emotional bond with you. Premature babies grow faster if held nestled in a sling (it mimics the womb) and it can make the transition from an incubator to the outside world a lot easier, more secure and more comfortable. Once a baby has achieved good head control (around 16–20 weeks), a carrier without head support can be used.

Feeding

Even after discharge from the SCBU, a prem baby may not yet have perfected the skills required to feed easily. In any event, he will feed more slowly and suck less strongly and efficiently than a full-term baby. Weakness in the oral muscles, poor coordination of the tongue and pharynx and the need to breathe frequently may further complicate feeding at first. Furthermore, the effort required to continuously suck at the breast or on a bottle can be exhausting for a small premature infant. Feedings will be slow and your baby may have to take several breaks to rest in the course of the 'meal'.

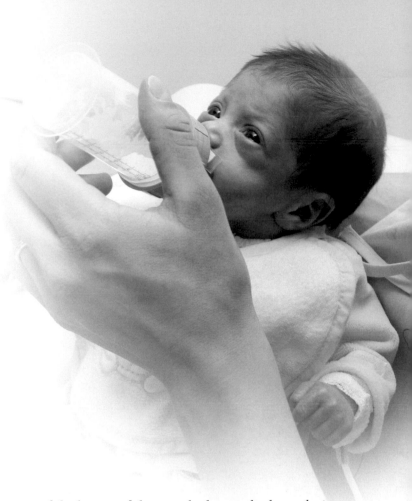

Part of the beauty of the way the human body works is that the breast milk of mothers who deliver premature babies contains more of the vital nutrients needed by a premature baby (protein, fat, calcium, phosphorus, vitamin D and iron). However, to ensure that a prem baby gets plenty of what he needs, a powdered breast milk fortifier is often added to expressed breast milk.

Bottlefed prem babies are initially given a premature infant formula (0.8 cals/ml [24 calories per ounce]) and extra nutrients, and usually require a multivitamin and iron drops.

As a rule, premature babies are not very good at knowing when they are hungry, so feeds must be given at regular intervals, as directed by the caregivers in the SCBU. Once your baby is able to ingest sufficient calories, he will grow remarkably quickly – typically, he will gain 20–30 g or more per day.

Development

While there are growth charts specifically for small premature infants (of greatest use for infants still in hospital), most of the time a standard growth chart is used. However, instead of your baby's chronological age, his corrected age is plotted against his weight,

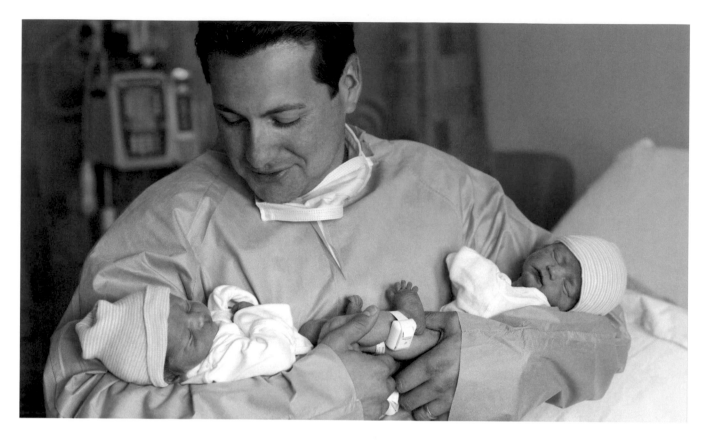

height and head circumference and it is likely that your baby will start off in the lowest percentiles for height and weight. With catch-up growth, however, he will soon approach a level of growth more typical for full-term infants of similar corrected, and eventually chronological, age.

Doctors always pay particular attention to the developmental milestones of premature infants. And as is the case with physical growth, your baby's corrected age will be used when he is assessed for attainment of milestones. So if your baby was born 2 months prematurely, the expected time for him to start smiling would be at a chronological age of 3½–4 months (6–8 weeks of corrected age).

Although there can be great variation in when prem babies 'catch up', a healthy premature infant usually enters the range of normal without correction for prematurity by a chronological age of 12–18 months in both his growth and the mastery of developmental skills. What should be most important to you as a parent is not when your baby reaches a milestone, but that he does reach it.

TWIN CONSIDERATIONS

Parents of twins face particular challenges due to the babies' closeness in age, their special relationship – which is often more intense than is normally found between siblings – and their underlying need to develop as distinct individuals despite their being part of a twosome.

Although identical twins look the same to most other people who don't see them daily and therefore don't get to know them so well, you may notice some subtle physical differences. Given their similarities (if identical), it's important that each child develops as a unique individual with his or her own skills and personality and that you encourage each twin's individual interests and talents. Try to spend a few minutes alone with each of your twins every day; don't only spend time with them together.

Managing two at once

Twin buggies may have made transporting twins easier, but it can be hard to juggle the needs of two small individuals. In addition to securing extra help, it is very important to create and stick to a schedule, which allows you (at least in theory) to have some free time. With two babies, it's difficult to get through the day without a rest period, especially if you are breast-feeding, but if your babies regularly have a long afternoon nap, it should be possible for you to sleep at the same time.

While some twins may have very different metabolisms and/or personalities, which leads to different eating and sleeping habits, a routine will certainly add more structure to the day and be an improvement on simply muddling through. Imposing a feeding and sleeping timetable will ensure that your babies follow the same or similar body clock. And once your babies get into the habit of eating and sleeping at certain set times, it will be easier to spot if something is wrong. If they invariably sleep every afternoon for 2 hours and one day for just 20 minutes, you will be alerted to a possible problem that has kept them awake.

Another vital aspect is to organise your home so that you can find everything you need quickly and easily. If your home is on two floors, make sure you have vital equipment – a changing mat and infant chairs – for example, on each floor. It is also a good idea to have somewhere for the babies to sleep on each floor. Two cots aren't necessary; you could use a pram and Moses basket on the lower floor.

It's not vital that you give both babies a bath every day; as long as you top and tail your twins regularly, you can alternate bath days.

Starting a routine

The best way to start a routine is to get your twins feeding at the same time. Choose times and stick to them. Newborns will need feeding every 3–4 hours, depending on their birth weights. If your babies were in the SCBU, they were probably fed at regular intervals from the start, and it is a good idea to maintain these times when your babies come home.

Whether or not you put your babies in the same cot (some parents find their twins sleep better this way, other parents think one twin keeps the other awake), it is important to put them to bed at the same time. It's also vital to follow the same bedtime routine every day. Bathing and feeding your twins immediately prior to putting them into bed is ideal, since a bath will both tire them out and relax them. If twins associate bathtime as being the precursor to bed, they will, hopefully, soon learn to settle without a fuss. Similarly, before their afternoon nap, if you create a little ritual – nappy changing, swaddling or putting into sleeping bags – you will set up a pattern.

If I do nothing else I will ...

I WILL CREATE AND STICK TO A ROUTINE

Having set times to do things is very important when bringing up twins because it:

✓ **Makes life more predicable.** You know when you have to do things for the twins and what time you have available to do things for yourself.

✓ **Helps the day run more smoothly.** No need to think about what to do next.

✓ **Synchronises** the twins' body clocks.

✓ **Enables you to recognise illness** more easily. Any interruption in the twins' normal pattern may be a cause for concern.

✓ **Creates time for relaxation.** If both twins sleep at the same time, you can nap as well.

✓ **Makes for happier babies.** Babies generally like a regular pattern in their lives.

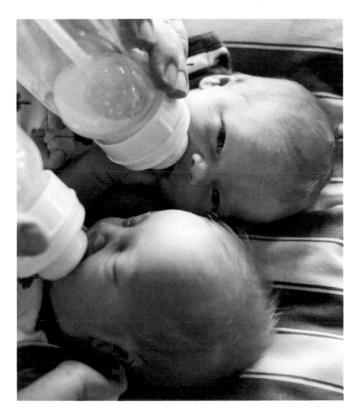

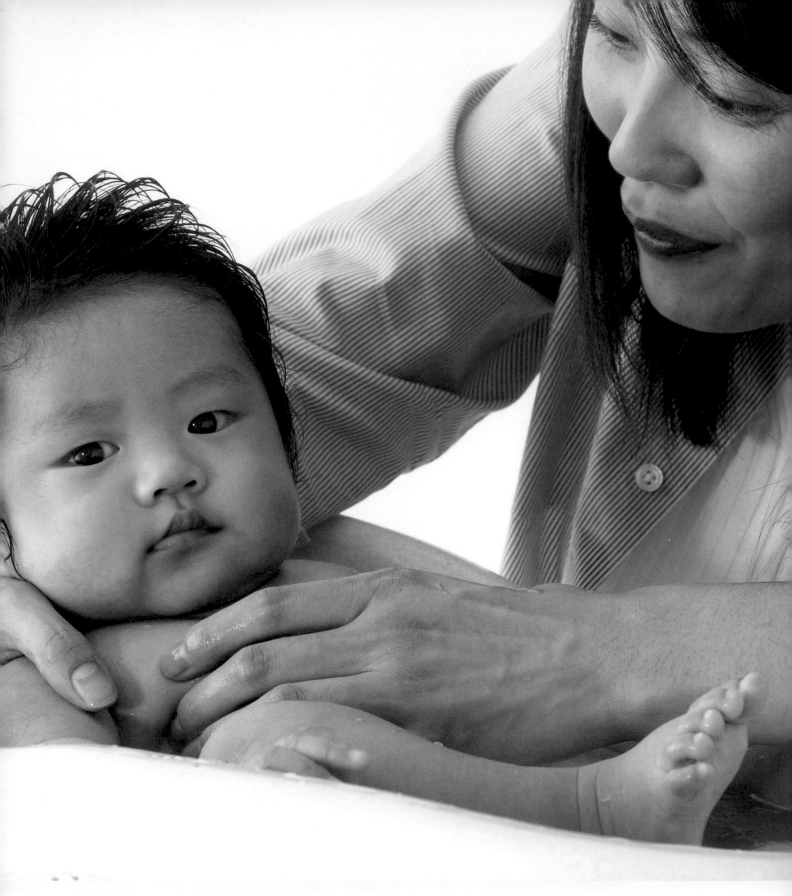

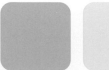

PART II My baby

Caring for my older baby

Now that baby and I have made it through the first 6 weeks or so, things have begun to settle down. I am better able to predict and meet her needs and she is beginning to sleep more and become more responsive. Now I'm looking forward to the many skills she is going to master. I've established the basic routines of sleeping, bathing, going out, etc., but soon there will be some extras to introduce, such as solid foods. One constant concern is to ensure her safety, particularly as she becomes more mobile.

Keeping up with baby's development

As my baby grows, she will replace the reflexes with which she was born with a great variety of skills. From being a fairly helpless infant, she will become a walking, talking and thinking being, able to manipulate things, experience many sensations, make friends and enjoy family life. How and when she acquires these skills may not conform to specific guidelines but should be within the range of normal. My baby, like every other, is unique and will develop at her own pace. As long as she seems to be progressing well, there won't be any cause for worry. However, if she starts to lag behind other babies of a similar age, I won't hesitate to discuss this with my GP just to make sure that everything is all right.

While my baby may achieve certain skills at a different age from other babies, she will be similar to them in the way she acquires her skills – she will practise a skill, say turning over, until she perfects it and then will build on that skill to achieve another, for example, sitting up. However, it is only when her body

and brain are sufficiently mature that she will master specific skills. She won't, for example, be able to stay dry until she is mature enough to recognise when she has to urinate and can control her bladder muscles.

MONITORING MY BABY'S PHYSICAL GROWTH

During the first 3–4 months of my baby's life, she grew remarkably rapidly but now the pace slows down for the remainder of her first year and slows down even more between 12–24 months. After the first two years, growth will continue at a relatively constant rate until puberty, when there will be another huge burst. The growth charts doctors use reflect these patterns.

That said, many healthy children do not grow as the typical pattern suggests and different factors – such as genetics – account for how big or small a child is. My doctor uses growth charts to track my baby's growth over time. What is important is not that she gains a percentile of a higher number, but that at each visit her height and weight percentile is consistent. A baby who

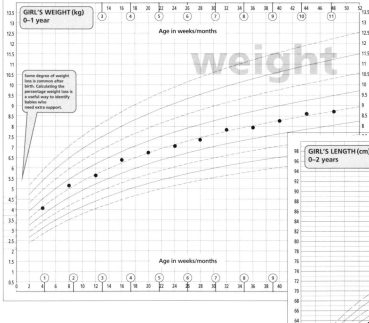

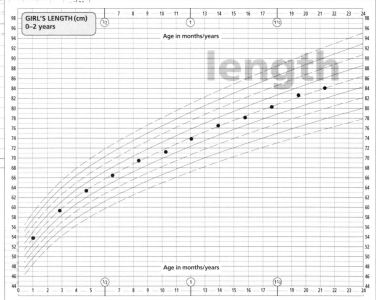

By plotting a child's measurements over time, a growth curve emerges, which tells doctors and health visitors whether her progress is normal. Boys and girls have different charts because their growth rates and patterns differ. On these growth charts there are nine lines, which represent the 0.4th, 2nd, 9th, 25th, 50th, 75th, 91st, 98th and 99.6th percentiles. The 50th percentile line represents the average for a particular age group.

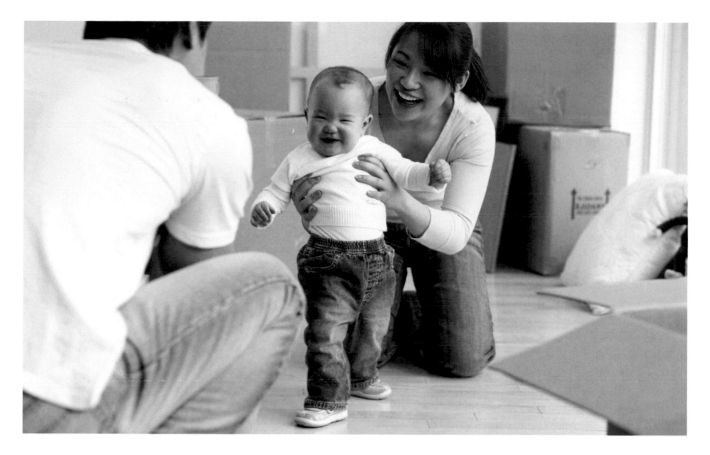

grows healthily has a growth curve that keeps pace with one of the percentiles, while a baby who has problems thriving will 'fall off' the curve.

One thing to bear in mind is that a higher percentile is not better than a lower one. A child can be healthy and growing well even if her percentile value for height or weight is below average; half of all children are at or below the 50th percentile.

HELPING MY BABY ACHIEVE THINGS

Although my baby has an in-built desire to keep achieving skills by performing them again and again, I can help the process by providing her with a safe and supportive environment (see also Making sure my home is safe, page 188) and appropriate activities (see also Suggested activities and toys for baby page 200 and for my toddler 220).

Most importantly, I try to make it fun for her to practise her skills and to always praise her efforts, whether or not she succeeds at what she attempts. Although I aim to provide encouragement and an environment in which she can succeed, I'm not pushing my baby to learn – she will do things when she is ready. Our daily play time needs to be enjoyable for us both.

If I do nothing else I will ...

KEEP AN EYE ON BABY

The achievement of milestones is individual but there are recognised time frames in which they generally are mastered. Certain problems can keep baby from achieving her potential, so I must contact the doctor if I notice:

✓ **After 3 months,** baby seldom looks at objects in the distance or to the side or appears cross-eyed.

✓ **By 4 months,** she doesn't turn towards me when I speak to her.

✓ **At 5 months,** she doesn't grasp objects.

✓ **Before 12 months,** she shows a preference for using one hand.

✓ **By 18 months,** she can't walk.

MILESTONES

Specific steps in a baby's development are commonly known as 'milestones'. These are markers in a child's progress to achieving maturity. However, variations exist not only in the time that a baby achieves certain skills but also in the order – some babies may skip a particular skill, such as rolling over or crawling, before going on to more difficult tasks. (Of course, all children will eventually come back and learn to roll or crawl.) As long as a new skill occurs in the interval reflecting the range of normal, it is normal, and even if a single skill is late (for example, sitting up) but other related skills (i.e. lifting one's head) are completely normal, there is little reason for concern.

Each of the body's systems and normal functions mature at different times and at different paces and such maturation is vital for the accomplishment of every developmental skill and milestone. Every baby will accomplish some tasks early, some at an average pace and others a bit slower than average. I'm using this checklist to monitor my baby.

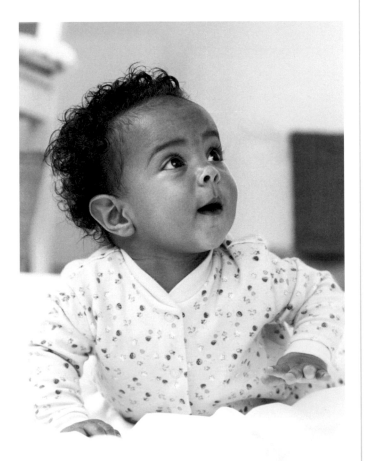

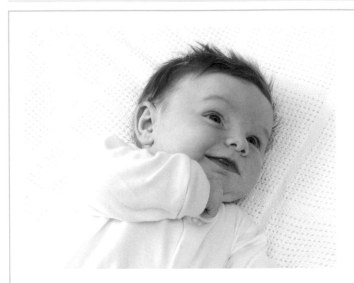

BABY'S SKILLS ACQUISITION

0–3 MONTHS

- [ ] Lifts head when held at shoulder.
- [ ] Moves arms and legs.
- [ ] Has a growing ability to follow objects and focus.
- [ ] Vocalises sounds (coos).
- [ ] Smiles spontaneously and responsively.
- [ ] Likes to be held and rocked.
- [ ] May hold a rattle for a few minutes if placed in her hand.

3–6 MONTHS

- [ ] Rolls over from stomach to back.
- [ ] Lifts up knees.
- [ ] Reaches for objects.
- [ ] Sits with support.
- [ ] Looks at objects in hand.
- [ ] Grasps with both hands.
- [ ] Can shake but not pick up rattle.
- [ ] Follows a moving object with eyes.
- [ ] Coos/gurgles.
- [ ] Chuckles/squeals.
- [ ] Smiles responsively.
- [ ] Laughs aloud.
- [ ] Has expressive noises.

- [ ] Recognises primary caregiver.
- [ ] Anticipates food on sight.
- [ ] Holds bottle in both hands.
- [ ] Can self-feed with finger foods.

6–9 MONTHS

- [ ] Rolls from back to stomach.
- [ ] On back, can lift head up.
- [ ] Learns to crawl.
- [ ] Pulls to standing for a few seconds.
- [ ] Starts eating with spoon.
- [ ] Reaches for a toy that is dropped.
- [ ] Bangs toys to make noise.
- [ ] Curious, puts everything in mouth.
- [ ] Responds to name.
- [ ] Speaks single consonants (da-da, ba-ba).
- [ ] Imitates sounds.
- [ ] May cry when strangers approach.
- [ ] May cry when mum or dad leaves the room.

9–12 MONTHS

- [ ] Crawls well.
- [ ] Stands holding on to furniture with hands.
- [ ] Sits down from standing.

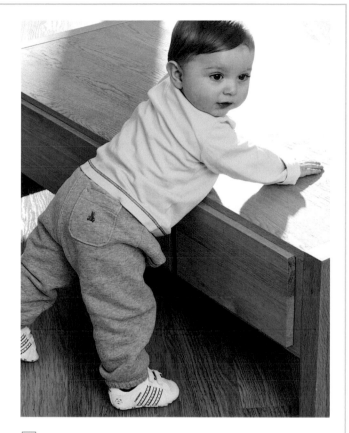

- [ ] Cruises round furniture.
- [ ] Walks with support.
- [ ] Learns to grasp with thumb and finger.
- [ ] Points to things that are wanted.
- [ ] Puts things in and takes them out of containers.
- [ ] Builds a tower of 2 blocks.
- [ ] Can throw things deliberately.
- [ ] May hold 2 objects in one hand.
- [ ] Interested in pictures.
- [ ] Drops objects on purpose.
- [ ] Understands "No".
- [ ] Says "Mama" or "Dada" correctly.
- [ ] Knows own name.
- [ ] Knows meaning of 1–3 words.
- [ ] Cooperates in games.
- [ ] Plays peek-a-boo and pat-a-cake.
- [ ] Waves bye-bye.

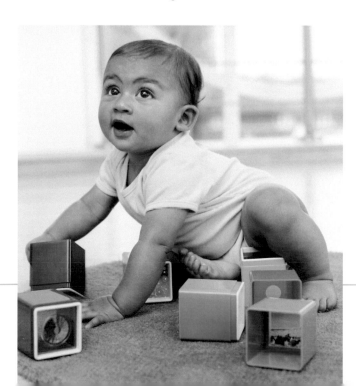

Making sure my home is safe

Young children are particularly at risk of accidents, especially once they start moving. This checklist will help me guarantee a safe environment at home and while out and about or in the garden. However, no home will ever be completely hazard-free, so I must ensure my baby is under constant supervision and that I know the first aid measures to take should anything go wrong (see Treating minor injuries, page 254 and Emergency first aid, page 264) as well as having a first-aid kit available. Also important is to make sure that I practise good kitchen hygiene (see page 208) and teach my toddler good hygiene habits (see page 227).

MY FIRST AID BOX

I need to make sure the container fastens securely and is kept locked away for safety.

☐ Thermometer.

☐ Paracetamol or other painkiller for children.

☐ Calamine for itching.

☐ Ointment for insect bites.

☐ Antibacterial cream.

☐ Scissors.

☐ Plasters and bandages, dressings and a compress.

☐ Adhesive tape.

☐ Sterile gauze.

☐ Disposable latex gloves.

SAFETY CHECKLIST

GENERAL

☐ I don't smoke or allow anyone else to smoke near baby or in my home.

☐ I know how to take baby's temperature.

☐ I make sure baby is never left alone unsupervised when awake and never left alone on a bed or changing unit.

☐ I always put bouncy chairs on the floor not on a table or worktop.

☐ I always use a safety harness in the buggy.

☐ I always use a safety harness with the highchair.

☐ I don't use tablecloths when my baby's highchair is by the dining table.

☐ When I cook, my baby is in her playpen, cot or highchair (with restraints).

☐ Hot drinks and food are kept out of reach of my child.

☐ I don't allow anyone to give my child peanuts, popcorn, nuts or hard sweets.

☐ All my babysitters are responsible and know what to do if anything happens; I keep a list of emergency phone numbers by the telephone.

HOUSEHOLD

☐ At least 1 smoke detector is fitted on every floor; batteries are checked every 6 months.

☐ Fire extinguishers are to hand in all areas where there may be open flames: kitchen, basement, garage and near fireplaces.

☐ Any flammable items, such as paraffin, gasoline and fertilisers, are kept in their original containers in a locked storage area separate from my home.

☐ Fireguards are placed around all fireplaces and heaters.

☐ Room thermometer is fitted in baby's room.

☐ Boiler is regularly serviced to prevent carbon monoxide poisoning; fixing a detector is a good idea.

☐ Any domestic animals are never left alone with baby, are wormed regularly and inoculated yearly.

- [ ] Emergency numbers are placed next to the phone.
- [ ] Safety locks or catches are fitted to all windows.
- [ ] Glass in low-level panels of doors and windows is toughened or laminated.
- [ ] Barriers or safety rails have been installed on landings and balconies.
- [ ] A guard has been placed over the slots in our DVD player.
- [ ] Electric sockets are covered by protective covers.
- [ ] All household chemicals, such as cleaning supplies are locked away.
- [ ] All tablets, medicines and alcohol are locked away; medicines are kept in child-resistant containers.
- [ ] A cooker guard is in place or I use the back two rings and position the pan handles away from the front of the cooker.
- [ ] The kettle is on a short lead or coiled flex and well out of reach of my child.
- [ ] No shade and blind cords dangle low off windows or hang in a loop.
- [ ] All furniture, including changing tables, cots and playpens, is positioned away from the windows to prevent falls.
- [ ] Small items such as buttons, safety pins, coins, batteries and jewellery are kept away from my child.
- [ ] The rubbish bin is covered with a lid.

SLEEP

- [ ] I always put baby to sleep on her back, with feet touching the foot of the cot.
- [ ] I have removed all pillows from baby's cot and pram.
- [ ] No pictures, toys or decorations containing ribbon or string hang on or over the cot.
- [ ] I use a baby listening device when my baby is asleep.

BATH

- [ ] I always run cold water into the bath before adding the hot and then test the temperature with a thermometer before putting baby in.

- [ ] I have turned down the water thermostat to 54°C (129°F) to avoid scalding.
- [ ] I never leave baby alone in a bath or paddling pool or near other water.

CAR

- [ ] I have the correct car seat for my baby's weight.
- [ ] Baby always travels in the back seat.

TOYS

- [ ] I check all toys to ensure they are safe before giving them to baby. I make sure they don't have any small, removable parts, strings or are made of furry material.
- [ ] I check to see that all toys have the British Standard or Toy & Hobby Association marks and are bought from reputable dealers.
- [ ] I safely dispose of any plastic wrappings or bags.

GARDEN AND OUTDOORS

- [ ] My child is supervised at all times when out of doors.
- [ ] My child wears a hat and sunscreen when outdoors.
- [ ] Any pond or pool in the garden is covered or fenced off; I drain our kiddie pool and turn it over when not in use.
- [ ] All garden chemicals are kept locked away.
- [ ] My garden is secured so my child cannot walk out into the road.
- [ ] I have checked that there are no toxic plants in my garden.
- [ ] I will teach my child not to eat plants, fungi, berries and seeds.
- [ ] Barbecues are always attended while in use and kept away from play areas.
- [ ] Power tools are stored unplugged and gardening equipment is kept out of reach.
- [ ] The garage door is kept down and locked at all times.
- [ ] The door and opening mechanism are checked regularly.

Taking care of my baby's needs

Now that my baby is older, I'm better able to establish a routine for her care and to make care times occasions for having fun.

KEEPING HER CLEAN

Bath times, for example, are very pleasurable now and it's often hard getting baby out the tub. From a hygiene point of view, it is not necessary to bathe her every day; a bath every 2–3 days is perfectly fine unless she gets especially dirty. A quick sponge bath outside the tub often suffices.

Once she can sit up, unsupported (about 6 months of age), she can be bathed in a bathtub. There doesn't need to be a lot of water – 5–7 cm or waist height is sufficient – and it needs testing to ensure it's not too hot or too cold. Baby should sit on a rubber non-slip mat and away from the taps, to prevent any possibility of her touching them and being scalded. Of course, I must never leave baby unattended in the bath, not even for a moment.

I use a non-soap cleanser (which is less likely to dry out or irritate baby's skin) or sometimes a soap with moisturiser; special baby soaps aren't necessary. Shampooing her hair can be a struggle, but there is a variety of gadgets – shields and pourers – that makes it easy to keep water and shampoo out of her eyes. I use baby shampoo, which stings less than an adult shampoo if it accidentally touches her eyes.

As well as supplying baby with water toys and playing gentle splashing games, I sometimes join her in the bath. However, I'm careful to keep her towel alongside the tub and to keep hold of her while I climb in and out.

SKIN CARE

Although my baby's skin is usually soft and moist, very occasionally it becomes dry or irritated.

Dry skin

When I gently rub my hand over my baby's skin and it feels rough to the touch or I can see fine white flakes or small bumps on the surface or even patches of dry, rough, slightly raised skin, I know that I have to adjust

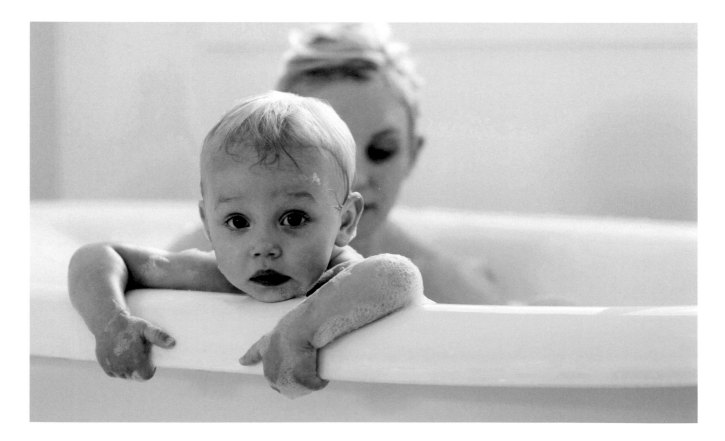

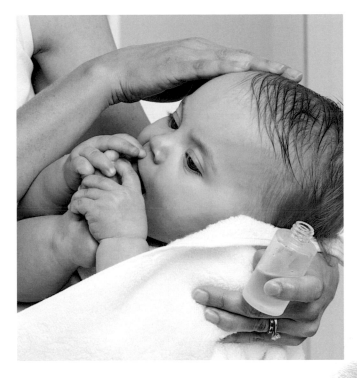

When my baby's scalp becomes flaky, I rub some baby oil into her scalp and let it remain there for at least several minutes (and sometimes overnight) before shampooing and gently rubbing away the skin flakes. I also have to shampoo her hair every day.

drooling a lot, I use a thick ointment on her cheek or chin such as Vaseline®, Aquaphor® or A+D®, as a barrier to prevent those liquids reaching the skin's surface. I can also use the ointment on her irritated skin to decrease friction between a sheet or blanket or clothing covering my shoulder.

If wind is the problem, I apply the ointment before going outside in cold weather. To prevent wetness in the neck folds, I put on a bib.

HAIR CARE

Although my baby was born with a lot of hair, much of the hair, especially on the top of her head, has fallen out. And, because she spends plenty of time on her

my care. Dry skin results from lack of moisture in the air of my home (most commonly in winter when the heating is on) or from being in water too long. Chronically dry and itchy skin is called eczema (see page 262), which can require medical treatment.

Because having dry skin can be uncomfortable and itchy for baby, when she does suffer from it, I bathe her a little less often, and when bathing her, I use a moisturising soap. Immediately after she has been towel dried, I apply a moisturising lotion to her skin. If the air in her room is dry, I turn on the humidifier.

Irritated skin

Rubbing and wetness occasionally cause irritated skin on the face and nappy area. Friction caused by rubbing her face against the sheet of her cot or against my shoulder (when she is being held) results in pink-red patches of irritated skin. Other causes are windy or cold weather.

Sometimes, a nappy rash (see page 164) becomes secondarily infected with yeast or a yeast infection can appear in her skin folds, where the warm, moist environment favours its growth.

Cheek and chin rashes also are quite common and usually caused by saliva. At about 3 months of age, my baby began drooling much more than previously as a result of her salivary glands maturing.

Treatment depends on my trying to alleviate the predisposing factors. When my baby is posseting or back, there is a bald spot at the back, where she rests her head. But I'm sure it will grow back as soon as she spends more time upright. Aside from shampooing and gentle brushing with a soft baby brush, it needs little attention, unless it becomes excessively flaky, a condition known as cradle cap. In this case, I massage in some aqueous cream or warmed baby oil into the white or yellowish scales and then leave it overnight before brushing the scales away the next day.

NAIL CARE

Although baby's nails needed frequent cutting when she was newborn, now I have to do so less often. The best time to cut her nails is after her bath, when the nails are at their softest.

Because her fingers are still quite little and it's hard to access the nail without involving the fingertip, I find the easiest and safest method is to use baby scissors,

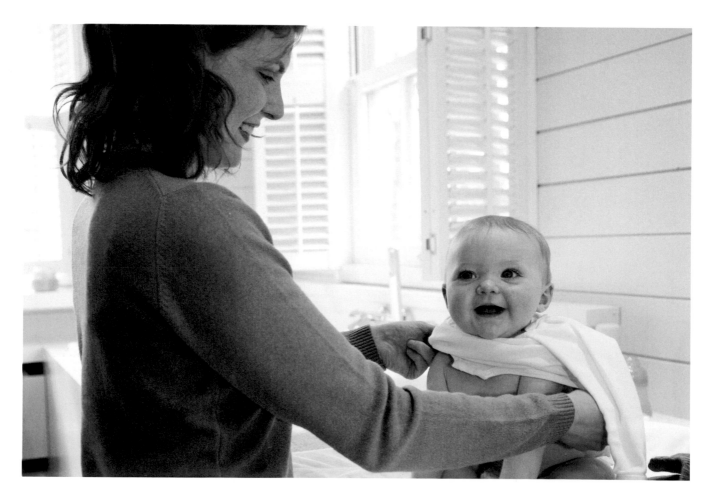

which have one sharp cutting blade and one dull, rounded blade. When I use the scissors, I place the dull blade facing downwards and the sharper blade on top so that the lower blade protects the skin of the finger, while the upper blade cuts the nail. By the time baby is 6–9 months old, her fingers will be bigger and I can use baby nail clippers.

Her toenails grow much more slowly than her fingernails and don't need to be kept quite as short nor trimmed so frequently. I always check for sharp edges, as if these catch on her clothing it will be painful for baby. Should I spot any redness, inflammation or hardness around a nail, I need to mention it to my doctor, as it may indicate an ingrowing toenail.

DRESSING MY BABY

Although buying clothes for baby is very enjoyable, I try to keep the more stylish, expensive clothing to a

If I do nothing else I will ...

CREATE A GENDER-NEUTRAL WARDROBE
In case I have another baby of a different sex later on, it makes sense if clothing can suit both boys and girls. I try to:

✓ **Choose colours that are appropriate for both sexes** such as white, yellow, light green and beige.

✓ **Select garments with gender-neutral patterns** such as stripes, checks or prints composed of animals, teddy bears, shapes or letters.

✓ **Buy all-in-ones**, T-shirts and pull-on trousers.

✓ **Choose black or dark blue leggings.**

✓ **Look for modified jean-style denim.**

✗ **Avoid designs and prints that are too gender specific** such as flower motifs or aliens.

✗ **Avoid gender-specific clothes** like dresses and obvious boy wear to a minimum.

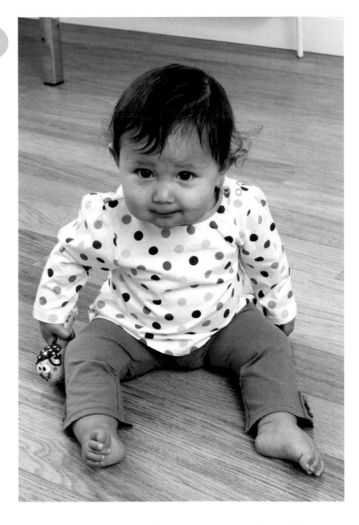

Leggings are a versatile choice. They are good underneath short skirts or dresses, as skirts will end up climbing around baby's waist as she kicks up her feet, and can be used with tops for boys.

minimum. It's more important to choose clothing that stands up well after multiple washes – since my baby can get a lot dirtier now than when she was younger – and not to spend too much on garments that she will quickly outgrow or are too seasonal.

Her everyday wardrobe includes bodysuits (some footless), hats, booties, socks and sleepwear, as well as warm outerwear, tops and trousers or leggings. She also has a few items of special occasion clothing. She still doesn't like to have shirts or jumpers pulled over her head, so I always pick garments with wide or button openings and tend to prefer elasticised waists.

She won't need shoes until she starts to walk so I put on soft booties or socks on her feet as she spends a lot of time with her feet in the air. I generally buy pairs of identical matching socks as baby often kicks off her socks and one goes missing.

As when she was smaller, I dress her in layers, which makes it easier to adjust to temperature changes. In cold weather I first put on a lightweight vest and top then something heavier if she goes outside or she's in a

chilly environment. I always make sure she has a warm hat on when outdoors. I have to remember to remove some layers when it gets warmer or we're indoors, as perspiration will dampen clothing and makes baby cold when we go back outside.

Dressing does not always go smoothly as baby often squirms or moves about and may resist getting dressed – which is why now it's vitally important never to leave baby alone even for an instant on the dressing table.

I try and make dressing fun by talking to her throughout saying things like "This is baby's arm and it needs to go into the sleeve..." or playing hide-and-seek with the garments. When I pull a top over her head, I'll say, "Oh, oh, where did baby go?" and once I pull the top down, I say, "There she is!"

Tooth care and teething

Around 6 months of age, my baby's first tooth appeared. Newly erupted baby teeth have not yet fully developed their protective toughened outer enamel surface so are prone to decay and erosion, hence it's important to take care of them properly. As well as brushing her teeth and having baby seen by my dentist, I also make sure she does not eat sugary foods or is left with her bottle, which can lead to 'nursing bottle cavities'. Teeth that are constantly bathed in milk, even breast milk, develop multiple cavities more easily.

FLUORIDE

Both paediatric dentists and paediatricians recommend that babies receive fluoride regularly as it results in stronger teeth, fewer cavities and stronger bones.

Fluoride can be obtained from a number of sources. Many, but not all, municipal water systems add tiny amounts of fluoride to drinking water to improve the oral health of the community. If yours doesn't, your doctor may prescribe a supplement or like me, you may be recommended to use a fluoridated toothpaste. As my baby is too young to spit it out (this will happen when she's around 3–4 years old), she gets sufficient fluoride by this route.

BRUSHING TEETH

As soon as her first tooth erupted, I began using a flannel or a wet gauze pad to wipe off the tooth after meals. Once she started on solid food, I switched to a small baby-sized toothbrush with soft bristles on which

I sit baby on my lap, take hold of the toothbrush and brush gently but quickly. I can work up or down, side to side or use a circular motion, as long as I clean each tooth thoroughly both front and back.

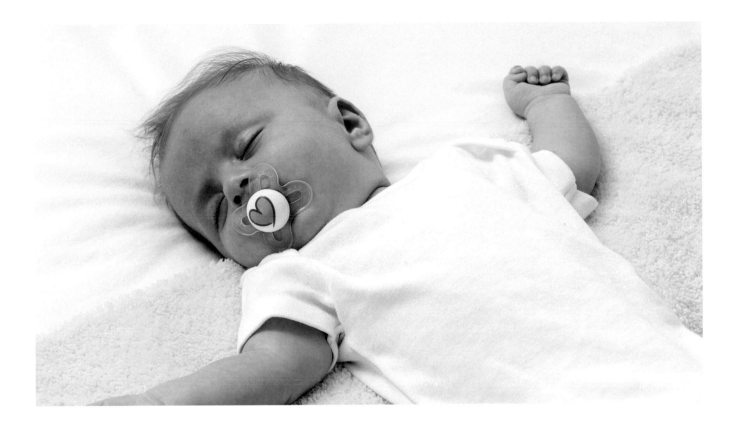

I placed a small, pea-sized dab of toothpaste. You need to ask your doctor or dentist if you should be brushing with toothpaste or only water. And if toothpaste is recommended, enquire if fluoridated or non-fluoridated toothpaste is preferred.

Most experts recommend brushing a baby's teeth twice a day – once after breakfast or in the morning and once in the evening. If food remains on the teeth, cavities start to develop, but tooth brushing will remove it. I find the best time to brush in the evening is before baby's final feed, as the bedtime feed is a relaxing part of her bedtime ritual. If I brush her teeth after this, it may undo her quiet, calm mood. It isn't true that giving only milk to a baby just before she goes to sleep will cause cavities; baby's saliva will wash away any milk that adheres to her teeth. Of course, what I mustn't do is ever allow her to sleep with a bottle of milk; in such a case the milk remains in her mouth overnight and isn't washed away, making cavities are a real possibility.

Toothbrushes

It is important to select one with soft, rounded bristles and to change it at least every 3 months. To keep it as free of bacteria as possible, I rinse it carefully after brushing and store it in a clean cup or holder.

WHEN TEETH ARRIVE

Eruption time varies but by the time your baby is 2–3 years old, all her primary teeth should be present.

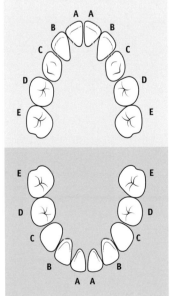

UPPER
A Central Incisors
 8–13 months
B Lateral Incisors
 8–13 months
C Canines (cuspids)
 16–23 months
D First Molars
 13–19 months
E Second Molars
 25–33 months

LOWER
A Central Incisors
 6–10 months
B Lateral Incisors
 10–16 months
C Canines (cuspids)
 16–23 months
D First Molars
 13–19 months
E Second Molars
 23–31 months

DUMMIES AND THUMBSUCKING

According to the British Dental Health Foundation, the longer a baby uses a dummy, the more chance there is of changes in the shape of the inside of her mouth, which can affect how her baby teeth, and later on her permanent teeth, meet when biting. Therefore, I always limit the times when baby uses a dummy (such as only for going to sleep) and I will try to wean her off her dummy when she is about 1 year old.

Thumbsucking, too, causes similar problems though it may prove harder to discourage as a thumb can't be as easily removed as a dummy. Most children, however, spontaneously stop sucking thumbs (between 2–4 years), so unless there are noticeable changes it might be best to adopt a wait-and-see attitude towards it.

TEETHING

Twenty baby teeth will erupt in the first 2–3 years, though the order and timing does vary (see page 195).

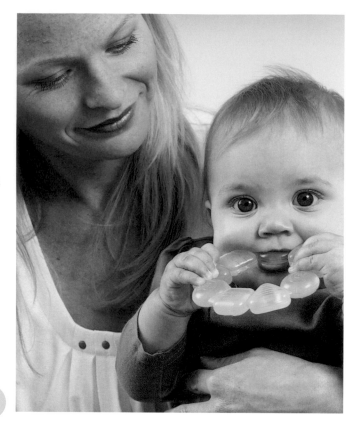

If I do nothing else I will ... ✓

PAY ATTENTION TO BABY'S TEETH

My goal is to help prevent damage to baby's teeth and ward off cavities, which will cause baby pain. I need to:

✓ **Remove baby from my breast between feeds;** cavities can result if baby's teeth are in constant contact with breast milk.

✓ **Encourage baby to drink water** as much as possible when she is not having milk and avoid sugary fruit drinks.

✓ **Dilute any fresh fruit juice** with a large amount of water and give it to her in a cup rather than a bottle.

✓ **Make sure all objects baby chews on are soft and firm,** not hard or sharp.

✓ **Alert my dentist** if I see any white, yellow or brown spots on her teeth.

✗ **Not leave baby's bottle in her cot** or allow her to use it as a dummy. If baby does need a bottle to settle down, I will fill it with water.

In the few weeks before a tooth arrives, many babies become fussy, drool heavily and enjoy chomping on hard objects – though this will happen even if a tooth does not appear for months. Like many things, tooth eruption occurs at the same time as various other developmental changes (such as the maturity of the salivary glands) or may overlap with a childhood illness, so that symptoms such as diarrhoea and fever, which are seldom a result of teething, are linked with it. Most teeth erupt without any detectable pain or discomfort, but always keep an eye on things.

Occasionally, however, there is some discomfort, so giving baby a safe, cold, firm object to chomp on will bring relief. Teething rings that contain liquid and can be frozen are available and, in a pinch, a frozen mini bagel is a good choice (but be sure to take it away before it becomes soft and pieces can be broken off).

If teething pain seems more severe, your GP may suggest giving paracetamol (Calpol® and others) or a topical anaesthetic (Bonjela). If using the latter, gently rub a small amount of the gel on to the sore area of gum with a clean fingertip.

Avoid any teething products containing benzocaine; in rare cases they can be absorbed into the bloodstream and cause problems.

Out and about with baby

Short trips to visit friends, the supermarket or to a restaurant now form a regular part of our day. Whether I take her in a carrier or buggy, I have to make sure I'm not carrying too many things other than my travel kit (see page 198). All the essentials fit into a large shoulder bag or backpack.

USING A CARRIER

Once baby was able to keep her head up – about 16–20 weeks – I started carrying her so that she faced outwards. Now that she's more active, getting her into and out of her carrier is harder. Of course, I still take care to protect her head when bending forwards. As she gets heavier or if I plan to do a lot of walking – particularly in crowded places or on rough lanes – I'll probably invest in a back carrier, in which she can sit up and look out. I need to choose one that distributes her weight evenly over my shoulders and across my back. The best ones have sturdy metal frames, adjustable seat heights and stand securely on the floor when baby is put inside. Backpacks and back carriers are aimed at babies from about 6 months onwards, when they can support themselves sitting up and their neck muscles are quite strong. One will enable baby to get a better view and it will be a lot easier on my back.

My getting ready to go out routine

It's important that I put the carrier on first. I put baby down in a secure place and once the carrier is properly fastened with the body opened out, I pick her up. Then we sit down on a chair and, holding baby under her armpits, I slowly lift her into the carrier.

I secure the body of the carrier and check that baby's comfortably seated, with her weight evenly supported. Then, if necessary, I adjust the straps.

To take baby out of the carrier, I reverse the process except that I sit down, then undo the body before lifting baby out. I lay baby down in a safe place before removing the carrier.

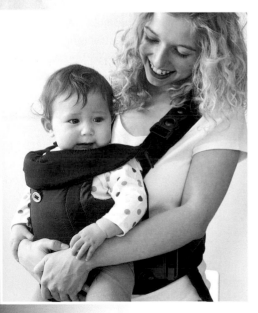

Playing with my baby

Play is not only fun, it also it helps baby develop all her vital skills – physical, intellectual, emotional and psycho-social. Play is most successful when the things we do together keep pace with her development. For example, when my baby was just some weeks old, I simply held her on my lap so that her face was close to mine (no more than about 20–30 cm away) and then I talked happily to her, giving her a chance to react – smile, gurgle, wriggle or move her mouth back at me. If I had tried to do this at a greater distance, she wouldn't have been able to see me and wouldn't have responded.

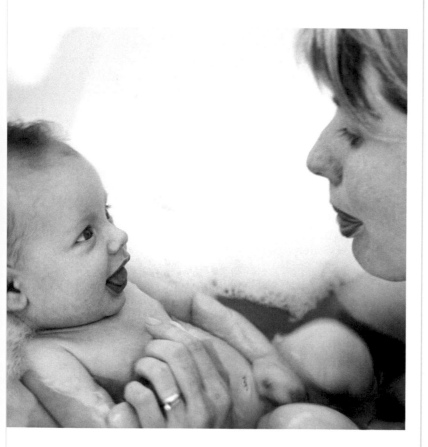

At one month, my baby started to imitate me – I tried smiling, sticking my tongue out, widely opening my mouth and giggling. It's important, however, if you try, that your baby is kept close so she can see you and that you do these things one at a time.

SUGGESTED ACTIVITIES AND TOYS

2 MONTHS

My baby still enjoys responding to expressions, but now she finds it interesting to look with me in a mirror. I change the angle of the mirror but allow baby plenty of time to watch the reflections. She also likes it when I sing songs and gently bump her up and down or move her arms and legs in time to music. I attached a brightly coloured moving mobile to her cot, sufficiently low down so that the movement will catch her eye.

3 MONTHS

Now that baby has started to enjoy brightly coloured items moved across her field of vision and differently textured materials moved over her hands, I use a variety of things that are hard and soft, warm and cool, furry and smooth. I also gently shake a rattle close to her face and play gentle rolling and rocking games – such as rolling her over a beach ball.

4 MONTHS

To encourage baby to reach for objects, I hold brightly coloured toys or rattles just in front of her. She likes rings and other moulded rubber toys that are easily graspable. If she gets them, she generally puts them in her mouth. I also sing to her or recite nursery rhymes; I still gently move baby up and down in time to the music or rhythm.

5 MONTHS

Now as I go about my activities, I point out familiar items to baby, letting her touch different things – furniture, cushions, drapes, flowers, pots and pans – to gain a sense of how different they feel. As baby enjoys looking at things – faces, objects and pictures in a book – we have started 'reading' board and bath books with large pictures.

6 MONTHS

Baby enjoys bouncing games and dancing – that is, being held in my arms and moved to a rhythm. She now makes greater efforts to reach a toy placed out of her grasp and if she gets it, can pass it from hand to hand. She also enjoys baby massage and when I play 'This Little Piggy'. She now has a variety of soft toys and balls that I can use when we 'sing' together.

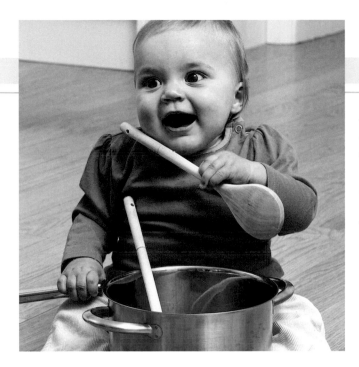

7 MONTHS

I read, sing and talk to baby as much as possible. She likes it when I play tickle games ('Round and round the garden [circle baby's belly button] Goes the teddy bear. One step. . . two steps . . . [walk your fingers up baby's torso] Tickle you under there!' [tickle your baby under her chin]) and laughs during the tickles. Now that she is able to sit on the floor unsupported, I've given her soft baby blocks and together we build things with them.

8 MONTHS

Because baby likes moving around a lot now, to keep her in one place. I stack different-sized cushions on the floor and hide some of her toys in between. She enjoys searching for them and other hidden items as well as playing 'peek-a-boo'. Bath play has become more important and she likes pouring water from different-sized beakers.

9 MONTHS

My baby likes to play with pots and pans – banging them together – and I encourage her musicality by having her sing along with me to nursery songs. As she's crawling everywhere, I make it fun for her by letting her go over different surfaces – carpet, wood and tile – and furnish her with push-and-pull toys. Hand games, such as 'pat-a-cake', are enjoyable for both of us.

10 MONTHS

Baby is standing up now and likes to climb over me, so we engage in some simple, soft gymnastics. She likes putting things into and taking them out of containers, so as well as her shape sorter, she finds a box that I have filled with a variety of safe objects – soft balls, large cotton reels, clothespins, socks and blocks – fun to empty while I watch. She also likes to shake things that make noise and I've attached a rattle to her feeding table, which she enjoys taking swipes at.

11 MONTHS

We read together a lot now. I make expressions that my baby copies and she repeats more of the words that she hears. She also enjoys nursery rhymes with movements and songs that include animal noises – 'Old MacDonald Had a Farm' – is a favourite. We have started some simple ball play – rolling a ball between us. She enjoys stacking objects.

12 MONTHS

Baby is very interested in toys that move, like small plastic or rubber vehicles, and ones that allow her to do things that I do – toy telephones, hammers, dust pan and brush, for example. Our activities involve more role-playing – exchanging calls or feeding teddy together. She also enjoys scribbling with crayons on paper.

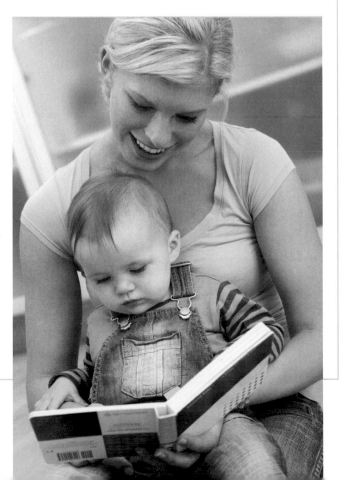

Baby's naps and bedtime

Baby is awake for more of the day and sleeps more at night now. As a newborn, she slept for almost 22 hours a day whereas starting at around 3 months, her time asleep began to diminish to 14–16 hours and now she spends at least 4 hours asleep at any one time. She has both a morning and afternoon nap – which gives me time to do things for myself or around the home. In the evenings, she does sleep through the night (roughly 6 hours) as long as she has a feed just before bedtime.

NAPS

Having some short sleeps during the day helps baby to make the most of her activities and, if timed right – not too close to bedtime, doesn't interfere with her sleep at night. I don't like to interrupt her nap pattern by keeping her awake in the hope that she will sleep better at night, as she only becomes overtired, is fretful during the day and sleeps less soundly at night.

Like most babies, mine prefers a routine for her naps. Now that she is older, there is more of a pattern to her behaviour, and I'm better able to know at what points in the day she tends to become sleepy, and I time her naps accordingly. Of course, it's important that she's calm before naptime, so I make sure she is flagging before I put her into her cot. Sometimes, I have to do some of the things I do at night-time to get her settled (see below).

BEDTIME

Having a routine enables baby to know that she will soon go to sleep and helps me to organise myself. Part of my routine is to give baby her bath in the evening as she enjoys this and finds it relaxing. Other babies, however, get very excited or cry when in the bath, so bathing them earlier would be better. Once she's had her bath, I change her nappy and put on her nightclothes. Then I talk, read and/or sing to her and give her a cuddle. Although her room is dimly lit and quiet, I don't worry about her hearing background noise – like the TV or radio or appliances elsewhere in the house.

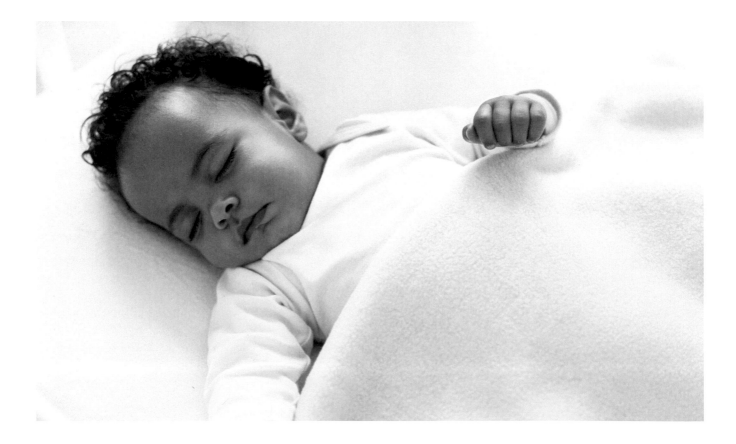

TWIN BABIES

As they get older, the twins may start to disturb each other, particularly if they have different sleep patterns and tend to wake at different times. At the age of 3 months or so, you will probably find your twins need more space anyway, so this may be a good time to put them in their own cot. Keep the cots in view of each other so that the babies can still communicate and keep each other company.

SLEEPING PROBLEMS

I've been told that babies who have slept well in the past can start to wake at night from about the age of 6 months. Because my baby is now more mature, she may be bothered by things that didn't affect her when she was younger. Some common situations are:
• Being hungry or thirsty.
• Having a dirty nappy.
• Being too hot or too cold.
• Teething (from around the age of 6 months).
• Illness.
• Being bored or lonely.
It is important that when baby wakes I try and ascertain the cause, remedy it and give her the chance to go back to sleep on her own. If I don't think my baby needs a feed when she wakes, I won't give her one just to help her settle, but if she's thirsty I'll give her water. I don't want baby to develop a pattern of waking for feeds that she doesn't need. If she is using a dummy, I'll leave several in the cot so that she may be able to find one if she wakes up.

Sometimes, however, baby has trouble settling down to sleep initially. If she can't settle, then I don't wait too long to return to her. Left for too long, she can become distressed and find it more difficult to sleep. Just as with the bedtime routine, however, it is important that I'm consistent in my approach.

If, after saying good night and leaving her room, she starts to cry, I wait for a few minutes to see if she'll fall asleep by herself before returning to check on her. I try not to disturb her by turning on the light or taking her out of her cot. I simply talk gently and soothingly to her for a minute or so to reassure her that I am still nearby and reassure myself that she is well, then leave again making the intervals between checks a little longer each time.

If this doesn't work for you, you could try taking your baby out of his cot and rocking him for a few minutes to settle him. However, there still needs to be a routine in place for bedtime and your baby should be

If I do nothing else I will ...

STICK TO MY BEDTIME ROUTINE
Doing the following helps baby to recognise that it is time for sleep. Just before putting her in her cot, I:

✓ **Tell baby it is time for bed.** I talk to her soothingly while I get her ready. Although she does not yet understand my words, they are familiar and pleasurable.

✓ **Share a story** or some nursery rhymes. Although she doesn't understand the words, she loves being held close to me and listening to my voice.

✓ **Sing a lullaby.** I generally choose one particular song that baby will associate with bedtime and sleep. Sometimes, however, I play some soothing music; she often falls asleep to the sound of music playing softly.

✓ **Give her a cuddle.** I cradle her in my arms then kiss on the cheek while lowering her into bed. This tells baby I love her.

able to get himself off to sleep when he first goes to bed. However, this approach goes against the advice of minimal disturbance and there is a chance that your baby will become reliant on your being there when he wakes at night.

It is to be expected that a young baby will wake early, and some babies always will wake earlier as they need less sleep, but it may be possible to have an older baby (over 6 months) sleep for longer in the morning. In the summer months, I plan to put dark curtains or black-out blinds in the windows in my baby's room to prevent sunlight waking baby before she is ready.

Gradually making bedtime a little later (up to an hour later) may help, although some babies may wake just as early as they did previously but instead of being refreshed, may feel grumpy and tired. Shortening naps or even eliminating one if a baby needs a little less sleep during the day may be effective (as long as she doesn't become overtired). When my baby first wakes, I leave her for a few minutes to see whether she'll settle back to sleep or is able to amuse herself happily in her cot for a while.

Feeding my baby

For the first year, breast or formula milk remains a vital source of nutrients for baby, and even when she starts eating more solid foods, she will still have at least four bottles of formula or the equivalent number of breastfeeds a day. Feeding bottles still need sterilising (see page 155), as warm milk is an ideal breeding ground for bacteria.

INTRODUCING SOLIDS

Weaning – the process of replacing a baby's total dependence on milk with food of a wide range of tastes and textures – is an exciting stage in baby's life and a natural part of her development. However, this is a gradual process and foods need to be introduced at the proper time and one at a time to ensure they are good for baby.

Timing

Breast or formula milk meets all of a baby's dietary needs for the first 6 months and there are no nutritional advantages to weaning before this age. However, there are wide individual variations in developmental maturity between infants and yours may start to need solid food some while before. Weaning prior to 4 months (17 weeks) is not recommended, as a baby's digestive system is too immature to cope with anything more than milk, and it may also make your baby fat and more prone to allergies, but neither should it begin much later than 6 months (26 weeks), unless

EXPERTS ADVISE

Non-formula milk

Cow's (also sheep's and goat's) milk can be included in cooking from 6 months of age but is not recommended as a main drink until your baby is 1 year old. Cow's milk contains too much salt and protein and insufficient iron and other nutrients for a baby's needs. Soya-based milks should only be given on the advice of your GP.

BABY IS READY FOR WEANING

- [ ] She seems unsatisfied after a milk feed and is hungrier than usual.
- [ ] Can sit up with support and hold her head up well.
- [ ] Can move her tongue back and forth.
- [ ] Makes chewing motions.
- [ ] Can close her mouth around a spoon.
- [ ] Shows an interest in adult food.
- [ ] Is teething.

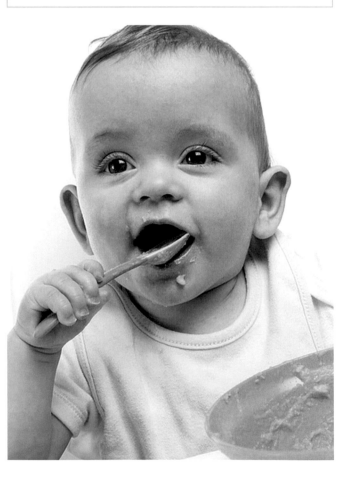

recommended by a GP, as by then a baby needs non-milk sources of nourishment to provide sufficient calories, vitamins and minerals – particular iron. Learning to bite and chew is also important for an infant's speech and language development.

Babies who are born pre-term need to be weaned depending on their individual needs, and a health visitor, GP or dietician will be able to advise on the best time to begin.

Starting baby off

When I began feeding my baby solids, I did so when I was not feeling too rushed or baby was too tired; mid-day is a good time. Eating was a new skill for baby and it took time to get it right; she spat out much of the food at first, which is perfectly normal. It was important to talk to baby throughout the feed, encouraging her and being positive.

I began by simply familiarising my baby with taking food from a spoon; the quantity eaten being largely immaterial and, in any event, no more than 1–2 teaspoons (although some babies do take more). Some mums miss out feeding purées and follow baby-led weaning offering finger foods right from the start (see page 208).

At first, I found it was a good idea to give baby a little milk first to curb any hunger pangs but, as feeding became more established, I offered the food before milk. Any first solids are supplemental to baby's milk feed. Once she took the food or was no longer interested, I continued with milk.

For the first few weeks, I gave baby the same food for around three days at a time to allow her to get used to the taste and to check there was no sign of an allergic reaction such as a rash, diarrhoea, bloated tummy or increased wind.

What did change were baby's stools; their colour and odour was different.

Very first foods

While most foods are suitable for baby from 6 months (see box page 206 for the exceptions), the following mild-tasting single ingredients are recommended:
• Fruit such as banana, pear and apple.
• Vegetables such as potato, yam, squash and carrot.
• Dry infant cereal prepared with some breast or formula milk.
• Home-cooked puréed white rice or dry baby rice mixed with breast or formula milk.

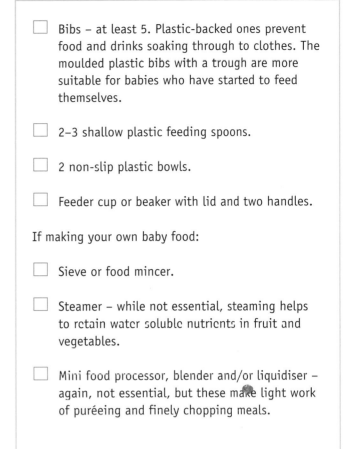

FEEDING EQUIPMENT

- ☐ Bibs – at least 5. Plastic-backed ones prevent food and drinks soaking through to clothes. The moulded plastic bibs with a trough are more suitable for babies who have started to feed themselves.

- ☐ 2–3 shallow plastic feeding spoons.

- ☐ 2 non-slip plastic bowls.

- ☐ Feeder cup or beaker with lid and two handles.

If making your own baby food:

- ☐ Sieve or food mincer.

- ☐ Steamer – while not essential, steaming helps to retain water soluble nutrients in fruit and vegetables.

- ☐ Mini food processor, blender and/or liquidiser – again, not essential, but these make light work of puréeing and finely chopping meals.

Adding new foods

Once my baby was happy with the foods offered, I gradually increased the number of meals and the variety of foods.

Once she ate a few tablespoons at one meal, then I started serving solids at a second meal and eventually, over the next few months, at the third. I started combining different ingredients then added additional foods. Once she was eating a wide variety of fruit and vegetables and baby rice I added more carbohydrates, such as pasta, and protein foods including chicken and fish. Children exposed to a variety of foods, flavours and textures from an early age are less likely to be fussy eaters later on in life. Between 6–9 months of age, children are very receptive to new tastes and textures and their experiences during this period are thought to define their palate.

There are no hard-and-fast rules as to how much a baby should eat, but around 1–4 tablespoons per meal is the general guideline once weaning is established. I always responded to my baby's appetite; if she was still hungry, I gave her a little more but if she ate only a small amount, I didn't force her to eat.

Do bear in mind that all babies are different – mine took to weaning readily, happily accepting new foods, but your baby may take longer. Don't panic or rush things; most importantly, try to ensure mealtimes are as happy and relaxed as possible and not occasions for power games.

For the first year, breast milk, formula or follow-on milk continues to be baby's main source of nutrients, including iron. Around 500–600 ml daily is recommended. Continuing to breastfeed ensures that a baby gets milk designed for her needs, so giving other milk is superfluous. If your baby becomes ill and loses her appetite, breastfeeding can keep her well nourished, giving her important antibodies to tackle bugs, as well as comforting her.

However, once feeding is established, the lunchtime milk feed can be replaced with water (see below) and, at other mealtimes, milk should be offered after the solids to prevent your baby becoming too full or preoccupied with the bottle before she has eaten any solid foods.

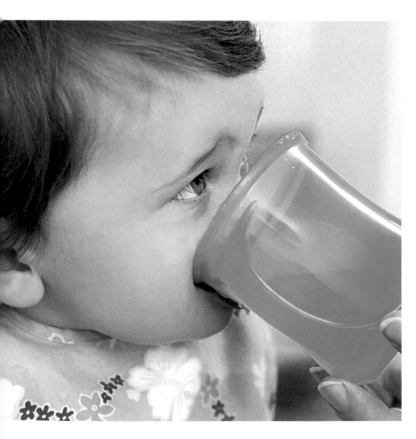

Off the menu ✕

The following foods should not be given to young children.

✗ Whole nuts because of the risk of choking and no nuts at all if there is a history of food allergies within the immediate family.

✗ Sugar.

✗ Honey.

✗ Cow's, sheep's or goat's milk as a drink.

✗ Raw or undercooked eggs.

✗ Salt and naturally salty foods such as bacon, cheese, stock and yeast extract should be limited.

✗ Shellfish, such as prawns and mussels.

✗ Marlin, shark and swordfish.

✗ Foods high in saturated fat such as butter, cheese, margarine, fatty meat and meat products, biscuits, pastry and cakes.

Water

When my baby started eating solids regularly, she needed fluids other than milk. So instead of her lunchtime milk feed, I gave her cooled, boiled tap water; some mineral waters are too rich in minerals for babies and bottled water is not sterile so will still need boiling and cooling beforehand. I never give her concentrated fruit juice, cordials or syrups as they are high in sugar and can damage teeth, even those that have not yet appeared. I started with 15 ml of water in a cup and increased the amount gradually in line with the number of meals she ate a day.

Supplements

If, like me, you are still breastfeeding your baby after 6 months, the UK Department of Health recommends giving him a liquid supplement of vitamins A, C and D, which is particularly important if your baby is dark-skinned and you live in an area with limited sunlight.

If your baby is drinking at least 500 ml of formula milk or follow-on milk, supplements are unnecessary as these milks are already fortified with these vitamins. However, if your baby is drinking less than 500 ml, he should be given a supplement.

INTRODUCING A CUP

Learning to drink from a cup should be part of the weaning process and can be started from about 6 months of age. While some babies happily accept the change, others take more time, having become strongly attached to a bottle. Open cups or free-flowing feeders are the recommended choices. Lidded and spouted cups can harbour bacteria and encourage frequent sipping (which is bad for baby's teeth). At first, to familiarise baby with this new method of drinking, I tried offering some milk in a cup.

COOKING FOR BABY

Making your own baby food is simple to do and it ensures that baby gets only the best ingredients – no unwanted additives or preservatives.

I wash or scrub all fruit and vegetables thoroughly before peeling and removing any core, seeds or pips. Then I roughly chop the food – whether fruit, vegetable, meat or fish – before placing it in a saucepan with a small amount of water and cooking it until tender. Finally, I purée it in a blender until smooth. Depending on baby's age and likes, I can adjust the texture from a runny purée to more chunky purées or I can mash or mince foods. Lumpier foods are of a challenge to eat and baby may spit them out at first.

Some babies prefer individual ingredients in their meals to be kept separately so that they can 'log' and identify each taste and texture; in this is true for your baby, his food has to be presented in a form with which he can cope.

It find it a good idea to prepare baby meals in bulk and freeze them in single portions for future use. When I prepare meals for later use, I cool the food as quickly as possible (ideally within 1–2 hours) then place it in the fridge. I can then divide the food into single portions for kee[omg in the fridge for up to two days.

To freeze prepared food, I wrap single portions in freezer cling film or food wrap or place them in ice-cube trays. I always label and date the food parcels and defrost the oldest ones first. When defrosting, I remove them from the ice-cube tray and store covered in the

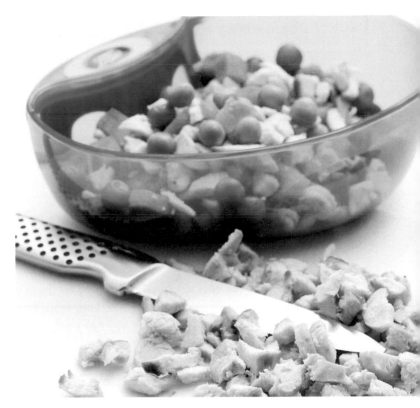

fridge overnight; if I'm in a hurry, I use the defrost setting on my microwave.

Once the food has defrosted, I heat it thoroughly. When it is piping hot, I stir it well to remove any hot spots and allow it to cool until it is the right temperature for your baby to eat. I discard any leftovers immediately; I do not reheat, refreeze or reuse under any circumstances, to avoid the risk of food poisoning.

Going organic

While I may have to pay a bit more for organic meat, fruits and vegetables, to me, the benefits are numerous. There is good evidence to suggest a connection between pesticide residues and allergies and hyperactivity in children. Non-organic food may also contain hormones and other harmful chemicals.

Fresh organic products tend to taste better because they are not intensively grown to absorb excess water and are usually grown in better quality soil and left to ripen for longer. Studies have shown that the lower levels of water in organic produce mean that it has higher concentrations of nutrients.

COMMERCIAL BABY FOODS

Colours, flavourings, stabilisers and emulsifiers are added to baby food to make it more attractive, tasty and long-lasting. However, it's a rare parent who doesn't use

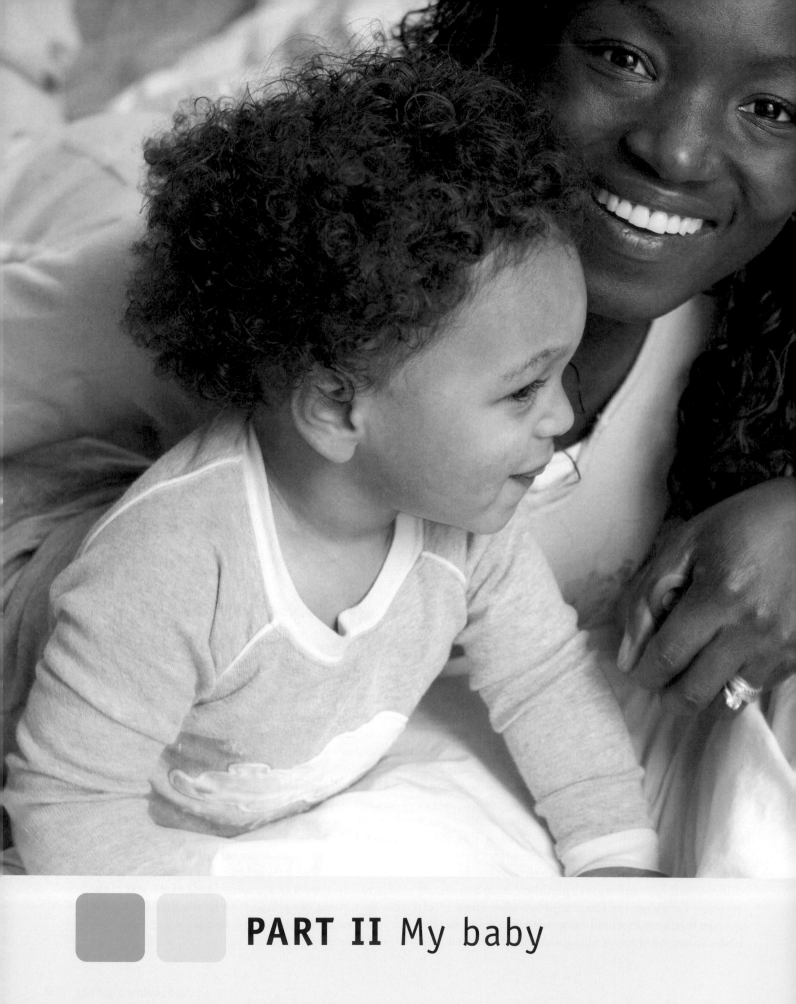

PART II My baby

Caring for my toddler

It seems like only yesterday that my baby was this tiny, helpless being completely dependent on me. Now I'm living with someone who is constantly getting into things and not shy of telling me what to do! She's definitely her own person and not a day goes by when I'm not thrilled with what she's acheived and amazed by the interesting person she's become. Yes, I know things will be more difficult to manage now that her wishes need to be catered for, but it's also a great time to share experiences and grow closer.

Monitoring my toddler's development

As my baby gets older, she will be acquiring skills at an ever-more rapid rate and my main concerns are that her development is within the range of normal and that her home environment remains safe for her to try out new-found abilities such as walking and self-feeding. As well as perfecting her movement and manipulative skills, the toddler years are marked by the appearance of personality and a greater ability to communicate and socialise with others.

PERSONALITY AND EMOTIONS

There is no doubt that my child was an individual from an early age, but in acquiring locomotive and other skills, she is better able to manifest the type of person she is. Although certain aspects of personality are a result of genes, a child is equally influenced by the way she is brought up and treated by others. Even identical twins brought up in the same way will show differences in personality.

As a parent, I aim to provide the best environment I possibly can in which to nurture my child and help her reach her full potential. However, how she will respond to the world around her is, to a certain extent, pre-ordained, and my influence can only go so far.

Initially, like all babies, mine was out-going and friendly, pleased to meet new people as well as to see those she knew well. Then she became wary of strangers, looking to me for comfort and reassurance when meeting someone new. Sharing is also something she finds difficult.

As she reached toddler age, she also developed moods – being happy when things go her way and tearful and grumpy if frustrated. Her frustration often leads to tantrums. This is understandable as toddlers have to live with certain physical limitations – mine is not always able to move around as fast as she would like or is sufficiently dexterous to play as she would

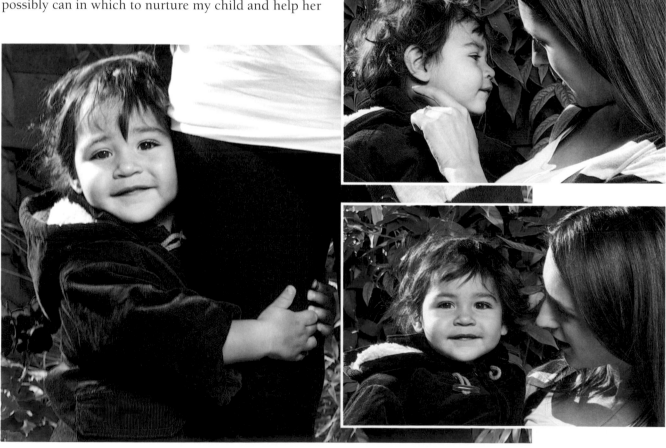

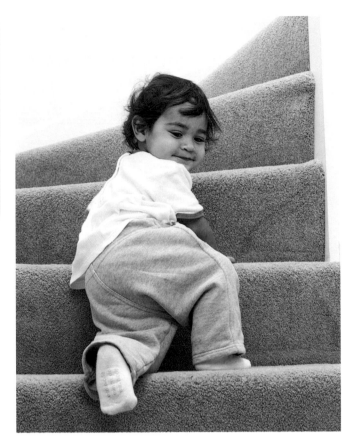

wish. Moreover, her speech is limited, too, so she is not always able to make me understand what she wants.

On the other hand, her growing sense of humour – she does funny things to gain attention – and the way she increasingly demonstrates affection – she'll give me a kiss, if asked – make her a joy to be with.

In order to help my child fit in with the world around her, I must learn to understand and accept her temperament and develop strategies to prepare her for and give her the confidence to cope with any situation.

GROWING INDEPENDENCE

Using her ability to walk is one way of showing her growing independence – she's as likely to walk away from me as to come when I ask!

She also tries to take some control of what is happening to her. She is better able to demonstrate her desires – through pointing and words – and often wants to get her own way. In fact, if she doesn't get what she wants, she is likely to start screaming and shouting.

My task is to encourage her growing abilities (see page 216) but at the same time managing her displays of temper (see page 234).

KEEPING HER SAFE

My baby's growing abilities and curiosity can put her in danger. Standing up on a chair or in the buggy, climbing downstairs standing up, missing a step, walking on busy roads or playing outside – all can be potentially hazardous so it's important not only to be constantly vigilant but also to teach her about the dangers. As well as taking the necessary precautions of putting unsafe things out of her reach and not exposing her to possible hazards (see page 188), I also need to start inculcating certain safety lessons. I must ensure that I set a good example, such as always putting on my seat belt in the car and crossing at the lights.

If I do nothing else I will ... ✔

HELP MY CHILD REMAIN SAFE

A mobile toddler is able to meet more dangers than a young baby. I need to educate my baby about:

✔ **Roads and traffic.** Even when she's in her buggy, I need to explain about crossing on the green, to look both ways and to hold onto someone's hand when walking.

✔ **Strangers.** I need to teach my toddler to check with me first before talking to someone she doesn't know.

✔ **Food and treats.** My toddler must learn to accept food only from someone she knows well and to check with me before eating any sweets.

✔ **Medicines.** I must explain that medicines are not sweets and that only I will give them to her.

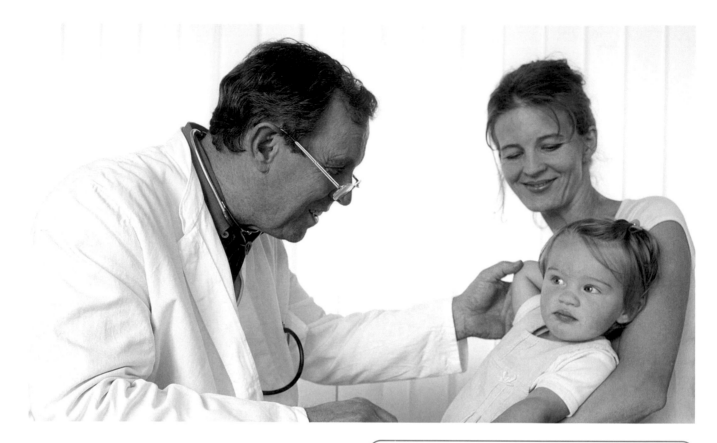

DEVELOPMENTAL CONCERNS

There are a number of conditions – developmental delay and sensory impairment, for example – that could hold my toddler back from achieving her potential. Since many conditions are treatable, it is vital that I report any concerns to my doctor. Although my toddler will have regular check-ups, as a parent, I'll probably be the first to notice if something is not as it should be. The checklist on page 215 should help me to note when she acquires anticipated skills.

If I suspect she has any developmental issues at all, it's important that I mention them as soon as possible – not wait for a regular check-up. In addition, I need to report any problems she may have with vision or hearing, as either a visual or hearing impairment will result in certain milestones being delayed.Situations that commonly arise and can indicate a problem include delay in:
• Sitting unsupported.
• Walking.
• Speech and language development.
I should report any aspects of my toddler's behaviour or personality – such as a lack of affection, disruptive behaviour or signs of vulnerability (withdrawal, tearfulness, timidity) – that I find troubling. Further investigation may be required to ascertain whether a

problem actually exists. The sooner a potential problem is diagnosed, the sooner it can be treated and the less impact it will have on a child's acquisition of skills. Many types of special help and/or support are available to assist children in developing to their potential.

Delayed Milestones ✗

Although every child develops at a different rate, there is a range of normal with milestones. Therefore, I must notify my doctor if my baby:

✗ Isn't crawling or scooting by 12 months.

✗ Doesn't walk by 18 months.

✗ Isn't talking by 2 years old.

TODDLER'S SKILLS ACQUISITION

12–15 MONTHS

- [ ] Uses spoon more expertly.
- [ ] Picks up cup and drinks from it.
- [ ] Interested in self-feeding.
- [ ] Picks up small object with either hand.
- [ ] Watches objects that are thrown or dropped to the ground.
- [ ] Starts to crawl upstairs.
- [ ] Walks unaided.
- [ ] May learn to walk backwards.
- [ ] Can stoop to recover an object.
- [ ] Recognises objects in books and will point to at least one picture.
- [ ] Can make animal sounds.

15–18 MONTHS

- [ ] Throws purposefully.
- [ ] Plays with push toys.
- [ ] Can build a 3-block tower.
- [ ] Cooperates in dressing.
- [ ] Can imitate a drawing stroke.
- [ ] May attempt a few chores.
- [ ] May follow a simple command.
- [ ] Knows a few body parts.
- [ ] Knows 3–5 words.

18–24 MONTHS

- [ ] Climbs into chairs and sits.
- [ ] Walks more steadily.
- [ ] Shows hand preference.
- [ ] Will be able to scribble.
- [ ] Can ask for toys, food and potty.
- [ ] Can fold paper if shown how.
- [ ] Pulls a person to show something.

- [ ] May be able to understand more complicated requests.
- [ ] Knows and uses about 50 words.
- [ ] May be able to play alone for short periods.
- [ ] Will like to help with household tasks.
- [ ] Turns pages of a book.

2–3 YEARS

- [ ] Can climb onto and off furniture.
- [ ] Runs and jumps.
- [ ] Climbs up and down stairs with 2 feet per step.
- [ ] Builds tower of 67 blocks.
- [ ] Throws and kicks a ball.
- [ ] Uses a fork.
- [ ] Can hold a small glass in both hands.
- [ ] Is starting to dress and undress.
- [ ] Can draw a circle.
- [ ] Can thread large beads.
- [ ] Can do simple puzzles.
- [ ] Opens boxes to find out what is inside.
- [ ] Recognises own image in photograph.
- [ ] Closely studies pictures in books.
- [ ] Listens attentively to conversations.
- [ ] Can follow many two-step commands.
- [ ] Has rapidly increasing vocabulary of at least 200 words.
- [ ] Points to and names familiar objects.
- [ ] Knows some nursery rhymes and colours.
- [ ] Plays alongside others.
- [ ] Enjoys 'let's pretend' play.
- [ ] Plays meaningfully with toys.
- [ ] Is aware of having to pee and poo.

Toddler activities and play

The toddler years are ones of constant learning – best done through play and activities. Toys and games not only enable my baby to hone manipulation and locomotion skills, build her imagination and practise her social skills, they also contribute to the loving bond between us.

From about 12–18 months of age, my toddler began to need less sleep, particularly as she found more exciting activities to do around the house and outdoors. This sometimes lead to night-time sleep problems (see page 203).

NAPS

Most toddlers have a day-time nap up to the age of 2, and some may need a short sleep up to the age of 3–4. A nap will last as long as a baby needs to sleep, and usually occurs at a regular time each day. I try to ensure my toddler naps when it's most beneficial to me – fitting into my schedule and not too late in the day. When my toddler refuses to nap, I allow her to play quietly in her bed with some toys or put on an audio story or some music so she still gets some rest.

If I do nothing else I will ...

ENCOURAGE MY TODDLER TO TAKE NAPS
Without sufficient rest, my toddler will become overtired and fretful. If she naps, however, I'll also be able to do things for myself or around the house. I try to do the following:

✓ **Ease her away from over-strenuous activity** some time before nap time.

✓ **Offer her a soporific snack,** for example milk and unsweetened biscuits.

✓ **Make sure her room is darkened.**

✓ **Settle her down much as for bedtime.** If necessary, spend a short time with her reading or just relaxing.

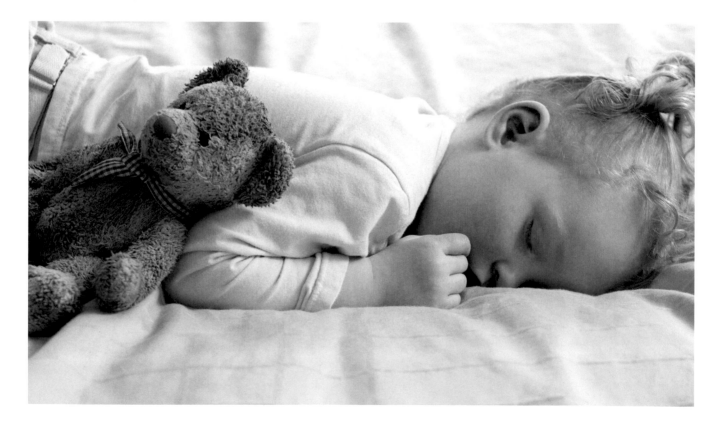

The amount of sleep a toddler needs varies; some toddlers need more than others. A bad temper and fretfulness can indicate a lack of sleep. Be realistic about how much sleep your own toddler needs. Generally, including naps, a 1 year old sleeps 12–14 hours, a 2 year old 12–13 hours, and a 3 year old around 12 hours.

TOYS

Young babies don't need many toys and even toddlers can make do with a small number of inexpensive ones. It's important to choose toys that are age appropriate (a baby finds it fun and engrossing) and safe. Often, the simplest toys or common household objects are favourites because a child's imagination can dream up multiple uses. From around 15 months, my baby enjoyed paper and drawing materials, while she used pots and pans to make noise and to fill with and carry all sorts of interesting things. Toys that leave more to the imagination – puzzles, building blocks and shape sorters – are generally more popular than those that are full of realistic details.

TELEVISION AND DVDS

TV and DVD viewing is not an important activity in my home. I know that many parents permit it in order to make some time for themselves, but any small benefit to language development that educational programmes claim is outweighed by the disadvantages. Time spent watching TV or DVDs is time not spent on more worthwhile pursuits like physical activities (to prevent obesity) or reading, and many children become upset by screen violence. Experts agree that if allowed at all, 'screen time' should be limited; children under 3 should have no screen exposure, while those aged 3–7 could watch 30–60 minutes a day. As long as my toddler has played outside, used her imagination, been read to, participated in other activities (drawing, building with blocks, etc.) and played with toys, then – and only then – do I permit limited screen time. I also make sure I choose calm, quiet programmes and try to watch them with her – so I can assess their suitability and change the channel if necessary.

INDOOR ACTIVITIES

There are many home-based activities that my child finds enjoyable. She happily sits in front of a low-level cabinet in the kitchen and plays with pots and pans. In the bath, she enjoys pouring water into cups, blowing bubbles and floating boats.

Successful shopping ✓

Shopping for food or other essentials with a lively or bored young child in tow, is an experience many of us would prefer to miss, but can't avoid. I have several strategies to prevent it being a hassle.

✓ I always stick to certain rules such as never buying sweets in supermarkets.

✓ I try to go to the shops when they are quiet and neither of us is tired or hungry.

✓ I carry a suitable snack such as a bun or banana.

✓ Whenever I can, I let my toddler choose the food I buy – for instance, she can pick between red or green apples or our breakfast cereal. If she picks up an unsuitable item, I explain why I don't want it or put it back when she's not looking.

✓ I try and visit markets or centres with good toilet and changing facilities – and I make sure I know where they are.

✓ Sometimes we go to a specialist shop such as a butcher's or baker's, so that she can see close up how food is cut up or weighed.

✓ If I have a lot of shopping to do, I try to break up the time with a visit to a café or check if a crèche is available.

From about 18 months of age, my toddler wanted to help with the housework. Now that she is a bit older, she wipes off the table or, with my help, puts the clothes in the washing machine or adds the laundry soap (which I measure out). She also enjoys helping out with baking – and she happily models pieces of dough or decorates biscuits. Painting at an easel with water-based paints, drawing with crayons and working with clay are other favourite pursuits.

Other activities we enjoy together are dressing-up play, dancing to music and doing simple jigsaw puzzles. Role-playing games enable her to practise social interactions and to channel the frustration and anger she keeps within. This is helpful to both of us as, the more often she expresses her negative feelings through play, the less severe and frequent are her temper tantrums will be.

LOCAL VISITS

Everyday outings are great learning experiences for my child. Visits to the shops, park, zoo, petting farm, activity class or a children's museum provide lots of new things to see, do and talk about. When taking everyday walks, I try to vary familiar routes so that my toddler sees new things. Having her sit facing me in her buggy means we can talk more together. I keep the visits short to avoid boredom.

En route to our destination, there are opportunities to discuss the things we pass, such as dogs, buses or goods in shop windows. While walking, we look out for things to collect to use later to make collages or leaf prints, or as a nature display. Horse chestnuts, stones, pebbles, shells, seaweed, driftwood, acorns, feathers, leaves, pine cones or grasses are all collectable.

Even when it's raining or snowing we go outside – dressed in suitable clothes – for some play or a short

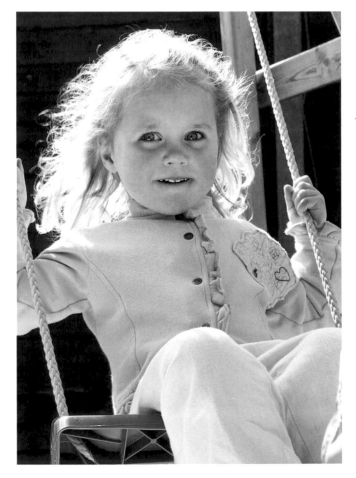

EXPERTS ADVISE

Car sickness

Motion sickness with associated nausea and vomiting results when the eyes make rapid movements to follow and refocus on moving objects. A good way to avoid it is to position your child in the middle of the back seat and put blinders – cut from cardboard and taped to the side of the seat – on her seat to stop her from looking out of the side window. By looking straight ahead, through the front window, the rapid eye movements can be avoided. An antihistamine can also prevent motion sickness. Ask your GP.

walk. In wellington boots, she's happy to go on a puddle hunt in the rain and splash through them or to look for her reflection. If it has snowed, we throw snowballs at a wall or have a mock snowball fight or possibly make a snow angel.

PLAYGROUND AND PARK

Visits to the playground are important to satisfy my toddler's in-built physicality in a safe and convenient environment. Here she can enjoy the slide, swings and climbing equipment; when she is happy sitting still, she joins in the fun in the sandpit. Of course, I make sure she plays carefully on roundabouts and waits until they have stopped before she climbs on or off. I also teach her that she should never climb up the front of a slide and that she must wait until the child in front of her slides off at the bottom before she goes down.

At the park, she enjoys feeding the ducks, playing in the fountains or just running around. If she's riding her tricycle, I make sure she wears a helmet.

GOING FURTHER AFIELD

Travelling long distances from home with a toddler requires a fair amount of time and effort – not only getting to where we are going but once we are there. Time away together is less restful than when I travel on my own, and my daily plans are strongly influenced by my toddler's routines. I try to be on the road during the hours she typically naps and we eat our meals at her usual times.

If we're going by car, I stop every two hours to allow her to use her potty (or change nappies) or to give her

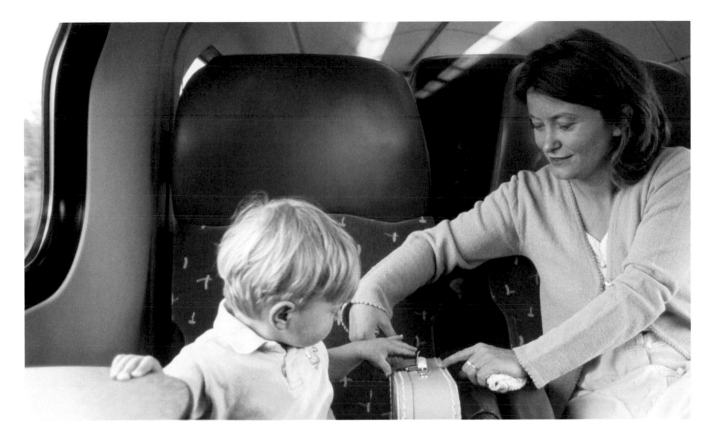

a chance to move around and burn off energy. On a train, I'm often able to vary things by taking her to another carriage – the dining or snack car– which offers a change of scene, more activity to watch and a place for a treat. She needs to hold my hand at all times and not run up and down in the aisle, as a sudden jolt of the train may throw her off balance. I sometimes load a movie or cartoons onto my laptop or take a portable DVD player.

Travelling by plane can lead to earaches and jet lag. To help ward these off, when the plane ascends and descends, I give my toddler something to chew on. However, I also carry a suitable painkiller. Jet lag seldom occurs in a trip with a time zone shift of less than 3–4 hours and is much less likely to occur when travelling from east to west than when going west to east. Where possible, I arrange flights to suit my child's normal sleep patterns. An overnight stop along the way also helps. I make sure she drinks plenty of water on the flight and that she is exposed to sunlight at our destination (if possible). This can help reset her internal clock. On brief excursions (less than 3 days) into a different time zone, I try to follow routines according to our original time zone. But for longer stays, I immediately adjust my toddler's eating and sleeping schedules to the new time zone.

If I do nothing else I will ...

ENSURE MY CHILD'S TOYS ARE SAFE

The age range given on the packaging is less important than my baby's state of development. It's essential that my young toddler's toys are:

✔ **Chunky** with large pieces.

✔ **Well made** with no sharp edges.

✔ **Washable,** if soft, so they can be cleaned every so often.

✔ **Furnished with strings no longer than 30 cm,** to avoid the risk of strangulation.

✔ **Well maintained by me** to make sure small pieces, such as eyes, can't come away and cause a choking hazard.

✗ **Not too heavy** in case they fall on her.

13 MONTHS

Messy play with finger paints, sand, water or moulding material is what my toddler finds particularly enjoyable now. Some favourite books have different textures and lift-up flaps. She has started to take the lead in play, telling me what to do, so our games now are mainly me fetching what she throws at me.

14 MONTHS

Her finger control is much more developed, so she loves putting small things into and taking bigger things and kitchen items out of yogurt pots, plastic beakers and juice bottles. She has started building with bricks and we both find it fun to build a tower and then knock it down, or make a bridge for a car to go underneath. She has a few simple musical instruments – a tambourine and drum.

15 MONTHS

Hide-and-seek and other chasing games in which she can initiate the play and 'order' me about are on the

BOOKS AND READING

One of our favourite activities – whether at bedtime or while driving in the car or when rain keeps us indoors – reading has a vital role to play both in developing my toddler skills as well as entertaining her. Reading not only enlarges her language skills but, in time, builds manipulative skills as she will perfect holding the book herself, turning the pages and pointing to objects she recognises.

We've graduated from cloth and board books to simple picture and storybooks. My toddler enjoys abridged versions of fairy and classic tales and nursery rhymes. Reading need not take too long – 5–10 minutes is generally enough at this time.

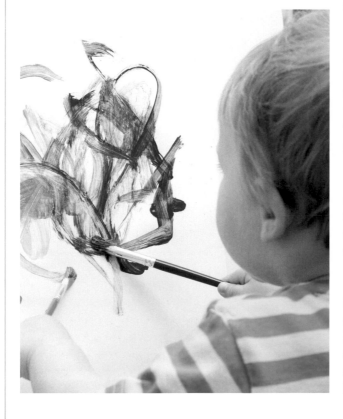

menu. She also likes activities with commands or actions – 'Simon Says' – or reciting rhymes with gestures, such as 'Incy Wincy Spider'. She's now able to use simple nesting and stacking toys.

16 MONTHS

My toddler is capable of doing simple jigsaw puzzles with my help. Now that she is more steady on her feet, we play simple ball games outdoors and she likes to wheel her doll in a buggy or pull a small wagon or other push-and-pull toy. She now plays with more sophisticated vehicles, generally of wood.

17 MONTHS

An activity board with lots of moving parts holds her attention and she enjoys simple craft materials – crayons, stickers and paper. She enjoys being outdoors and discovering items from the natural world.

18 MONTHS

My toddler is now much more accurate at stacking and sorting, at fitting shapes through holes, and at using blocks for building. Making things with play dough is fun and she likes it if I ask her to make certain items for me such as a 'biscuit'. She also likes going to the dressing-up box and pretend play with teddy.

20 MONTHS

She enjoys playing with her doll – one that is spongeable and has an assortment of clothes – and other soft toys. In addition to books with lots of simple rhymes, she enjoys listening to recordings of simple stories and nursery tunes.

22 MONTHS

More sophisticated noise-making toys – like a xylophone and music box – are fun for her. She's also enjoying introducing other materials into her pictures, making collages with fabric, pasta and shiny papers.

24 MONTHS

Artistic activities now include the use of modelling medium. She's become adept at stringing spools and can work better with building blocks; she may engage in imaginative play with them – building a fort or other enclosure or tower. She joins in singing songs and repeating nursery rhymes and particularly likes those with actions, such as 'Wind the Bobbin Up'.

26 MONTHS

My toddler has become interested in pretend play – taking care of her ill teddy or getting teddy ready for bed – but often asks me to join in. Although she won't play with other children, she enjoys sharing activities with me at a toddler gym or swimming class.

28 MONTHS

Pretend games continue to be great fun and are endlessly developed, from playing at being the postman delivering letters to setting up shop with some mini provisions. I've put a cloth over a table so that she can 'camp out' underneath and let her use large cardboard boxes as a fire truck or car. She likes the stories I make up about someone she knows and will answer questions about the story.

30 MONTHS

My toddler wants to help join in with the housework and I've given her a dustpan and brush and a wooden drill. She likes it when I bake – she can add decorations – and I let her water some plants or sponge down her high chair and put her toys away. Together we create simple artwork projects – she helps decorate Christmas cards by colouring or adding glitter or stickers.

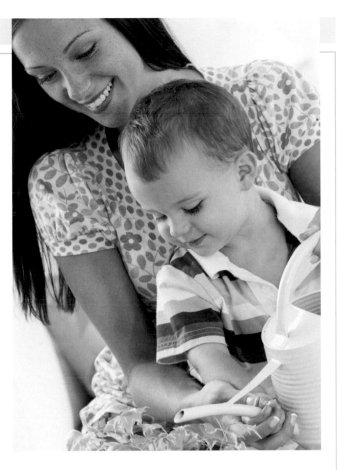

32 MONTHS

Art activities, such as drawing and colouring-in or painting, are endlessly attractive – particularly if they leave a mess! We also try making potato prints using poster paints and creating sticker books.

34 MONTHS

My toddler enjoys doing jobs, which are simple and easy. She joins in with baking – bringing ingredients from the larder, mixing flour, adding raisins or putting the spoons away – and can do a simple treasure hunt; if I show her a picture in a magazine or a book, she can find a similar one at home. Books are very important and she appreciates ones with 'proper' stories. I let her choose her bedtime book.

36 MONTHS

Playing together is the greatest fun. We make music, dance, play 'catch', do puzzles and even play simple board or card games. Even putting groceries or the laundry away together can be a game. We also spend time baking and creating artworks.

Helping my toddler become independent

Now that she is able to get about on her own (with some help), my toddler demonstrates a growing desire for independence – not just in where she wants to go but in feeding and dressing herself and expressing her opinions. The toddler years are characterised by a determination to achieve tasks alone, though this may be complicated by separation anxieties (see page 240)

SELF-FEEDING

As soon as my baby started on solid foods, I began to encourage her to feed herself. As well as providing her with a cup or letting her hold her bottle, I gave her finger-sized pieces of solid foods such as fruit segments, vegetable sticks, pieces of baby biscuits and bread sticks. Just after her first birthday, she started to try to feed herself using a spoon, though it was many months before she was able to get food into her mouth and chew it properly.

DRESSING AND SELF-DRESSING

Initially, once she reached toddler age, it became more difficult to dress her as she didn't want to stay still long enough for me to put on her clothes. To encourage her to get dressed, I tried making a game of it, such as hide-and-seek: "Where's your head gone then? Oh, there it is!" when I pulled a jumper over her head or sang her a song about dressing or the parts of her body.

Starting at about 18 months of age, however, she not only found it fun to discard her clothes, but she also became more cooperative when I dressed her. She first reached out her arms to go into sleeves and then was able to remove her hat, mittens and socks. Now that she's approaching 3 years, she's beginning to have very definite likes and dislikes about what to wear.

Learning to dress herself is an important step for my toddler so it's important that I not interfere with the process or laugh when she gets it wrong, otherwise she becomes angry or discouraged and her pleasure in learning is taken away. To minimise arguments, I put clothes that I want her to wear in accessible drawers and let her select from a suitable range of garments. Then I lay out the garments in a way that it makes it

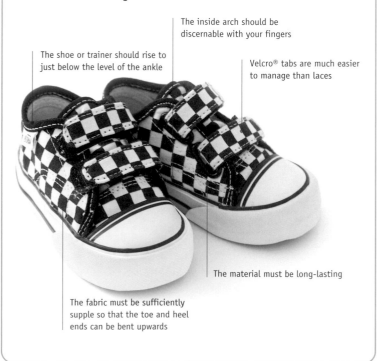

RECOMMENDED SHOES OR TRAINERS

You should just be able to place your index finger between the tip of your baby's big toe and the end of the shoe or trainer while she is standing.

The inside arch should be discernable with your fingers

The shoe or trainer should rise to just below the level of the ankle

Velcro® tabs are much easier to manage than laces

The material must be long-lasting

The fabric must be sufficiently supple so that the toe and heel ends can be bent upwards easy for her to put them on easily. For example, if a shirt or skirt has a picture on the front, I place it downwards so that the picture is facing away from her when she puts it on. If there are buttons on the back of the garment, I place these facing upwards. I lay out her trousers with the waist closest and the front upmost and her shirts and jumpers are placed downwards with the head furthest away. I show her how to burrow into these from the bottom. I've also bought her a 'learning to dress' doll, which gives her practise in doing up buttons, laces and zips.

I always give myself plenty of time for dressing – even if I have to get up a few minutes earlier. My toddler seems to know to slow down and resist more when I am in a hurry.

Shoes and socks

Once my baby began walking outdoors, it was time to buy her proper shoes. These need to sturdy yet flexible and of breathable material. Both shoes or trainer styles are suitable if they fit properly (see page 222). She needn't wear shoes at home, however, and letting her go barefoot or walking around in socks is fine.

It's also important she wear the right sized socks; if socks are too big, they can ruin a correctly fitted shoe by causing pressure; if they are too small, they will scrunch the toes and discourage straight growth. Socks need to be checked regularly to ensure they still fit. They should be made of pure cotton and not acrylic or wool. Cotton enables feet to breathe properly and it minimises the possibility of fungal infections, such as athlete's foot.

SLEEPING IN A BED

Once my baby can climb over the top of her cot, I need to introduce a bed for safety reasons; she can easily hurt herself climbing over the high rail. I understand that most toddlers don't object to changing over, but some children may be reluctant to leave a familiar environment. As space isn't a problem, I plan to keep both the cot and the new bed in her room for a few weeks, so my toddler can sleep part of the time in each.

The best time for the changeover is when times are fairly settled – no new siblings or holidays on the horizon – and a toddler is not ill or being toilet trained or weaned.

The new bed should be low to the ground to prevent injuries in case the toddler falls out. Initially, guard rails should be placed down the sides of the bed or cushions alongside the bed until she gets used to it.

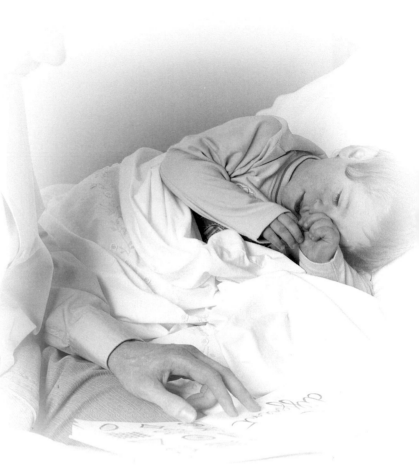

If I do nothing else I will ...

MAKE THE TRANSITION TO A BED EASIER

Involving my toddler in the process and being sensitive to her needs will help her take this big step. I plan to do the following:

✓ **Have my toddler help pick out** new bed linen as long as I narrow down the choices.

✓ **Cover the new bed with waterproof sheeting** in case of accidents.

✓ **Transfer a favourite blanket.**

✓ **Surround the bed with selection of her favourite cot toys.**

✓ **Buy her a new stuffed animal** as a 'big bed' companion.

✓ **Maintain our bedtime routine** with story and cuddles.

Daily care

My baby's growing independence impacts on aspects of her daily care. She wants to do a lot more for herself now – tooth brushing and hair combing, for example, so making sure these are done well is a lot trickier. I also have to teach her how to clean her hands before meals and after certain activities.

BATHS

My baby really enjoys her time in the bath, though she thinks a bath is for having fun not getting clean. I use the time she's in the bath to encourage her to wash herself; part of this involves teaching her the different body parts.

Some young toddlers, however, develop a dislike of bath time because they are frightened of being in water. If your child becomes fearful, try making it more fun by adding a mild bubble bath, soap crayons, a selection of water toys or singing appropriate nursery rhymes such as 'Rub-A-Dub-Dub, 3 Men in a Tub'. If your toddler is scared of getting her face wet, show her how to blow bubbles in the water. Taking a bath together can make

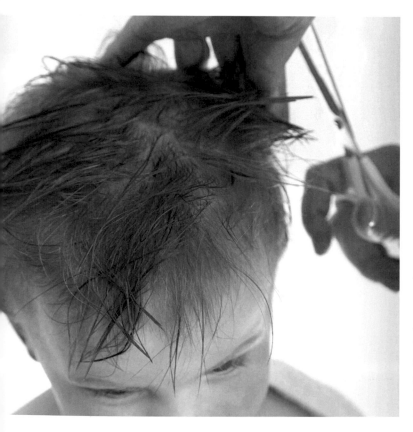

If I do nothing else I will ...

MAKE HAIR WASHING LESS STRESSFUL
My toddler is not alone in not liking to have her hair washed. There are a number of things to try. I:

✓ **Wash her hair while she's in the bath.** I get her to lie back and tilt her head backwards so that the water falls backwards away from her eyes. Using a spray attachment makes the direction of the water easier to control.

✓ **Or hold a dry face cloth, folded in two, against her eyes** and forehead to shield them from soap and water.

✓ **Sometimes she wears a shampoo hat or visor,** which goes across the forehead, just over the ears, and around the back of the head. Water poured on the top of baby's head will not land in her eyes.

✓ **Alternatively, there are rinse cups** that have a flexible edge, which fits against the forehead and forms a watertight seal to keep water and shampoo away from the eyes and face.

your toddler feel more at ease and it will be a good occasion to let her splash you or pour water over your head, then you do the same to her. If she is really making a fuss about bathing, revert to sponge bathing until she feels ready to go back into the water or try taking her into the shower with you.

HAIR CARE
Although hair cutting can be quite a challenge – many toddlers are uncomfortable and fearful when scissors or clippers are near them – I try and keep baby's hair short as it's then easier to care for. Hair is more easily combed if it is moist or wet, so I comb my toddler's hair straight after towel drying at bath time or spray on water before starting. It can help to use a detangler on toddlers with longer hair, which will need brushing more frequently. My toddler is keen to hold a brush but is not able to get

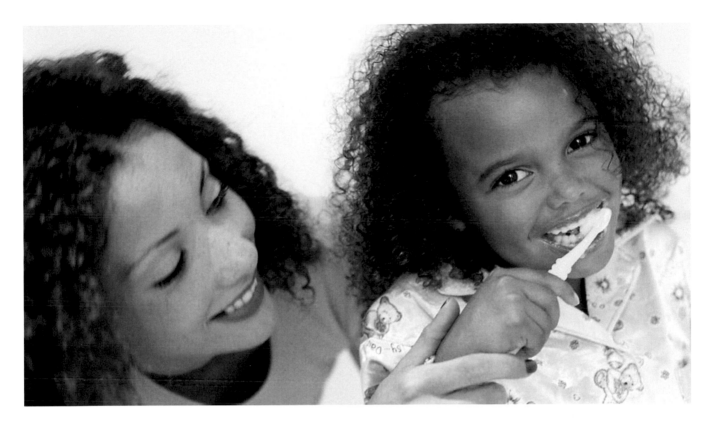

rid of any tangles. For haircuts, I use a salon that specialises in cutting children's hair.

Shampooing can be a bit of a battle because my toddler doesn't like water being poured on her head and she is afraid of shampoo getting in her eyes. It's not necessary to shampoo her hair every day, so I wash her hair 2–3 times a week at most. When I do shampoo, I have a number of strategies (see page 224).

TOOTH CARE

Although my toddler wants to brush her own teeth, she's not able to do it effectively; she'll probably need some help with brushing until she reaches the age of 7 or so. Although her milk teeth will eventually be replaced with her permanent set (from around the age of 6), I need to take good care of her first teeth.

Children's teeth have very deep fissures and I must take extra care to ensure I get into those grooves and clean them properly – 90 per cent of all tooth decay happens in a child's back molars. Dental decay can be painful and will require treatment, which is an unwelcome experience that can easily be avoided. Also, if teeth appear discoloured or contain fillings, a child may become self-conscious. My toddler and I brush our teeth together, which makes it more fun. I also try and floss her teeth – though not all toddlers are willing. I don't permit my toddler to have lollies and other

sweets on a regular basis, as these stick to the teeth and promote cavities. However, she is allowed the occasional treat, and I have to be vigilant to brush her teeth afterwards. Cheese is a great acid neutraliser and I encourage my child to eat it after meals or before bed.

Toddlers who use dummies or suck their thumbs may well be putting their teeth at risk. A toddler still using a dummy regularly by the age of 2–3 is likely to develop a crossbite (where the upper teeth are behind the lower teeth rather than in front of them), while thumbsucking also can affect tooth alignment and speech and introduces germs into the mouth.

I bring my toddler with me now to my dental appointments. Not only is my dentist able to take a quick look to check that everything is normal, but it helps my child get used to having her teeth checked.

BEDTIMES

A simple and soothing routine is important to create security for a toddler and to prevent possible sleep problems. A mainstay of my toddler's bedtime routine is her story.

Bedtime occurs at the same time each night. I give her plenty of notice and let her play a little beforehand so she winds down. After putting on her pyjamas and brushing her teeth, we dim the lights and both of us snuggle down in her bed ready for a story. Whatever we

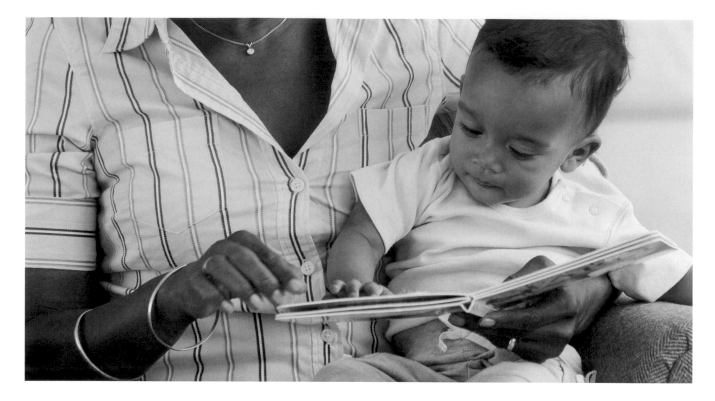

read has to be short – no more than 10 minutes – and have a happy ending. When it's over, we might have a little chat about the day's events, then it's a goodnight kiss and turn on the nightlight.

Sleeping problems

A child's need for sleep lessens as she gets older; once my toddler started waking very early, I put her to bed a little later, cut down on her daytime naps and made sure she had plenty of exercise and fresh air during the day. Because her imagination has become more active, aspects of night-time can be frightening. To prevent any fear of the dark, I ensure my child never sleeps alone in a dark room – especially when visiting relatives or is on holiday and she is sleeping in a strange bed. At home, I keep her door ajar and a nightlight on in the room and make sure it does not cast strange shadows.

Most children experience scary dreams at some time. Commonly, they begin between the ages of 18–36 months and are usually sparked off by a disturbing television programme or a frightening story. However, if they occur very frequently, they may be a sign that a child is anxious or upset about something. To help forestall bad dreams, it is a good idea to limit television – particularly programmes that contain lots of action – and loud music or noisy games before bedtime. If a child has a nightmare she will need comforting and reassuring upon waking.

Occasionally, you may be awakened by your toddler giving a piercing scream or crying in fright and find her sitting up and staring in terror but still asleep. This is what is called a night terror. Your child is not aware of your presence and in the morning she will not remember the dream. During a night terror, the best thing to do is not to wake your toddler but to tuck her in and stay with her until she falls into a calm sleep.

More commonly, a toddler may repeatedly come into her parents' room during the night. This happened with mine when she began sleeping in a bed. When she comes into my room, I tell her firmly that she has to go to her own room and I take her back to bed. I try to remain calm but firm. I remind her that she has toys in her room with which she can play.

HYGIENE

While I know it's impossible to protect my child from every illness and infection and in any case, she will need to build up her immunity against these, children are particularly vulnerable to stomach upsets such as diarrhoea and vomiting, as well as diseases picked up outdoors, so good hygiene habits are important.

As soon as my child began feeding herself, I tried to get her into the habit of washing her hands before eating or touching food. I gave her her own flannel and towel and supervised her hand washing so I could check she was doing it properly.

I also make her wash her hands or use a hand sanitiser when she goes to the potty, when she comes in from outdoors or plays with animals.

Toddlers are at particular risk from toxocariasis, a disease caused by roundworm infection, if they crawl or play on the ground or in sand pits and put dirty fingers in their mouths or eat dirt. For that reason, I also try to prevent my child eating dirt, sand or grass and discourage her from sucking dirty fingers.

⚠ EXPERTS ADVISE

Toxicariasis
This disease can cause asthma, stomach upset, listlessness and sight problems and affected children will need to be treated with steroids and anti-parasitic drugs. Toxicara eggs are found in the faeces of infected dogs and cats and these can remain in the ground for two years or more.

If I do nothing else I will ... ✓

HELP MY TODDLER WITH HYGIENE
To prevent her picking up dangerous bacteria, I:

✓ **Keep her nails short** to minimise dirt getting stuck under them.

✓ **Cover our sandpit** when not in use.

✓ **Wash her comfort blanket frequently** and not allow her to trail it around and then suck it.

✓ **Teach her not to eat** any fruit or raw vegetables before these have been washed.

✓ **Use sanitary wipes** when we are out and about.

✓ **Wash and disinfect the potty** every time she makes use of it.

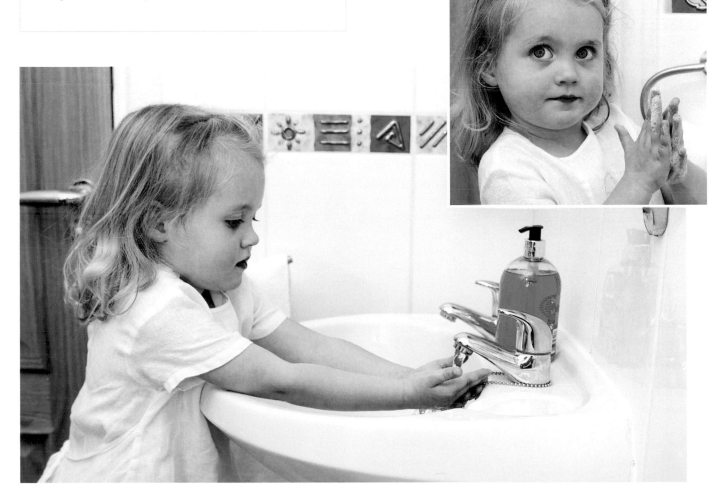

Toddler meals

Energy requirements increase from years 1–3 as a toddler grows and becomes more active. Although the need for good quality protein is much the same as when she was younger (2–3 servings a day), my toddler needs more vitamins and minerals. I aim to supply what she needs by serving her a varied diet from the different food groups. However, since mealtimes don't always go smoothly – occasionally a meal remains largely uneaten or she only wants to eat peanut butter sandwiches – I don't obsess about whether she gets what she needs on a daily basis but consider what she eats over a week. As long as my child eats a good mix of healthy foods on a regular basis, she will get all the nutrients she requires.

NUTRIENT NEEDS

Basically, the same building blocks of nutrition for younger babies form the basis for what a toddler needs to thrive. Toddlers, however, need a certain amount of fat for normal growth and development. Unsaturated fat is found in vegetable oils, oily fish and soft margarine, and I offer a small amount each day. Snacks, too, are increasingly important to cater to my toddler's high energy requirements and small stomach.

Carbohydrates/starchy food

Excellent sources of energy, fibre, vitamins and minerals, carbohydrates make up the main part of every meal, but as toddlers find it difficult to digest large amounts of high-fibre foods such as wholemeal bread and brown rice, I try providing refined (white) as well as wholemeal (brown) carbohydrates. So, for example, I serve white and wholemeal toast.

Protein foods

Meat, fish, poultry and eggs provide rich amounts of vitamins and minerals and are essential for growth and development. I also like to include vegetarian choices that contain a good mix of protein foods like beans, lentils, tofu and nuts.

Oily fish – tuna, salmon, mackerel, herring, sardines, pilchards and trout are rich sources of omega-3 essential fatty acids, which have been found to benefit the brain, eyes and skin. Lean red meat and liver are rich in iron.

Fruit and vegetables

Fresh, frozen, canned, dried or juiced fruit and vegetables provide a whole host of vitamins and minerals, especially vitamin C, vital for good health. Vegetables can be eaten raw or cooked, incorporated into dishes or puréed in sauces, stews, soups and pies.

Dairy products

Full-fat milk, cheese, yogurt and fromage frais provide protein for growth and development, calcium for teeth and, together with vitamin D, help make bones and teeth stronger. Crème fraîche, fromage frais and thick natural yogurt, which are lower in fat, can be used in cooking to flavour sauces.

SNACKS

My toddler usually needs a snack mid morning, mid afternoon and sometimes pre-bedtime. Instead of sugary, salty or fatty processed foods, I offer a range of healthy choices. However, I have to ensure she gets

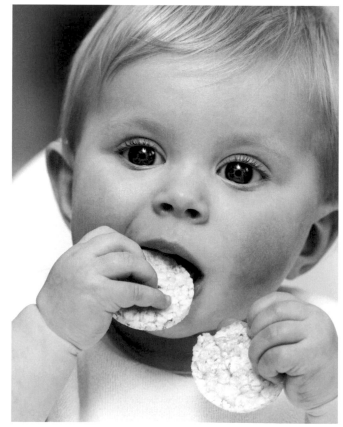

MY TODDLER'S DAILY DIET

PORTIONS	1–2 YEARS OLD	2–3 YEARS OLD
CARBOHYDRATE/STARCHY FOODS	3–4 servings	4–5 servings

- Bread (1 slice).
- Crackers (2–3).
- Cooked cereal (50 g).
- Dry cereal (75 g).
- Cooked pasta, noodles or rice (50 g).
- Potatoes (1 small).

	2 servings	2–4 servings
PROTEIN FOODS		

- Lean, red meat (25 g).
- Poultry (25 g).
- Fish (25 g).
- Pulses (25 g).
- Eggs (1).
- Peanut butter (1 tbsp).

	2 servings (1 veg 1 fruit)	5 servings (3 veg 2 fruit)
FRUIT AND VEGETABLES		

- Cooked vegetables (50 g).
- Chopped raw vegetables (50 g).
- Leafy raw vegetables such as lettuce or spinach (100 g).
- Tomato (1 small).
- Whole fruit, i.e. apple or banana (½).
- Grapes (handful).
- Glass of fresh juice (1 small).
- Canned fruit (50 g).
- Dried fruit (25 g).

	4 servings per day	2 servings
DAIRY PRODUCTS		

- Milk (120 ml).
- Yogurt (120 ml).
- Hard cheese (45 g).
- Soft cheese (60 g).
- Frozen yogurt (120 ml).
- Ice cream (150 ml).

Iron needs

Iron deficiency, which is not uncommon in children, can be prevented by giving a vitamin C-rich drink, such as orange juice, at the same time as an iron-rich food (such as red meat or if vegetarian, beans, lentils, green leafy vegetables, dried fruit (particularly apricots, raisins and sultanas), as well as fortified breakfast cereals. This will help with iron absorption.

most of her vital nutrients from her main meals and keep snacks to a minimum. Our favourite choices are:
• Sticks of cheese with apple slices or an oatcake.
• Toasted cheese muffin.
• Chunks of melon with ham.
• Humous and breadsticks.
• Rice cake with nut butter.
• Mashed banana sandwich.
• Pitta bread with yeast extract.
• Dried apple rings.

VEGETARIAN WEANING

With a little planning and attention, a varied vegetarian diet can provide all the nutrients a child needs for growth and development. Protein must be provided from a variety of sources – nuts (if there is no sign of an allergy within the family), seeds, eggs, dairy products, beans and pulses (including lentils and tofu) – and combined with vitamin C-rich fruit and leafy green vegetables to aid iron absorption. Pulses and beans should be a significant part of a toddler's diet as they are important sources of iron, but young babies should not be given large quantities of brown rice, wholegrain bread or wholemeal pasta. A child needs to get sufficient B vitamins, particularly B_{12} (found in eggs, cheese, textured vegetable protein and fortified breakfast cereals and yeast extract), iron and zinc. Iron is contained in beans, lentils, leafy green vegetables, dairy products, fortified breakfast cereals, dried fruit, brown rice and wholegrain bread, while zinc is found in nuts, seeds, dairy products, beans, lentils, whole grains and yeast extract.

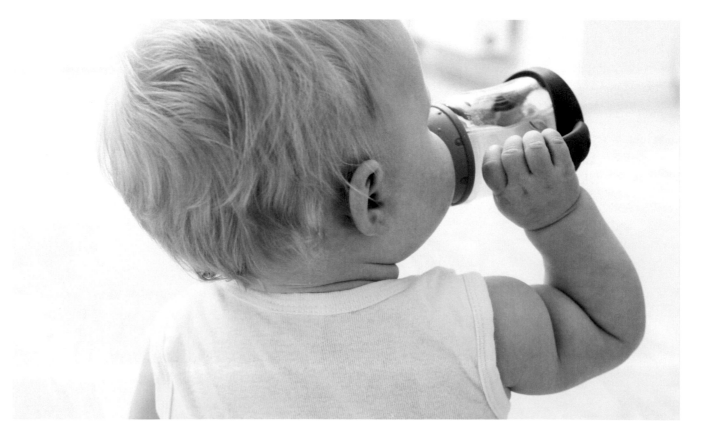

- Toasted fruit muffin or teacake.
- Natural yogurt with mango.
- Fruit scone.
- Chunks of fresh fruit.

MILK AND OTHER DRINKS

Whole cow's, sheep's or goat's milk can still be given to toddlers as a main drink (as part of the 500–600 ml milk needed a day) but, after age 2, if she's eating well, I will give my child semi-skimmed milk.

Water is always the best drink option but diluted fresh fruit juice provides vitamin C and, if served alongside a meal containing iron, can help absorption of this mineral. However, even fruit juice contains natural sugars, so I avoid giving it to my toddler other than at mealtimes to prevent damage to her teeth.

A minimum of 6–8 glasses of water per day is recommended for children aged 2 and over and even more for children who are very active. Dehydration can affect concentration as well as the transportation of nutrients around the body and brain.

SUPPLEMENTS

My doctor has recommended that my toddler continue to take a liquid supplement of vitamins A, C and D. You should check with your GP if your child needs to do the same.

FUSSY EATER

All children go through stages of picky eating and appetites can be equally unpredictable. If a toddler attends nursery or a playgroup, there may be peer pressure to eat certain things and not others, while keeping my child away from sugary treats becomes increasingly tricky as she interacts with other children, and becomes more aware of children-orientated brands.

Forcing my child to eat is a no-win situation. Conflict and tension only make a situation more difficult and may lead to her using mealtimes as a way of seeking attention. When my toddler refuses food, I try and gently coax her to try just a mouthful and when she does, I offer plenty of encouragement and praise. It's important not to offer an alternative, as it can become tiresome if a child cannot get used to eating what she is given expects endless alternatives.

Of course, I don't serve large portions, which can be off-putting for a child; if my toddler eats the food and wants more, there's always seconds. Sometimes, I combine untried or previously rejected foods with ones I know my child likes. Some parents find sticker charts

If I do nothing else I will ...

HELP MY TODDLER DEVELOP GOOD EATING HABITS

Although toddlers like to demonstrate independence at meals, instilling good habits will be beneficial in long term. I need to:

✓ **Remain relaxed about teaching manners.** While ideally I would like her to eat with a fork or spoon, my toddler will continue to eat with fingers or hands for a long time and make messes.

✓ **Encourage family meals.** Eating together encourages chatter and discussion between parents and children and parents can demonstrate good eating habits.

✓ **Be patient and persevere.** Children acquire a taste for foods over time and it takes an average of 10 "tastes" for a child to accept new foods.

✓ **Make the food tempting** by using different colours, tastes, textures and shapes when planning a meal. Interesting or colourful plates, bibs, cutlery and mats can also make a difference.

encourage their toddlers to try new foods, especially unfamiliar fruit and vegetables.

WEIGHT ISSUES

In the UK, the prevalence of obesity is increasing markedly among both adults and children. Today, more than 25 per cent of children are overweight as they are increasingly inactive and not burning enough calories. Most fat babies will start to slim down when they start to crawl or walk and become normal weight toddlers, but a few remain overweight.

The best way to prevent a child becoming fat is to breastfeed exclusively for six months and to teach good eating habits early on; prevention is much easier than cure. Young children should not be put on a diet unless advised by a doctor. However, developing a healthy family approach to food and exercise is important in weight management. I try to stick to a routine of three meals a day plus 2–3 healthy snacks. Many children are grazers, but constant nibbling is not ideal and makes them less likely to enjoy a proper meal.

Potty training my toddler

I began to think about potty training my toddler when she turned 18 months (physiological readiness occurs between 18–30 months). A girl is usually ready sooner than a boy and generally stays dry earlier. That being said, most children are dry during the day between the ages of 2–3. Usually, bowel control is learnt before bladder control because it is easier for the anal sphincter to hold in faeces than it is for the urethral sphincter to hold in urine. As the bladder matures, its ability to retain urine increases. Roughly speaking, a child will first indicate that she has a soiled or wet nappy, then that she needs to 'go potty' and, finally, is able to stay dry during the day and night.

STARTING THE TRAINING

Eighteen months is the earliest age to start toilet training, but 2 years old is a more realistic age. You can,
if you wish, get your toddler used to sitting on the potty from around 15 months after a meal (if he's sufficiently coordinated), but although he may empty his bowels, this is an involuntary reflex action, not toilet training. It is a good idea to wait until your child demonstrates some interest in the potty or refrains from having a bowel movement until he's in some special place (indicating he is aware that he has to poo).

Until your child is ready, trying to potty train him may result in frustration and frayed tempers for you, anxiety for your child and a lot of hard work for nothing. In order to become clean and dry, your child's nervous system must be sufficiently mature for him to recognise the signs of a full bladder and bowel. He then needs to be able to control the muscles that open the bladder and bowel long enough to get to the potty before emptying them.

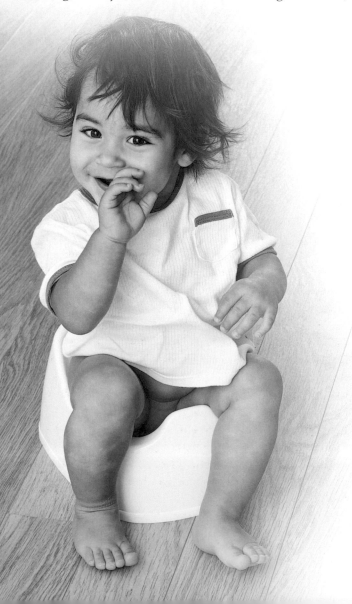

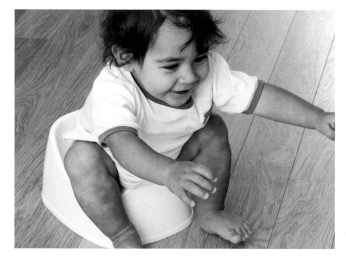

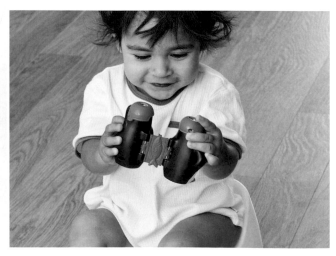

Boys are generally ready for potty training later than girls and take longer to be trained. If you have a boy, he should start off by sitting on a potty, which should have a splash guard. You will need to show him how to direct his penis so his wee goes into the bowl, but it's a good idea to keep a plastic sheet under the potty if he is prone to splashing. Later on, you'll have to teach him to use the toilet. Don't insist that he stands to wee – it is usually easier to sit at first. If he wants to stand, provide him with a block or step stool to reach the bowl. You will also have to show him how to take aim into the bowl. Some boys, particularly if they start late, may insist on using a toilet from the start. Letting your child copy his dad using it will get him used to the idea.

Choose a period when you can give him the time and encouragement needed. If there is a distraction, such as going on holiday, moving house, or you have just had another baby, leave potty training until things have settled down. It is also easier in warm weather, when a child has fewer clothes to cope with.

MAKING IT EASY

I began by taking my toddler to buy a potty. I let her pick one out in her favourite colour that had a rigid base to stop it tipping over.

I then explained in simple language what I wanted her to do. I used the words 'wee' for passing water and 'poo' for when she opened her bowels and let her know that she should wee or poo in her potty from now on. I kept the potty in a warm place, where she could get to it easily, and where it couldn't topple over. (In a home with more than one floor, it is a good idea to have potties on each floor.)

I made sure I dressed my toddler in easily removable clothes – trousers with an elasticated waist, for example – and taught her how to pull them down. Trainer pants are easier to remove than nappies and wearing them made her feel more 'grown up'.

I then put her on the potty regularly – particularly after meals and before going out – and stayed with her in the early stages. I encouraged her to sit for a few minutes looking at a book, or I read her a story. I also took her to the toilet with me hoping she would catch on to what I was doing. I never forced her to use the

potty or left her on it for more than a few moments. If she became bored or cried, I took her off.

When she used the potty successfully, I praised and encouraged her – but not too much, as she might have become disappointed if she didn't get a result the next time. I tried not to expect results too soon and didn't nag or force the issue or get angry when she failed to perform, refused to use the potty or wet herself. I expected the occasional accident and was matter of fact about cleaning up.

If she was successful with a bowel movement, I wiped her bottom carefully (she won't be able to do this effectively for some time) then made sure she washed and dried her hands thoroughly. Girls must be taught to wipe themselves from front to back.

GRADUATING TO A TOILET

I got my child used to using a toilet by letting her use those in public places or in people's homes. I showed her how to use the various toilet paper dispensers but carry sufficient tissues in case they are empty. I make sure she washes her hands extra thoroughly afterwards.

It is important that a child feels safe and secure when sitting on the toilet and a special child's lavatory seat is useful. A sturdy step stool or box is important to help him reach the seat. Some children are afraid of falling down the hole; if this is the case with your toddler, you will need to hold him on at first.

GOING THROUGH THE NIGHT

Learning to stay dry throughout the night usually takes children a little longer than staying dry during the day. A child has to recognise the feeling of a full bladder while asleep and respond either by 'holding on' until morning or waking up and going to the toilet. About 25 per cent of 3 year olds wet the bed and need to wear a night-time nappy, so don't be in any hurry to remove the plastic sheet and try not to lose your patience if your child has frequent nightly accidents. It is normal for a child up to the age of 5 to wet his bed.

I make it easier for my child to stay dry at night by making sure she doesn't have drinks and uses the potty before going to bed. Some parents take their children to the potty before they themselves go to bed – generally the child barely wakes – or keep a potty in the child's room. I minimised the outcome of accidents by putting a small rubber sheet on top of my child's ordinary sheet with a half sheet over that. When she had an accident, I quickly removed the half sheet and the rest of the under sheet was spared.

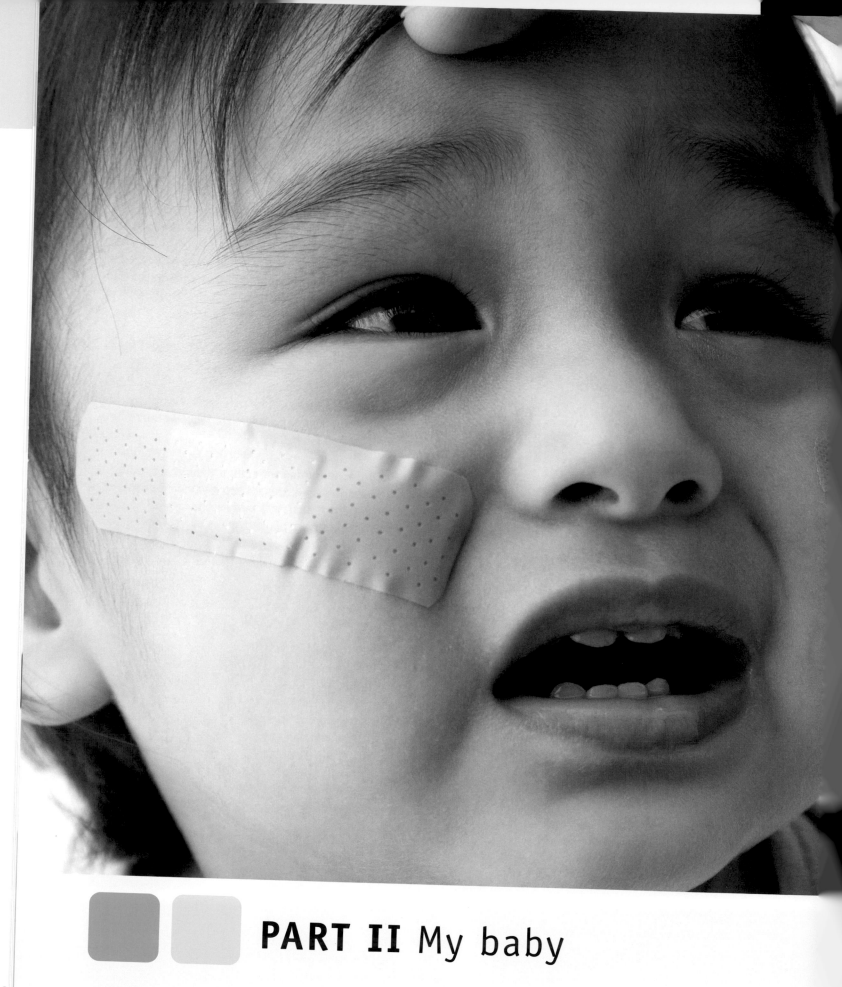

PART II My baby

Keeping my baby healthy

I need to ensure my child is has her regular checks and immunisations and that I'm alert to any signs of ill health. Knowing what to do when my child seems poorly, has a common childhood illness or suffers a minor accident will be vital for her wellbeing. Most importantly, I need to be able to recognise when a doctor's care is needed and how to perform first-aid procedures in case of an emergency.

Carers and checks

As a parent I'm in the front line when it comes to looking after my baby's health. Because I'm with her every day, I can observe her at close hand and should be able to pick up things that may indicate something isn't right. It's important that any potential problems are picked up as early as possible for the best chance of a successful outcome.

In the UK, normal screening checks are performed during early childhood as part of the Child Health Surveillance Programme. Some aspects of physical health, including weight gain and growth, are also continually monitored. In addition to seeing children at the scheduled check-ups, health visitors and doctors assess children informally at appointments made for other reasons, such as illness or vaccinations.

HEALTH VISITOR

My baby had her first medical assessment at birth (see page 110) and subsequently we were looked after by a health visitor. She gave me advice on all aspects of baby care and could allay my worries if baby cried all the time, didn't feed or wasn't gaining weight. She also monitored my baby's progress. If I had any worries about my child's development or behaviour, my health visitor was my first port of call. She could also have helped me if I felt low. Health visitors are very

experienced in such matters and, if additional help had been needed, mine could have put me in touch with local services available for babies and young children.

GENERAL PRACTITIONER

Once my baby was older, I took her to the baby clinic at my doctor's surgery for her regular check-ups. When she was ill, I sought advice from my GP. Sometimes, all I needed was being told what measures to take to ease her symptoms; at other times my GP had to see her to prescribe treatment. Before my baby was born, I checked on which of the GPs in the practice had a particular interest in caring for children and I try and take baby to see the same doctor on every visit. In this way, I'm building a rapport with the doctor and he is getting to know my child.

PAEDIATRICIAN

These doctors specialise in a child's care; some cover all aspects of child medicine, others focus on one particular area, such as heart disorders. If my GP has any concerns about my child's health that need further assessment or specialist treatment, he will refer me to see a hospital-based paediatric consultant, though there are community paediatricians who have a special interest in child development and care who practise outside the hospital environment.

If I have to see a paediatrician, he or she will send a letter to my GP setting out the diagnosis and describing the treatment given. In this way, my GP surgery keeps a full record of my child's medical history. I should be entitled to receive copies of any letters.

DENTIST

A paediatric dentist is important to find as not only will he or she be able to advise on the best dental care for a child and to check that all is well, but is more likely to have an office and chairside manner that appeals to children. Positive experiences at the dental surgery in early childhood are very important for a lifetime of good dental care. It's a good idea to schedule regular 6-monthly checks from the time a child is about 3.

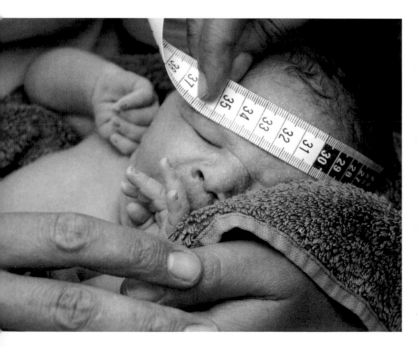

In the first weeks after a baby is born, a health visitor will perform vital checks at home, such as measuring head circumference.

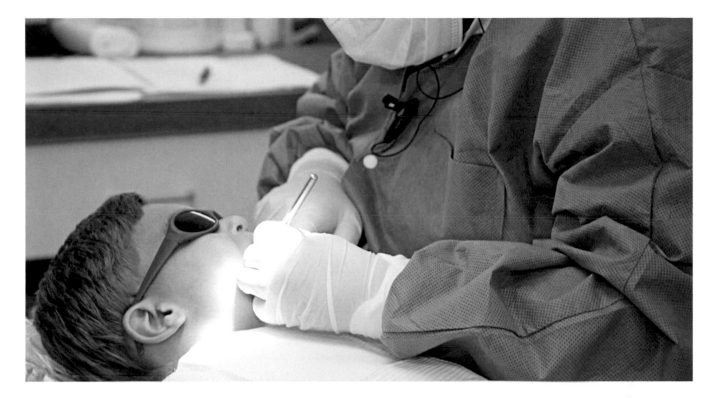

ROUTINE ASSESSMENTS

The purpose of routine checks is to assess both a baby's development and his physical health. Because these are closely related – learning to walk depends on the correct working of muscles and coordination, which both rely on a healthy nervous system – developmental problems may alert healthcare professionals to the presence of a medical disorder. Some medical conditions, such as a heart murmur, may be picked up during physical examinations when the doctor listens to a child's heart with a stethoscope. Other conditions may be uncovered with special tests.

After 6 weeks of age, early childhood assessments are usually carried out at the same time as necessary immunisations (see page 250). As well as assessing development, the doctor or health visitor takes these opportunities to make certain physical checks, including whether my baby's hips move normally and whether any heart murmurs are present when listening to her heart sounds. Measurements will be taken to assess weight gain and growth.

At each assessment I will be asked various questions about my baby's progress, including whether I think there are any problems with her hearing and vision. I also will have the opportunity to ask questions about her health and development as well as to voice any concerns. Should any problems be found, my baby will be referred to specialists for further assessment.

VISION CHECKS

At birth, my newborn was checked for abnormalities of the eye, such as cataracts. By the 6–8 week check, my baby will be tested to see whether she follows an object moved across in front of her face.

At 6 months of age, my baby will be checked to see whether she reaches out for toys. By 2 years of age, more formal tests can be carried out, such as asking her to pick out small objects on pictures and then, at age 3, by asking her to match letters on charts (a letter is held up across the room and my child will be asked to point to it on her chart).

HEARING CHECKS

Although these simple tests are not always accurate, they do give a good indication as to whether a child has a hearing problem. In addition, I can check on baby's hearing by being aware of her responses to sounds and to my voice. There are two tests that can be done on very young infants using earphones. If the results of these tests are abnormal, a baby will be referred for further assessment by an audiometrist.

Evoked otoacoustic emission involves clicking sounds being emitted into each ear in turn via the earphones. The vibrations in the cochlea should be picked up if the ear is functioning normally.

In auditory brainstem response audiometry, the earphones again emit clicks, which trigger impulses in

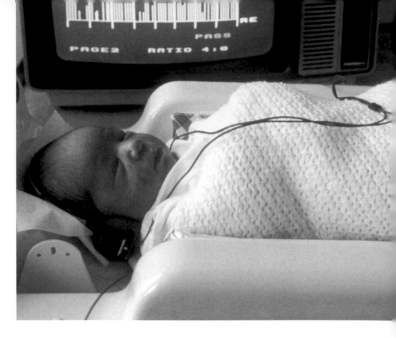

the ear that are carried to the brain where they trigger electrical responses. These responses are recorded and analysed by a computer.

From around 7–9 months of age, distraction testing can be done. A tester sits opposite a child and keeps his attention while an assistant makes sounds of high and low frequency just outside the child's field of vision. The child should turn towards the noises.

From around 18 months of age, the speech discrimination test can be performed. A tester sits opposite a child and names toys quietly with a hand placed in front of his or her mouth. The tester asks the child to point to each toy, all of which are laid on a table between them.

SCHEDULE OF BABY CHECKS

6–8 WEEKS
During this and subsequent check-ups, all the key aspects of development are assessed. I may be asked whether my baby has started smiling yet, when she cries and how she reacts to sounds (factors important in social development, language and hearing).

Baby's gross motor development will be checked by simple observation of her muscle tone and early head control. To assess her eyesight, the health visitor or GP will watch whether baby follows an object with her eyes when it is moved across her field of vision.

Some physical checks will be carried out, too, including examining the hips, listening to the heart sounds and, for boys, re-checking the position of the testes. My GP may also check baby's eyes for evidence of cataracts and other eye conditions that can affect young babies.

6–9 MONTHS
Gross motor skills really come on now and my baby will be assessed on all of these milestones – whether she has started to sit on her own, stand with support and, if 9 months old, pull herself up to a standing position. My baby may even start to crawl. Babies of this age also start to reach out for toys and pass them from hand to hand. The examiner will ask about these fine motor skills as well as speech as, from the age of 9 months, a baby may start to use the odd word. At this age, it is possible to perform the distraction hearing

test (see page 247). Social and self-care skills are starting to feature more in development; from 6 months, my baby may be able to feed herself with finger food.

10–12 MONTHS
I will be asked again about several key developmental milestones. By this age my baby should really be on the move, perhaps cruising (walking with the support of furniture) and even taking early steps. At around 10 months, she may have started to hold small items between her finger and thumb (known as the pincer grip). From around 12 months she may call "Mama" and "Dada". She may use a few other words, too. She may be starting to eat with a spoon and holding a cup using both hands.

18–24 MONTHS
Many skills will have been acquired by the age of 2 in all areas of development. The assessor (doctor or health visitor) will be able to engage my child in activities and see the great progress that has been made. My toddler will probably be a confident walker, may hold a pencil and scribble and build a tower of 3–6 bricks.

As far as language is concerned, my toddler will be able to communicate some of her needs and wishes with short phrases like "Want milk". She will probably feed herself well with a spoon by now.

IMMUNISATIONS

Immunisations protect babies from potentially serious diseases. An unvaccinated baby is a danger to himself and the children around him. Currently in the UK, babies are immunised against 11 diseases or the bacterium or virus that cause them, but if a child has a long-term condition or is otherwise at risk, he may be offered a seasonal flu jab as well.

Tuberculosis

This is a bacterial infection, which is passed on when people with the disease cough. It tends to start in the lungs, but can also affect other parts of the body. Babies who live in an area where there is a high incidence of the disease, or whose parents or grandparents were born in a country where TB is still a problem, are at particular risk. Effective treatments are available, but without treatment the disease can cause persistent symptoms and can be life threatening in some cases.

Diphtheria

This bacterial infection affects the throat and can cause breathing problems. It is transmitted when infected people cough or sneeze. The infection may also spread in the blood to cause potentially life-threatening problems, including heart failure.

Tetanus

This is a life-threatening bacterial infection that can affect the nerves that control muscles, resulting in severe muscle spasms. Sometimes the muscles of the throat and chest are involved, which will affect swallowing and breathing.

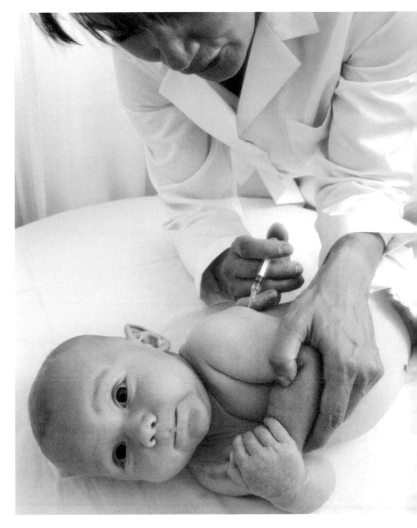

EXPERTS ADVISE

Immunisations

There are only two reasons why vaccinations should not be given. The first is if a baby is unwell and has a raised temperature (colds and coughs with no fever are not reasons for postponing immunisations) and the second is if a baby has reduced immunity (being treated for cancer, taking immuno-suppressant drugs or suffering from HIV).

Pertussis

Also known as whooping cough, this is a potentially life-threatening bacterial illness in the very young; it results in severe bouts of coughing.

Poliomyelitis

This disease is caused by a virus whose effects can vary from mild to very severe, resulting in problems affecting the nervous system, even paralysis. The virus is passed on by contact with infected faeces, often through contaminated water or food.

Haemophilus influenzae type b (Hib)

This is a bacterium, which can cause serious, often life-threatening, diseases including meningitis (see page 251) and septicaemia (see page 250). It also can cause epiglottitis, inflammation of the flap of cartilage that lies behind the tongue, which is a life-threatening condition.

Caring for my child when she is ill

All children become ill at one time or another and most suffer minor injuries. It is always worrying to me when my child becomes ill or has an injury because she is unable to tell me much, if anything, about what may be wrong and due to her young age and small size, she is probably at particular risk.

It's important therefore that I'm able to recognise early on when my child is ill and to be able to take appropriate steps in either seeking care or providing it myself. Knowing how to take a temperature, give medicines and create cold compresses and packs are vital in caring for a young child as is ensuring her environment is conducive to her getting better.

MEASURING BODY TEMPERATURE

There are two main types of thermometer for children – digital and sensor. When my child was a baby, I placed my digital thermometer, in her armpit of a baby and when she reached toddler age, I put it in her mouth. At all ages, I'm able to use a sensor thermometer in her ear – but not if she has an ear infection or earache.

A normal body temperature for children is 36–36.8°C (96.8–98.2°F). A raised temperature for children under the age of 5 is over 37.5°C (99.5°F), and for age 5 and over 38°C (100.4°F).

WHEN TO CALL MY DOCTOR

If my child does not seem her usual self – is not as active or responsive as normal – I shouldn't hesitate to get in touch with my doctor. I should contact my doctor or the emergency services (*) straight away if my baby is:

☐ Sleepier than normal and does not have her usual times when she is alert and active.

☐ More floppy than usual (*).

☐ Crying more than usual or her crying sounds different from her usual cry (*).

☐ Feeding (eating or drinking) less.

☐ Not passing much urine.

☐ Vomiting.

☐ Passing bloody stools (*).

☐ Suffering from a high temperature (over 39°C) or the temperature remains high after you have tried measures to bring it down (see page 256).

☐ Coughing persistently or brings up phlegm when she coughs.

☐ Having problems with her breathing or is wheezy.

☐ Exhibiting one or more purplish-red spots (*) (see also page 251).

☐ Is pulling on her ear.

GIVING MEDICINES

I give oral medicines using a syringe or spoon. When giving the medicine, I prop baby up or get her to sit so that her head is raised higher than her body. I have to hand her favourite drink for afterwards but I never mix the medicine in with a drink as I won't know whether she has had the full dose. If it fits in with the directions, I try to give oral medicines before a feed when my baby will be hungry.

When I give ear drops, I sit or lay my baby next to me her head resting on its side on my knee. I pull her ear upwards and back slightly to straighten the ear canal and allow the drops to fall straight in. I make sure she keeps her head on its side for 30 seconds or so to prevent the drops from trickling out again.

When applying eye drops, I lay baby across my knee on her back and support her head in the crook of my arm. I gently pull down her bottom eyelid so that the drops can fall between her eyeball and lower lid. This is hard to do by myself, so I wrap baby up in a blanket to keep her arms out of the way or wait until my partner or someone else can help to hold baby still in the correct position and open up her eye.

MAKING COMPRESSES AND COLD PACKS

To make a compress, I soak a flannel or other cloth in cold water then wring it out. I hold it firmly over the swollen or bruised area for around 5–10 minutes.

To make an ice pack, I wrap a bag of frozen peas – or other vegetables – in a towel or use a wrapped bag of ice cubes.

CREATING A COMFORTABLE ENVIRONMENT

Small changes to my child's room can make it easier to care for her when she is ill. It's important that she not be in my room or bed, if at all possible, so in order to keep tabs on her at all times, I make sure there's a baby monitor in her room. This keeps me in touch while cutting down on the number of times I need to go in and check on her. Similarly, keeping some tissues and hand wipes and the thermometer in her room saves me having to go and get things frequently.

If she has a fever, it's handy to have a cool box containing water beside her. This also can be used to hold cooled-down water for sponging. All medications, however, are kept locked up in place that is accessible to me but inaccessible to her.

To add some cheer, I put up some brightly coloured pictures and surround her with a supply of books and comics and some simple toys that will keep her amused. Audio tapes with stories and songs are entertaining as is a portable TV and/or DVD player.

Prevent infection ✓

Many childhood illnesses, including skin conditions such as allergic rashes and eczema, while distressing to both parent and child, are not infectious. However, colds and flu are easily spread from person to person in respiratory droplets of coughs and sneezes as well as being picked up from inanimate objects – doorknobs, tissues, towels, etc. When caring for a child with an infectious disease, it is important always to:

✓ Encourage your child to cover his nose and mouth when he coughs and sneezes. You should have plenty of tissues close at hand.

✓ Wash your hands with soap and water or use an alcohol-based hand rub often and especially after handling any used tissues.

✓ Clean hard surfaces, such as door handles, toys and equipment frequently using a normal cleaning product.

✓ Provide your child with his own towel and face cloths and keep these isolated from the others used by the rest of the family.

✓ Be prepared to keep your child somewhat isolated; the ideal 'sick' room should be free of clutter and lit well so you can easily spot signs of worsening health.

✓ Check with your doctor about any special precautions you might need to take such as wearing a face mask when close to your child.

Treating minor injuries

It is nearly impossible to prevent all minor accidents, so it's important that I know how to deal with cuts and bruises, bites and stings, minor burns and splinters. My first aid kit (see page 188) is readily to hand.

BRUISES
Falls and bumps often damage small blood vessels so that blood leaks out into the surrounding tissues causing discolouration and swelling.

To treat a bruise, I will:

✓ Apply a cold compress for 5–10 minutes over the area to help to reduce any swelling.

SCRATCHES, CUTS AND GRAZES
Infection can enter an open wound, so is important to clean the wound and help it close. Ideally, I should wear disposable gloves, but if these are not available I can wash my hands thoroughly before I start.

To treat a scratch, cut or graze, I will:

✓ Rinse the wound under cold running water to get rid of any dirt, then clean it with wipes or swabs, using a new one every time I wipe across the area. I start with the wound itself and then work on the skin around it so that I don't introduce bacteria from the surrounding skin into the wound. I use a piece of clean gauze to dry the area.

✓ Apply a plaster to small wounds or, for larger ones, a dressing that I keep in place by tape, or a bandage.

ANIMAL SCRATCHES AND BITES
Domestic animals can be sources of harmful bacteria. After treating an injury, I must consult my doctor as antibiotics or a tetanus booster may be needed.

To treat a cat scratch, I will:

✓ Wash the scratch carefully and apply disinfectant.

To treat a dog bite, I will:

✓ Carefully wash the area with soap and water.

✓ Pat the wound dry with clean swabs and cover with a sterile dressing or a plaster. However, if the area is bleeding, I apply firm pressure with a clean cloth or sterile dressing and raise the limb.

If the wound is deep or large or the bleeding continues, I must immediately take my child to my nearest A&E department.

NOSE BLEEDS
Bleeding from the nose most commonly occurs when tiny blood vessels inside the nostrils are ruptured, either by a blow to the nose or as a result of sneezing or picking or blowing the nose. A nosebleed can be dangerous if a child loses a lot of blood.

To treat a nose bleed, I will:

✓ Sit my child down with her head tilted forwards to allow the blood to drain from her nostrils. I'll tell

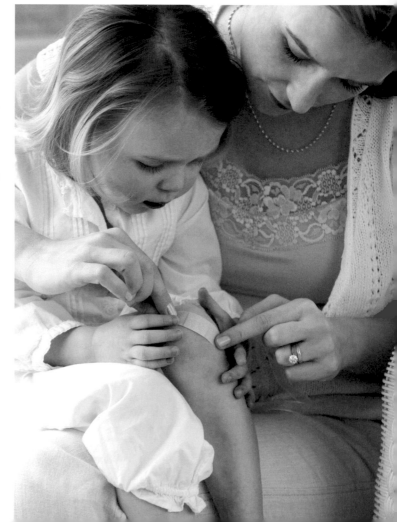

her to breathe through her mouth (which will have a calming effect) but not speak, swallow, cough, spit or sniff because these may disturb blood clots that have formed in her nose.

✓ Pinch the soft part of her nose and hold for 10 minutes. If the bleeding has not stopped, I reapply the pressure for two further periods of 10 minutes.

✓ Once the bleeding has stopped, and with her still leaning forwards, I clean around her nose with lukewarm water. My child needs to rest quietly for a few hours and try not to blow her nose.

If the nosebleed is severe, or if it lasts longer than 30 minutes in total, I must take my child to my nearest A&E department, making sure she maintains a head-down position.

SUNBURN

Although my child should always wear a hat and sunscreen when in the sun, if she should get burnt, I need to soothe the area.

To treat sunburn, I will:

✓ Use a clean, soft flannel to dab cold water onto the affected area then apply calamine or other soothing cream.

✓ Make sure my child drinks cool fluids as, if she has been out in the sun, she may be dehydrated.

If a large area is affected or the area is blistered, I need to seek medical advice.

STINGS

To ease the discomfort, I need to remove the sting.

To treat the sting, I will:

✓ Try scraping across the area with a credit card.

✓ Apply an ice pack to relieve any discomfort and swelling.

SPLINTERS

If a splinter is protruding from the skin, I need to try and remove it with tweezers. These need to be sterilised by holding them in the flame of a match for a second

before allowing them to cool. If possible, I should wear disposable gloves to reduce the risk of introducing infection into the wound.

To remove the splinter, I will:

✓ Run cold water over the area to remove any dirt.

✓ Using the tweezers, grasp the end of the splinter and pull it out firmly but gently in the same direction as it entered the skin.

If the splinter is embedded and there is no end to get hold of, I must seek medical attention. (Poking around will only cause pain and may cause the splinter to become more deeply embedded.)

FOREIGN OBJECTS

Children occasionally poke objects in their ears or nose or swallow things.

If my child pokes something into her ear, I will:

✓ Look in her ear to check whether the object is visible and tilt her head to the side to see whether the object falls out. If it remains lodged, I will seek medical attention as trying to remove it myself can damage the delicate structures inside the ear or push the object further into the ear.

If an object becomes lodged in my baby's nostril, I will seek medical help so that it can be removed.

If my child swallows an object, I should seek medical advice; I may be advised to let nature take its course and wait for the object to be passed in the stool or I may be told that X-rays are needed to monitor the progress of the object through the gut or a treatment may be needed to remove the object.

MY NEAREST ACCIDENT & EMERGENCY DEPARTMENT

_____

Treating common conditions and illnesses

I'll be able to look after my child without additional medical help when she suffers from many of the following – although I should let my doctor know if my child develops any of them. But some rare and dangerous conditions – meningitis (see page 251) and septicaemia (see page 250), for example – resemble less dangerous illnesses, so it's a good idea for me to be able to recognise their symptoms and to take appropriate action. In any event, if I have any worries about whether I'm treating my child correctly, I should seek medical advice (see also page 252).

FEVERS

Fevers are common during childhood and usually short-lived; a raised temperature is a sign that the immune system is working to get rid of an infection. However, high temperatures need treating as they cause children to feel unwell. In rare situations, they may result in febrile convulsions.

Fevers are often associated with shivering, headaches and dehydration. If my child has a fever (see

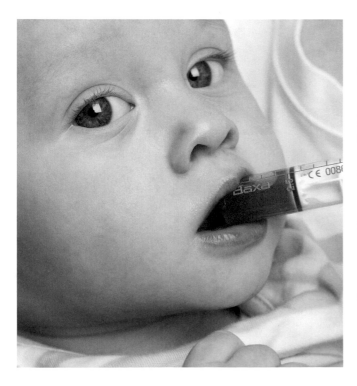

Measuring body temperature, page 252), she may be flushed and will feel hot to the touch. After checking her temperature and finding it raised, I need to follow the advice below. After I have followed these measures for around 30 minutes (and no sooner), I can retake my child's temperature. If it is lower, I can continue with the cooling measures but if it remains raised for more than 24 hours or if I am worried about any of her symptoms, I will seek medical advice.

If my child has a fever, I will:

✓ Make sure she drinks plenty of cold drinks.

✓ Sponge her down with a tepid, not cold, sponge to cool her down.

✓ Give a fever-reducing medication such as a child's preparation of paracetamol or ibuprofen.

✗ Not use too many blankets or clothes; although she may be shivering, too many covers and clothes will only increase a child's body temperature and make her feel worse.

✗ Not overheat her room; I need to be guided by whether I feel comfortable in my normal clothing.

If my baby exhibits signs of febrile convulsions – stiffening and then jerking her body – I must:

✓ Lay or gently roll her onto her side, ideally with her head at a lower level than the rest of her body.

✓ Call 999 if the fit continues for more than 5 minutes. Otherwise, I must seek urgent medical advice once the fit has stopped.

✗ Do not hold her still but let the fit take its course.

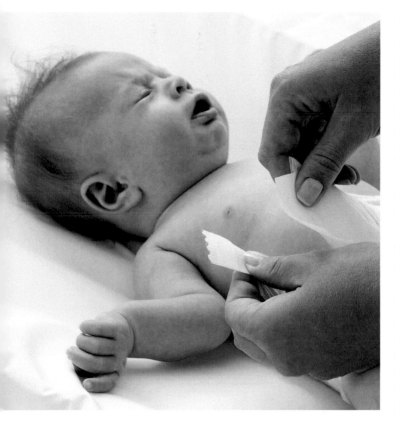

COLDS

Many different viruses cause colds and snuffles. My toddler will become particularly vulnerable if she attends playgroups or a nursery, as she will come into contact with infections that her immune system has not encountered before. My child can catch cold viruses if someone suffering from a cold coughs and sneezes near her or if a cold sufferer wipes his hand across his nose and then touches my child. Colds are not caused by going out without a coat or with wet hair.

When suffering from a cold, my child may have a runny or blocked nose, sneeze and sometimes have a raised temperature. Other symptoms may include a sore throat, a cough that is often worse at night, loss of appetite, lethargy and tiredness.

Colds last for a week or so, but some affected children go on to develop chest and ear infections.

If my child has a cold, I will:

✓ Keep her comfortable – making sure she has an adequate fluid intake.

✓ If necessary, give a fever-reducing medication such as a child's preparation of paracetamol or ibuprofen.

EAR INFECTIONS

Acute infections of the middle ear (otitis media) are common. Many children have recurrent episodes because a child's eustachian tube, which connects the outer ear to the middle ear, is short and positioned horizontally so that that infection-causing secretions present in colds cannot drain away. Recurrent episodes of otitis media can cause a chronic condition known as 'glue ear' to develop.

In addition to cold-type symptoms (including a runny nose, snuffles, cough and fever), if she has infection, my child may pull on her ear, which will usually be painful. She may be off her food. Because a young child may not be able to describe ear pain, she can just be generally miserable.

If the eardrum becomes very inflamed, it may perforate (pressure causes a hole to develop), allowing fluid to drain to the outside. The perforation should eventually heal.

I need to seek my doctor's advice for the condition to be diagnosed and treated. If an infection is present, my doctor may prescribe antibiotics and/or a pain-killing medication.

If I suspect my child has an ear infection, I must take her to the doctor.

INFLUENZA (FLU)

This highly infectious viral illness is easily passed on in the secretions of those affected. The symptoms develop within a couple of days of contact and are similar, but more severe than those of a cold.

I should suspect my child has the flu if she has a fever that often goes above 37.5°C (99.5°F), or 38°C (100.4°F) if over 5, and the shivers; she also may have a runny nose, dry cough and sneezing. She may complain of a sore throat and have swollen glands. She also will probably lack an appetite.

Symptoms usually tend to settle over a few days but because babies and young children are particularly vulnerable to secondary bacterial infections, she may require medical treatment.

If I think my child has the flu, I will:

✓ Follow the recommendations for bringing down a fever (see page 256).

✓ Take my child to the doctor if she is very young or the fever is very high (over 39°C/102.2°F); if the symptoms persist for more than a few days; if my baby has breathing difficulties or wheezing, earache or discharge from the ear, a very sore throat or a persistent cough or a cough that brings up phlegm.

CROUP

In this common condition, a viral infection affects the larynx (the voice box) and the trachea (windpipe). Croup may be caused by a number of viruses and is particularly common in the autumn. It affects children between the ages of 6 months–6 years, but those aged 1–2 years are most likely to be affected.

The illness will often start with a fever and cold-type symptoms, such as a runny nose and snuffles. The main symptoms will then develop – a barking cough, noisy breathing (particularly when breathing in) and hoarseness. These symptoms tend to be worse during the night. The inflammation and swelling of the lining may, if severe, cause breathing difficulties.

If my child has mild symptoms, I may be happy to care for her at home. However, if I have any worries, I'll seek medical attention, particularly if my child continues to breathe noisily or draws in her chest when she breathes.

To treat my child with croup, I will:

✓ Make sure she drinks plenty of fluids.

✓ Give a fever-reducing medication such as a child's preparation of paracetamol or ibuprofen.

✓ Use a vaporiser or place a bowl of water over a radiator.

CONJUNCTIVITIS AND STICKY EYES

Particularly prevalent in the first week or two after birth, I should suspect conjunctivitis if the tissue that covers my child's eyeball and lines her eyelid (the conjunctiva) becomes red and possibly sticky. A common condition, it often settles without medication but sometimes antibiotic treatment, in the form of drops or ointment, is needed.

To treat my child's conjunctivitis, I will:

✓ Wipe her eyes with cotton wool and cooled boiled water (using a fresh piece of cotton wool for each eye) to clear the stickiness.

✓ Ensure my child does not share her face cloth or towel to prevent transmission to others.

✓ Seek medical advice if redness and stickiness persist.

GASTROENTERITIS AND FOOD POISONING

Babies and young children are at particular risk from the effects of stomach upsets as they can quickly become dehydrated (see box). Gastroenteritis may result from a variety of bacteria and viruses, some of which are transmitted as a result of poor hygiene techniques when handling food. The most common cause of infective gastroenteritis is the rotavirus infection. It is particularly common in the winter.

I should suspect gastroenteritis if my child suffers from diarrhoea and perhaps vomiting, fever, listlessness and signs of dehydration. She may also complain of abdominal pain.

If I think my child is affected, I will:

✓ Make sure she has an adequate fluid intake,

Dehydration

This is common when children become unwell. If your child exhibits one or more of the following, he is dehydrated:

- Passes less urine than usual.
- Eyes are sunken.
- Skin and lining of the mouth are dry.
- Lethargy.
- Breathing more rapidly than usual.
- Drowsier and less alert than usual.

particularly of oral rehydration solutions (recommended by my doctor or chemist).

✓ Give a fever-reducing medication such as a child's preparation of paracetamol or ibuprofen.

✗ Not omit milk from her diet or give it in a watered-down form.

I must see the doctor if:

✓ The vomiting or diarrhoea persist for more than 24 hours.

✓ My child has any signs of dehydration.

✓ There is blood in her stool.

✓ My child has a very high fever.

CHICKEN POX

In this common illness, the varicella zoster virus spreads around the body to cause a characteristic rash. The red spots, which tend to appear first on the head and trunk before spreading out to the arms and legs, soon develop into small blisters. An affected child also may have a slight fever. The spots take up to 5 days to appear and then over the next few days crust over. Sometimes there are only a few spots.

Chicken pox rash is very itchy, so a skin-soothing lotion such as calamine will provide relief.

For most children, the main problem is the itchiness of the spots; if present in the mouth, the spots may cause sore areas. However, in a few cases, complications can develop, such as a bacterial infection of the spots. Most children will be over the worst within 10–14 days.

The illness is no longer contagious when all the lesions have crusted over.

To treat chicken pox, I will:

✓ Apply calamine and other anti-itching creams to the spots.

✓ Give a fever-reducing medication such as a child's preparation of paracetamol or ibuprofen.

✓ Seek medical advice if my child has impaired immunity or her symptoms are severe.

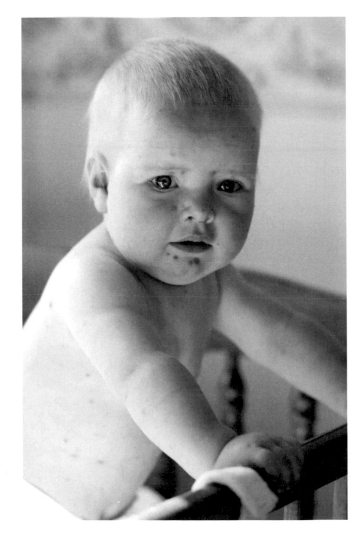

FIFTH DISEASE

Caused by a type of parvovirus, this condition can occur at any time of the year, but is particularly common in the spring and can may be contracted at any age. The virus is often passed in the secretions of those affected. Complications are rare in children, but may include joint pains and inflammation.

The illness may begin with a fever (which may be slight) and/or a headache. A week or so later, the cheeks will become red followed by a rash on the trunk, arms and thighs, which may be itchy, and persist for up to 6 weeks.

No specific treatment is required as the symptoms are very mild, so if my child is affected, she can, if appropriate, continue to go to nursery.

HAND, FOOT AND MOUTH DISEASE

This common viral illness results in blisters in the mouth (including on the tongue) and on the hands and feet. These blisters are painful, but settle within a week or so. The illness can occur at any age, but children under 10 years are most commonly affected. If my child is affected, she will feel generally off colour, possibly with a fever, for 1–2 days before developing a sore throat and then small spots in her mouth, which soon develop into painful ulcers. Within 1–2 days, spots will develop on her hands and feet, as well as her legs and buttocks and other areas of the body in some cases. The spots look similar to those that occur in chicken pox, but are smaller in size and less itchy (though more sore).

This is generally a relatively mild illness with the blisters settling within a week or so. The biggest problem for a child with the disease tends to be a sore mouth, which can cause her discomfort when eating and swallowing.

To treat hand, foot and mouth disease, I will:

✓ Give a fever-reducing medication such as a child's preparation of paracetamol or ibuprofen.

✓ Offer cool drinks and ice lollies to help soothe my child's mouth.

✓ Encourage her to drink even though she may find it uncomfortable for a few days.

✓ Be sure my child washes her hands after going to the toilet and before eating. Good hygiene measures are important because the disease is infectious, particularly while the spots and ulcers are present, and may be passed in the faeces.

MEASLES

This potentially serious viral disease has become less common thanks to the measles vaccination but it still occurs, and is currently on the rise due particularly to the fall in uptake of the MMR (measles, mumps, rubella) vaccine. Children with impaired immunity, such as those being treated for cancer, are particularly at risk.

Children suffering from measles feel miserable and unwell, but a small number can suffer from life-threatening complications; in about 1 in 5,000 cases, inflammation of the brain tissue (encephalitis) and hepatitis (inflammation of the liver) occur.

Of the common childhood diseases, measles is among the most serious and affected children can become quite ill. Make sure your child is vaccinated against the disease.

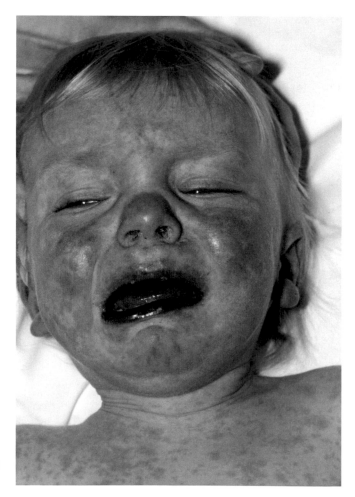

The illness starts with a fever and cold-type symptoms, including snuffles, a cough and sometimes conjunctivitis. The rash appears after 3 days or so – first on the face, then behind the ears before moving down the rest of the body. The rash begins as groups of spots, but after another 3 days or so, the spots join together to form a blotchy rash. Ear infections and pneumonia can develop.

A child is infectious from before the rash appears until day 5 of the rash.

To treat my child's measles, I will:

✓ Give a fever-reducing medication such as a child's preparation of paracetamol or ibuprofen.

✓ Make sure she has an adequate fluid intake.

✓ Consult my doctor if my child develops an ear infection or her condition worsens; antibiotics may be needed.

MUMPS

Mumps tends to be a mild illness during which a child may have no particular symptoms or she may have a fever lasting 3 days or so and the characteristic inflammation and swelling of the parotid glands that lie in front of her ears. Occasionally complications occur; there may be problems with hearing after mumps, but this is usually on one side and temporary, but for a few children, the mumps virus can result in meningitis and encephalitis.

In the wake of the fall in uptake of the MMR (measles, mumps, rubella) triple vaccine, more unimmunised children have once again been affected by mumps. Mumps tends to occur in winter and spring. It is spread through the secretions of those affected.

The primary symptoms are swelling of the glands beneath the ears, which may begin on one side, but in most cases the other side will also be swollen within a few days. The swollen glands may be painful and there may be discomfort on swallowing and earache. The swelling lasts for 5–10 days. The disease is infectious for a week after the parotid glands begin to swell.

To treat my child's mumps, I will:

✓ Offer her plenty of fluids and soft foods if swallowing is painful.

✓ Give a fever-reducing medication such as a child's preparation of paracetamol or ibuprofen.

✓ Contact my doctor urgently if my child becomes seriously ill, has a headache with a stiff neck, swollen testicles, abdominal pain or persistent earache.

ROSEOLA INFANTUM

This common viral illness causes a rash and a high fever. It is particularly common between the ages of 6 months – 2 years.

The first symptoms to appear are a high fever, dry cough, earache and swollen glands in the neck; some children will have mild diarrhoea. After a few days, a rash of tiny spots develops on the face and trunk. Usually the condition settles on its own within a week or so.

To treat my child's roseola infantum, I will:

✓ Give a fever-reducing medication such as a child's preparation of paracetamol or ibuprofen as a high fever may be associated with febrile convulsions.

✓ Make sure she has an adequate fluid intake.

RUBELLA OR GERMAN MEASLES

This viral illness is usually mild in those affected and may pass unnoticed, but it can damage an unborn baby during pregnancy. The infection is passed in the secretions of sufferers.

A rash of tiny pink spots develops on the face and trunk before moving down the body. This rash lasts for up to 5 days. There may be swelling of the lymph glands and a mild fever, but otherwise no particular signs of the illness. Inflammation of the joints (arthritis) and brain (encephalitis) may occur, but these are rare.

To treat my child's rubella, I will:

✓ Give a fever-reducing medication such as a child's preparation of paracetamol or ibuprofen.

✓ Notify my doctor immediately if I am pregnant and have not been vaccinated against the illness or tested for antibodies to the disease.

IMPETIGO

This common skin condition is caused by a bacterial infection and is passed on very easily. Impetigo is particularly common in early childhood and tends to develop in areas of skin that are already damaged, for example by eczema (see below).

A child's face and hands will develop reddened patches and blisters and soon other areas of skin will be affected. The contents of the blisters leak out leaving crusted areas, which are typically honey coloured.

If I suspect my child has impetigo, I will:

✓ Consult my doctor. He will most likely prescribe antibiotics, sometimes in the form of ointments for mild cases, but usually as oral drugs.

✓ Keep my child at home until the areas have dried completely as the condition is highly contagious.

ECZEMA

Eczema is a chronic illness that may need specialist medical attention. It is a common condition – up to 20 per cent of children are affected – though the symptoms can usually be relieved to a great extent by the measures described below and the condition tends to decrease in severity as affected children get older. Eczema often appears during the first year of life. Often, family members of affected children will have other allergic conditions, such as asthma and hay fever, to which children with atopic eczema are at increased risk. Some affected children may have allergies to a particular food or a constituent in food.

Reddening and itching of the skin can be intense, causing those worst affected to have problems sleeping at night. A hot environment can make the itching worse. The areas children scratch will be weepy and form crusts. Repeated scratching may lead to thickening of the skin. The skin tends to be dry all over and needs frequent applications of fragrance-free moisturiser. Sometimes, patches of eczema will become infected when bacteria enter the damaged skin. Viral infections, such as herpes, also may cause skin infections in those affected. Some children find their condition worsens when they are stressed.

The areas of the body on which the eczema rash appears tend to change as an affected child gets older.

Eczema causes reddening and itching of the skin. It can occur quite early on in life but often decreases in severity as the affected child gets older.

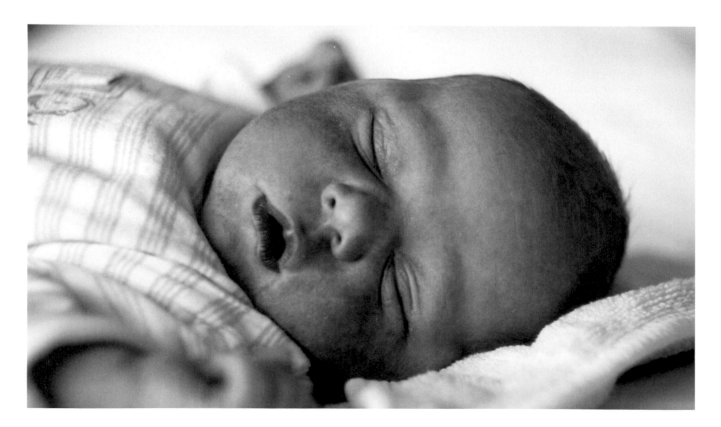

The face, neck and sometimes the scalp of an infant, are most commonly affected whereas, with an older child, it's the creases of joints that tend to have patches.

If my child develops eczema, I need to see my doctor who may prescribe an ointment or steroid cream or oral drugs such as antihistamines to relieve itching. He may prescribe further medication if a bacterial or viral infection arises. Occasionally, eczema requires treatment in hospital.

I will treat my child's eczema by:

✓ Keeping her nails short and avoiding substances that can irritate the skin, like soap and perfumed lotions (I can use soap substitutes), and clothing made from synthetic fibres.

✓ Using sparingly any ointment or steroid cream my doctor has prescribed and according to his instructions.

THREADWORMS

This infestation is common in childhood and particularly in preschool children. The worms live in the gut, but during the night the females work their way down to the end of the bowel and lay their eggs in the area around the anus. (The tiny worms may be visible in the anal area.) The eggs are picked up on the fingers when scratching and then are passed on to others and ingested, starting the cycle over again.

Threadworms can be spread easily and strict hygiene measures are needed to eradicate them permanently. The worms can cause intense itching around the anus and sometimes in the genital area. There may also be pain. However, some children affected with worms have no symptoms at all and the condition may go unnoticed for some time.

If I suspect my child has worms, I need to see my doctor. He can prescribe a number of different medications and each member of my family should be treated. These medications do not kill off the eggs, so hygiene measures need to be continued for six weeks, which is how long threadworms live.

Even with medication and hygiene measures, threadworms may persist. If this is the case with my child, my doctor will be able to give me advice on additional medication and further hygiene methods.

To treat my child's threadworms I will:

✓ Cut her nails short and encourage her to wear cotton gloves to prevent scratching. As much as possible, I'll try to prevent her sucking her thumb or biting her nails.

✓ Ensure my child washes her hands frequently and thoroughly and that she does not share her towel or face cloth with other family members.

✓ Change my child's underwear and nightclothes daily.

✓ Thoroughly wash all her bedding, towels, underwear and nightclothes.

HEAD LICE

These are common in nurseries and schools where children are in close contact with each other. I should suspect she has head lice if my child's scalp becomes intensely itchy. I may actually see lice on her scalp or the empty eggs on her hair. These eggs are known as nits. They stick to the hair and so move away from the scalp as the hairs grow.

Precise treatment recommendations vary as lice can become resistant to certain drugs. However, all involve the application of a lotion or hair rinse and often the use of a fine-tooth comb to comb out the lice.

If my child has nits, I will:

✓ Seek advice from my GP or local chemist as to the best treatment to use.

✓ Make sure my child's brushes, combs and towels are thoroughly cleaned and not shared with other family members, as lice can be transmitted through their use.

Emergency first aid

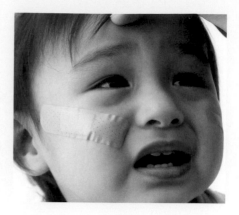

Certain situations are life threatening and, if one occurs, I must seek urgent medical attention from a doctor or NHS Direct (0845 4647) or ring 999 or 112 for an ambulance. However, I also need to know basic first aid techniques should my child become unconscious, choke or stop breathing. These techniques differ depending on my child's age. In case of a serious accident, I should put my child in the recovery position, with a warm covering if necessary.

RECOVERY POSITION

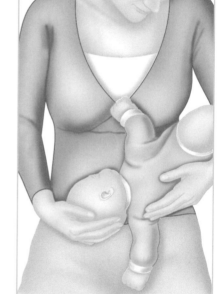

This position can help safeguard my child's breathing. If my child ever loses consciousness but is still breathing, I must hold her or place her in this position. Until medical help arrives, I would need to monitor her vital signs – determine her level of response (conscious or not), the presence of a pulse and that she is still breathing. If she should stop breathing, I must follow the advice for choking (see page 265).

Baby
I must hold my baby as if I was giving her a cuddle but she must be on her side, with her head lower than her tummy and tilted.

Toddler
I must place my child on her side so that the arm underneath her lies at a right angle. Then I have to move her other arm, so that the back of her hand is underneath her cheek. I need to pull her top knee up until her foot is flat on the floor and the leg is positioned at a right angle. I can ensure that her airway remains open by lifting her chin. I must keep checking she is breathing until help arrives.

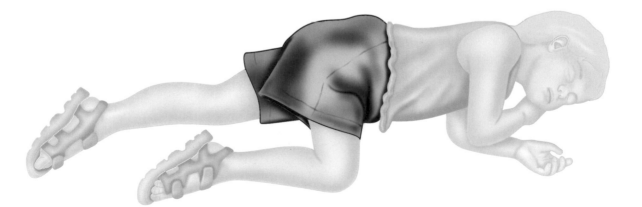

TREATING CHOKING

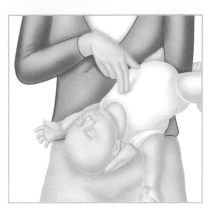

If my child starts choking but is able to talk or cry, she may have something obstructing her airway that might clear on its own. However, if she can only signal or looks in distress, back blows and chest thrusts (see below) will be necessary. If the obstruction doesn't clear with 3 cycles of each, I must dial 999 or 112 for an ambulance before continuing. If her condition deteriorates (she becomes unresponsive), I must resuscitate her (see page 266). After administering abdominal thrusts, I must seek medical advice for her.

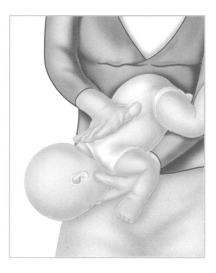

Up to 1 year

1 I must lay my baby face down along my forearm, with so that her head is held low. With the heel of my hand, I will give up to 5 back blows between her shoulder blades (as shown). I must check her mouth quickly after each one and remove any obvious obstruction. If the obstruction is still present...

2 I need to turn baby onto her back and give her chest thrusts. Using 2 fingers, I will push inwards and upwards in the middle of her chest up to 5 times. After each thrust, I will check her mouth quickly. If the obstruction does not clear with 3 cycles of back blows and chest thrusts, I must call for an ambulance then continue cycles of back blows and chest thrusts until help arrives.

Over 1 year old

1 Using the heel of my hand, I will have to give up to 5 back blows between my child's shoulder blades and check her mouth quickly after each blow to remove any obvious obstruction. If the obstruction is still present...

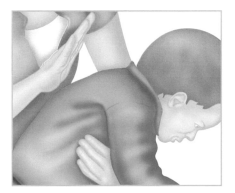

2 I need to give up to 5 abdominal thrusts. I will place my clenched fist between her navel and the bottom of her breastbone and pull inwards and upwards, checking her mouth quickly after each thrust. If the obstruction does not clear after 3 cycles of back blows and abdominal thrusts, I must call for an ambulance then continue cycles of back blows and abdominal thrusts until help arrives.

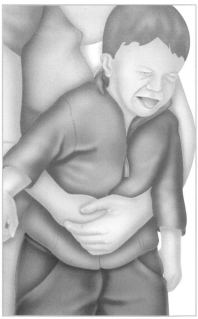

GIVING CPR (CARDIO-PULMONARY RESUSCITATION)

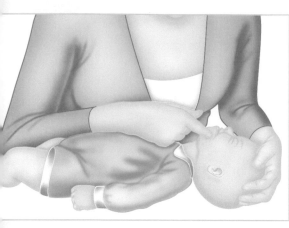

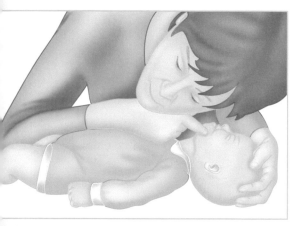

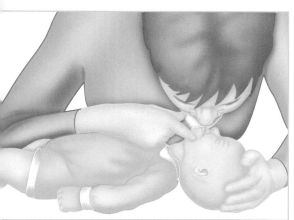

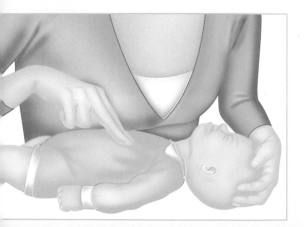

If my baby or child isn't responsive – doesn't react to my calling her name or gently tapping her foot, I need to do the following:

Under 1 year old

1 I must place one hand on my baby's forehead and gently tilt her head back and lift her chin. With my finger, I'll remove any visible obstructions from her mouth and nose.

2 Then I'll check to see if she's breathing by looking, listening and feeling for breathing on my cheek for up to 10 seconds. If she is not breathing normally, I must follow steps 3 and 4 for 1 minute then call 999 (or 112) for an ambulance. If another person is present, I'll ask him or her to call an ambulance straight away.

3 Then I must fill my cheeks with air and place my mouth over baby's mouth and nose and blow gently and steadily 2 times. I must look along her chest and stop blowing when baby's chest rises; the I'll allow it to fall.

4 I next have to place 2 fingers in the middle of her chest and press down one-third of the depth of her chest. After 30 chest compressions (at the rate of 100 per minute) I will give 2 breaths (as in step 3). I must continue with cycles of 30 chest compressions and 2 breaths until help arrives.

Over 1 year old to puberty

1 I must place one hand on my child's forehead and gently tilt her head back and lift her chin. I'll remove any visible obstructions from her mouth and nose.

2 Then I'll pinch my child's nose. Placing my mouth over her mouth, I'll blow gently into her lungs 2 times, looking along her chest as I breathe. I need to take shallow breaths and not empty my lungs completely. As my child's chest rises, I'll stop blowing and allow it to fall.

3 With my arm held straight, I will place my hand on the centre of her chest and, using the heel of my hand, press down one-third of the 30 times (at the rate of 100 compressions per minute). Depending on her size, I might need both hands. After every 30 chest compressions, I'll give 2 breaths (as in step 2).

4 I must continue with cycles of 30 chest compressions and 2 breaths until help arrives.

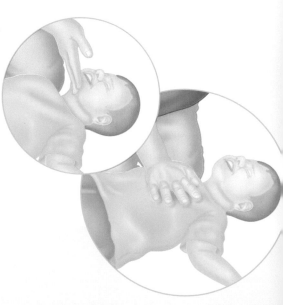

POISONING

If my child ingests something harmful or I suspect that she has, or a potential poison has come in contact with her skin and eyes, I need to call 999 (or 112) for an ambulance immediately.

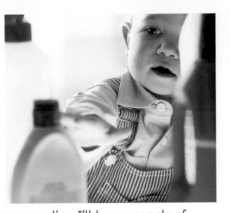

I'll need to try and find out what she took, how much and how long ago, so that I can inform the doctor or paramedics. I'll keep a sample of any vomit she produces – but I won't try and make her sick. She can have sips of water but not large amounts to drink. If she is breathing but unconscious, I'll put her in the recovery position (see page 264).

BURNS AND SCALDS

Babies with burns, even small or superficial ones, should get urgent medical attention.

I'll cool the burn as quickly as possible by placing the affected area under cold running water for at least 10 minutes.

I won't apply any creams that may introduce infection, just cover the injury using a sterile, non-sticky dressing such as a clean handkerchief or other clean covering such as cling film. I'll use a loose bandage to hold the dressing in place. I'll get her to raise the limb to reduce swelling.

BLEEDING

If I find my child bleeding, my main aim will be to stem the flow while waiting for an ambulance to arrive (call 999 or 112) or while taking my child to hospital. If possible, I should wear disposable gloves to reduce the risk of cross-infection. I need to check whether there is an object embedded in the wound.

If nothing is embedded, I'll press on the wound with my hand, ideally over a clean pad, and secure with a bandage. If the wound is on an arm or leg, I'll raise the injured limb above the level of my child's heart.

If I think something is embedded, I won't press on the object but press firmly on either side of it and build up padding around it before bandaging to avoid putting pressure on the object itself.

ELECTROCUTION

I'll need to call 999 for an ambulance immediately.

Then I'll break the contact between my child and the electrical supply by switching off the current at the mains.

If I can't reach the mains I'll need to stand on some dry insulation material, such as a telephone directory, to protect myself. Then, using something made of a non-conductive material (e.g. a wooden broom), I will push my child away from the electrical source or push the source away from her.

If at any time my child stops breathing or becomes unconscious, I'll follow the instructions for giving CPR (see page 266), then put her in the recovery position (see page 264) until help arrives.

DROWNING

If I find my baby under water, I'll lift her out immediately and hold her so her head is lower than her body. This will help prevent water, or vomit if she throws up, getting into her lungs. If she is unconscious but still breathing, I'll put her in the recovery position, while I call 999 (or 112). If she is not breathing, I'll begin resuscitation (see Treating choking, page 265). Water in the lungs means I will have to breathe more firmly than usual to get the lungs to inflate properly.

Index

Acknowledgements

ILLUSTRATIONS
Amanda Williams

SUPPLIERS
Thanks to the following companies for supplying
products/photography:
Mothercare, for equipment shown p80-81, p82, p91 and p198.
Babybjorn p176 and p199.

PHOTOGRAPHS
Professor Stuart Campbell p26-27 and p29.

PHOTOLIBRARY.COM
Jacket, p6, p7, p8-9, p12, p14, p15 (top right and middle left),
p18-23, p26, p33, p34, p35, p37, p40, p41, p42, p52, p54, p61,
p62, p70-71, p73, p87, p98-99, p100-101, p102, p104, p105,
p107, p109, p110, p112-113, p114, p116, p117, p131, p133
(left and middle), p134-135, p136, p141, p144-145, p160, p164,
p171, p177, p178, p179, p180, p182-183, p185, p186 (bottom
left), p187 (bottom left), p190, p192, p201, p204, p206,
p210-211, p214, p216, p219, p220, p221, p224, p225, p226,
p228, p230, p234, p241, p242, p243, p244-245, p246, p247,
p248, p249, p254, p259, p262, p263, p264, p267.

SCIENCE PHOTO LIBRARY
p15 Saturn Stills (top left) Mendil (middle right), p111 Mark
Clarke, p122 Dr P. Marazzi, p137 Mike Devlin (top left),
Dr P. Marazzi (top right), Dr P. Marazzi (bottom left) Dr P.
Marazzi (bottom right), p151 Tek Image, p251 Gustoimages,
p260 Dr M.A. Ansary.

GETTY IMAGES
p27, p200 and p181.